Quality and Performance Improvement in Healthcare

A Tool for Programmed Learning

Fifth Edition

**Patricia Shaw, MEd, RHIA, FAHIMA,
and Chris Elliott, MS, RHIA**

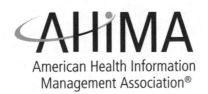

AHiMA
American Health Information
Management Association®

ISBN: 978-1-58426-310-4
AHIMA Product No.: AB102711

AHIMA Staff:
Claire E. Blondeau, MBA, Senior Editor
June E. Bronnert, RHIA, CCS, CCS-P, Technical Reviewer
Katie Greenock, MS, Editorial and Production Coordinator
Ashley Sullivan, Assistant Editor
Ken Zielske, Director of Publications

For more information, including updates, about AHIMA Press publications, visit http://www.ahima.org/publications/updates.aspx

American Health Information Management Association
233 North Michigan Avenue, 21st Floor
Chicago, Illinois 60601-5809
http://www.ahima.org

Contents

Part I   *A Performance Improvement Model*

The model used for performance improvement activities is defined. How this model is applied to organization-wide and team-based performance improvement is discussed.

The principal aspects of continuous improvement targeting healthcare performance are described. The QI toolbox techniques of brainstorming, affinity diagramming, and nominal group technique are defined.

The effective use of teams in performance improvement activities is introduced. The composition of the PI team and the use of team charters; team roles; ground rules; and mission, vision, and values statements are discussed. Effective listening and questioning techniques within performance improvement team activities are discussed.

Various data types, data display techniques, and aggregation and analysis methods to support the performance improvement process are discussed.

About the Authors

Patricia Shaw, MEd, RHIA, FAHIMA, earned her master's degree in education in 1997 and has been on the faculty of Weber State University, where she teaches in the Health Information Management and Health Services Administration programs, since 1991. She has primary teaching responsibility for the quality and performance improvement curriculum in those programs. Pat maintains contact with practice settings as a consultant specializing in the areas of reimbursement and coding issues. Prior to accepting a position at Weber State University, Pat managed hospital health information services departments and was a nosologist for 3M™ Health Information Systems.

Chris Elliott, MS, RHIA, holds a master's degree in information systems and has pursued significant graduate study in medical informatics at the University of Utah. He recently retired as director of Health Information Services and privacy officer designee at San Francisco General Hospital Medical Center after 40 years of public service in hospitals and health professions education settings.

Acknowledgments

Dawn Booth, who for the fourth edition served as a reviewer for chapter 12, "Managing the Environment of Care."

Jeb Brown, PhD, who for the fourth edition served as a reviewer for chapter 7, "Refining the Continuum of Care."

Lloyd Burton, DM, who for the third edition served as contributing author for chapter 17, "Managing Healthcare Performance Improvement Projects," and chapter 22, "Predicting the Future of Performance Improvement in Healthcare."

Kathy Murphy, JD, who for the third edition served as contributing author for chapter 21, "Understanding the Legal Implications of Performance Improvement."

Anne B. Casto, RHIA, CCS, who served as technical reviewer for the entire text for the third edition.

Special Acknowledgments

Special thanks to Polly Isaacson, RHIA, CPhT, and Elizabeth Murphy, M.Ed, RN, who were part of the primary author team for the first through the fourth editions. Their contributions to the manuscript over the years have been immeasurable.

Preface for Students

You will soon be entering your chosen profession in the healthcare field. The issues involved in the management of quality in healthcare span the various clinical and administrative disciplines and must be approached from a variety of perspectives. Many improvements for healthcare services are developed through team-based activities. Employers also will expect you to be able to apply performance improvement (PI) data analysis and presentation tools. Prepare now for the possibility that at some point in the future you will be asked to facilitate a PI team meeting.

The authors of this text hope that this tool for programmed, incremental learning of the PI process will prepare you well for the challenges you will face in your new career. If you use this text carefully, you will probably find yourself miles ahead of your fellow students in preparation for today's healthcare environment.

Preface for Educators and Practitioners

This textbook from AHIMA presents a comprehensive introduction to the theory, practice, and management of performance and quality improvement processes in healthcare organizations. Parts I and II are intended for use by students in technology-level health professions programs of all kinds and provide a basic background in performance improvement (PI) philosophy and methodology for healthcare practice today. Each chapter has real-life examples and case studies from healthcare settings that bring home the importance of quality in healthcare services. QI toolbox techniques are presented both in theory and in practice so that your students can see how the techniques can actually be used in PI activities. Healthcare information management students will find the textbook's unique step-by-step and case-study-based approach to the subject easy to use and understand. Students also will gain hands-on practice applying the analytical and graphic tools used in performance and quality improvement. Integrated into the chapter discussions are student projects that range from designing specific improvement projects to ongoing quality monitoring and managing quality improvement programs and staff.

Part III is intended for use by students in management-level programs in the health services. Its chapters focus on the issues inherent in the management of quality and PI programs in healthcare. Each chapter presents the issues and their backgrounds and concludes with a case study to reinforce student learning and encourage critical thinking about the issues.

Instructor materials for this book include lesson plans (for students in both two-year and four-year programs), lesson slides, and other useful resources. The Instructor Guide is available to instructors in online format from the individual book pages in the AHIMA Bookstore or through the Assembly on Education (AOE) Community of Practice (CoP). Instructors who are AHIMA members can sign up for this private community by clicking the Help icon on the CoP home page and requesting additional information on becoming an AOE CoP member. An instructor who is not an AHIMA member or a member who is not an instructor may contact the publisher by e-mail at publications@ahima.org to request instructor resources. The instructor materials are not available to students enrolled in college or university programs.

Introduction

People naturally expect their world to improve over time. This expectation affects everything people come into contact with: food, housing, cars, education, and healthcare. Such expectations stimulate general social progress. Progress may take considerable time to develop, and the desire for progress sometimes takes a counterproductive path, as during times of war and political upheaval. Still, the objective of making the human situation better is a constant in human endeavors.

Progress is commonly accomplished in one of two ways. First, progress can be achieved through an understanding of the scientific basis of the natural world and its constituent parts. Understanding the way the human body functions through biochemistry, for example, facilitated the development of the pharmaceuticals in use today. Second, progress can be achieved through improvements in the ways that people perform their work. Understanding the procedures that healthcare professionals must perform to help people get well, for example, facilitated the development of one of the best healthcare delivery systems in the world. This textbook examines the second type of progress.

The focus of this textbook is healthcare quality and performance improvement (PI) in the United States and the means by which progress is accomplished in healthcare organizations. Every healthcare professional needs to understand the issues surrounding quality and PI in healthcare, because society expects that progress will result in better healthcare products and services. But there are other reasons why healthcare professionals should be concerned about quality improvement. There is a tradition to be upheld and carried forward.

Early Quality Improvements in Healthcare

There is a long tradition of quality improvement in healthcare. (See figure I.1.) From colonial times to the present, healthcare in the United States has undergone a series of developments and reforms, from the creation of hospitals in the 18th century and the scientific discoveries of the 19th century, to the professionalization of medical and nursing practice in the early 20th century and the technological advances of the late 20th and early 21st centuries. Healthcare institutions, professional associations, individual leaders, and political visionaries all laid the foundations of modern healthcare.

Healthcare Institutions

During the mid-1700s, before the American colonies became a nation, the citizens of Philadelphia, PA, recognized the need for a place to house the mentally ill and to provide relief to the sick and injured. They also recognized the need to sequester newly arrived immigrants, who often contracted diseases during their long voyages to America. Thousands of people immigrated to the Pennsylvania colony in an attempt to improve their lives. Although most healthcare was provided in people's homes at that time, established inhabitants, particularly the poor, sometimes required a place to rest and mend during times of illness and injury. Recognizing these needs, Dr. Thomas Bond, with the help of Benjamin Franklin, persuaded the Pennsylvania legislature to undertake the organization and development of a hospital for the community. The famous Pennsylvania Hospital was the first in the growing nation (Morton 1973).

Over the next 150 years, the Pennsylvania Hospital became a model for the development of hospitals in other communities. It even attempted to standardize its care processes by publishing rules and regulations for its physicians and staff (Morton 1973). These regulations represent early attempts at healthcare improvement.

The annals of Massachusetts General Hospital provide an early example of an action taken by a hospital board of trustees to ensure the quality of care provided in the institution. In 1837, the trustees became aware that the son of a resident surgeon (a surgeon who had not attained appointment to the hospital) had practiced in the hospital during his father's

Figure I.1.   Historical perspectives on PI in healthcare

1700s	1800s	1900s	2000s
Mid-1700s Pennsylvania Hospital becomes the model for the organization and development of hospitals. **1760** New York State begins the practice of medical licensure. **1771** New Jersey begins the practice of medical licensure.	**1837** Massachusetts General Hospital sets limitations on clinical practice in the first granting of clinical privileges. **1853** Massachusetts General Hospital establishes the first disease/procedure index by classifying patient disposition. **Mid-1800s** Medical licensure is deemed undemocratic and is stopped. **1872** New England Hospital for Women and Children organizes a general training school for nurses. **1874** American Medical Association (AMA) encourages the creation of independent state licensing boards.	**1903** North Carolina passes the first nurse registration bill in the United States. **1910** Flexner Report indicates unacceptable variation in medical school curricula. **1917** American College of Surgeons (ACS) establishes the Hospital Standardization Program. **1920** Most medical colleges meet rigorous academic standards and are approved by the Association of American Medical Colleges™. **1946** Hill-Burton Act establishes funding to build new hospitals. **1952** Joint Commission on Accreditation of Hospitals (JCAH) was formed by the AMA, the American College of Physicians (ACP), the American Hospital Association (AHA), and the Canadian Medical Association (CMA). **1965** Public Law 89-97 establishes Medicare and Medicaid. **1972** Local peer review organizations are formed. **1980s** Prospective payment system is established. State and regional peer review organizations contract with Health Care Financing Administration (HCFA). **1990s** JCAH becomes JCAHO. Deming's total quality management (TQM) philosophy begins to spread in US healthcare. JCAHO integrates quality improvement into the accreditation process.	**2001** Ambulatory payment classification system is initiated. **2002** HCFA becomes the Centers for Medicare and Medicaid Services (CMS). **2003** JCAHO implements the National Patient Safety Goals. **2005** JCAHO begins unannounced and tracer methodology surveys. **2007** JCAHO renames itself the Joint Commission. **2008** Medicare-Severity diagnosis-related groups (DRGs) are implemented. **2009** HITECH legislation is passed. **2013** ICD-10-CM and ICD-10-PCS scheduled for implementation.

absence. The trustees reiterated to all of the medical staff the need for allowing only those accorded privileges at the institution to practice there (Bowditch 1972, 135):

> The Trustees have recently seen with great pain, that a violation of the rules of the institution by one of its officers has become the subject of newspaper animadversion. In an institution like this, to which it is so difficult to attract, and in which it is so important to command, public confidence, the strictest and most scrupulous adherence to rules, of which the propriety is unquestioned, is required by a just regard as well to its usefulness to the public, as to the character of those who have any agency in its direction and control. Where many persons are connected in different departments, the reputation of all is more or less affected by the conduct of each; and all are therefore bound, by respect for others as well as themselves to conduct in such a manner as to give no reasonable ground of complaint.

It is also interesting to note that the trustees believed that the expectations of the members of their community—their customers—should be considered.

The annals of Massachusetts General Hospital include other examples of the hospital's concern about service quality. For example, in 1851, the hospital hired a watchman to guard against the danger of fire during the night (Bowditch 1972, 367). In 1853, the hospital commended one of its surgical staff members for compiling an analytical index for the surgical records of the institution and reflected on the quality of the surgical services provided (Bowditch 1972, 483). In 1872, the trustees decided to regulate the use of restraints at the institution, and they identified each by type and set the conditions under which the restraint could be used (Bowditch 1972, 679–680). Throughout the history of the institution, the trustees received regular reports on the number of patients treated as well as the classification of each patient's outcome at discharge—"well," "relieved," "not relieved," or "dead" (Bowditch 1972, 447).

Medical Practice

Human anatomy and physiology were not well understood before the 20th century. At one time, it was believed that four basic fluids, called humors, determined a person's temperament and health and that imbalances in the proportion of humors in the body caused disease. The therapeutic bleeding of patients was practiced into the early 20th century. Early physicians also treated patients by administering a variety of substances with no scientific basis for their effectiveness. The science of medicine began to evolve in the late 19th century but was not fully realized until the second and third decades of the 20th century.

Early on, the medical profession recognized that some of its members achieved better results than others, and attempted to regulate the practice of medicine. At first, the regulation took the form of licensure, beginning in New York in 1760 and New Jersey in 1771. The New Jersey law stated that "no person whatsoever shall practice as a physician or surgeon, within this colony of New Jersey, before he shall have first been examined in physic and surgery, approved of, and admitted by any two of the judges of the Supreme Court." The examination was to be performed before a board of "medical men" appointed by the state medical society (Trent 1977, 91). Various states developed similar legislation over the following decades.

By the middle of the 19th century, however, medical licensure had been repudiated as undemocratic, and the penalties for practicing medicine without a license were removed in most states. "Buyer beware" was the rule of thumb because the title of "doctor" could be used by anyone who wanted to sell medical services (Haller 1981). During this period, medical education consisted primarily of an apprenticeship with an already-established practitioner of some kind. After the apprenticeship, the new doctor could hang out a shingle and begin to treat patients. Some trainees did attend schools that claimed to teach them how to become physicians, but there was no established medical curriculum. Many people received diplomas just by paying a fee. Many others with no education, apprenticeship, or license just hung out a sign and began collecting fees. Effectively, doctoring had become a commercial enterprise. Any man with sufficient entrepreneurial talents could enter the practice of medicine. The emphasis was on making a living rather than joining a true profession. The result was an overabundance of "medical men" who provided medical care based on all kinds of traditions, and at times, no tradition at all.

The American Medical Association (AMA) was established in 1840 to represent the interests of physicians across the United States. The organization was dominated by members who had strong ties to medical schools and the status quo. The organization's ability to lead reform was limited until it broke its ties with the medical colleges in 1874. At that time, the association encouraged the creation of independent state licensing boards (Haller 1981).

In 1876, the Association of American Medical Colleges™ (AAMC™) was established. The AAMC was dedicated to standardizing the curriculum of US medical schools and developing the public's appreciation of the need for medical licensure.

Together, the AMA and the AAMC pushed for medical licensing. By the 1890s, 35 states had established or reestablished a system of licensure for physicians. Fourteen states granted medical licenses only to graduates of reputable medical schools. The state licensing boards discouraged the worst medical schools, but the criteria for licensing continued to vary by state and were not fully enforced (Haller 1981).

By the early 20th century, it had become apparent that promoting quality in medical practice required regulation through curriculum reform as well as licensure. The membership of the AMA, however, was divided on this issue. Conservative members continued to believe that the organization should stay out of the regulatory arena. Progressive members advocated the continuing development of state licensure systems and the development of a model medical curriculum.

The situation attracted the attention of the Carnegie Foundation for the Advancement of Teaching and its president, Henry S. Pritchett. Pritchett offered to sponsor and fund an independent review of the medical curricula and the medical colleges of the United States. The review was undertaken in 1906 by Abraham Flexner, an educator from Louisville, KY.

Over the next four years, Flexner visited every medical college in the country and carefully documented his findings. In his 1910 report to the Carnegie Foundation, the AMA, and the AAMC, he documented the unacceptable variation in curricula that existed across the schools. He also noted that applicants to medical schools frequently lacked knowledge of the basic sciences. Flexner reported how the absence of appropriate hospital-based training limited the clinical skills of medical school graduates. Perhaps most important, he documented the huge number of graduates produced by the colleges each year, most with unacceptable levels of medical expertise.

Several reform initiatives grew out of Flexner's report and recommendations made by the AMA's Committee on Medical Education. One of the reforms required medical college applicants to hold a baccalaureate degree. Another required that the medical curriculum be founded in the basic sciences. Reforms also required that medical students receive practical, hospital-based training. Most important, Flexner recommended the closing of most medical schools in the country. These former recommendations were instituted over the decade after the release of Flexner's report, but only about half of the medical colleges actually closed. By 1920, most of the colleges met rigorous academic standards and were approved by the AAMC.

Nursing Practice

During the 19th century and throughout the first part of the 20th century, more than half of the hospitals in the United States were sponsored by religious organizations. Nursing care at that time was usually provided by members of religious orders. As the US population grew and more towns and cities were established, hospitals were built to accommodate the healthcare needs of new communities. Older cities also were growing, and city hospitals became more and more crowded.

In the late 19th century, nurses received no formal education or training. Nursing staffs for the hospitals were often recruited from the surrounding communities, and many poor women who had no other skills became nurses. The nature of nursing care at that time was unsophisticated, and ignorance of basic hygiene often promoted disease rather than wellness. In 1871 at Bellevue Hospital in New York City, for example, 15 percent of patients died while hospitalized, and hospital-acquired infections were common (Kalisch and Kalisch 1995, 71). Even simple surgical procedures and maternity care often resulted in death due to infection.

In 1868, the president of the AMA, Dr. Samuel Gross, called the medical profession's attention to the need for trained nurses. During the years that followed, the public began to call for better nursing care in hospitals.

A small group of women physicians working in the northeast area of the country created the first formal program for training nurses. Dr. Susan Dimock, working with Dr. Marie Zakrzewska at the New England Hospital for Women and Children, organized a general training school for nurses in 1872 (Kalisch and Kalisch 1995). The school became a model for other institutions throughout the United States. As hospital after hospital struggled to find competent nursing staff, many institutions and their medical staffs developed their own nurse training programs to meet staffing needs.

The responsibilities of nurses in the late 19th and early 20th centuries included housekeeping duties such as cleaning furniture and floors; making beds; changing linens; and controlling temperature, humidity, and ventilation. Nurses also cooked the meals for patients in kitchens attached to each ward. Direct patient care duties included giving baths, changing dressings, monitoring vital signs, administering medication, and assisting at surgical procedures (Kalisch and Kalisch 1995). Nurses generally worked 12-hour shifts, 7 days per week.

During this time, nurses were not required to hold a license to practice. Because licensure was not required and because it was difficult to attract women to nursing staff positions, many women who had no training at all continued to work as nurses in the nation's hospitals and as private-duty nurses.

In the years immediately following the turn of the 20th century, nurses began to organize state nursing associations to advocate for the registration of nurses. Their goal was to increase the level of competence among nurses nationwide. Despite opposition from many physicians who believed that nurses did not need formal education or licensure, North Carolina passed the first nurse registration bill in the United States in 1903. Many other states initiated similar legislation in subsequent years. Today all the states have carefully developed boards of nursing registration that maintain basic standards for nursing practice, promulgate advanced standards for clinical and managerial nurse specialists, license the professional membership, and require ongoing education for maintenance of nursing skills.

Allied Health Professions

Other healthcare professions in the United States developed as specialized areas of practice over the course of the 20th century. Each underwent periods of formalization in similar ways. Each became regulated either by the states or by national professional associations as membership and professional responsibilities grew and the public demanded that they document their professional competence. These developments made important contributions to the quality of healthcare delivered in this country. The allied health professions include radiologic technology, respiratory therapy, occupational therapy, and physical therapy, among others. For example, health information management professionals today are certified and registered by the American Health Information Management Association (AHIMA).

Contributions of Individuals

Many individual healthcare professionals have made significant contributions to the early improvement of healthcare delivery in the United States, including the development and implementation of a variety of improvement strategies. A small sample of these individuals and their contributions is included here. It is important to recognize the progress that can be made when healthcare professionals care about the quality of their work.

Maude E. Callen, an African American public health nurse-midwife, undertook the training of midwives in coastal South Carolina in 1926. A registered nurse, Callen recognized that the midwives' lack of training contributed to high infant and maternal mortality rates in the region, and she traveled extensively throughout the region to assist at deliveries and improve the expertise of midwives (Hill 1997).

Robert Latou Dickinson, an obstetrician and gynecologist practicing in New England around the turn of the 20th century, developed a standardized patient questionnaire. He used the patients' answers on the questionnaire to structure his examinations. His questionnaire represents one of the first uses of a structured health assessment tool in the United States (Bullough 1997).

Lavinia Lloyd Dock, a nurse and early nurse-educator, developed important approaches to disaster nursing at the end of the 19th century. After graduating from a nurse training program, Dock worked to institute appropriate nursing practices during the yellow fever epidemic in Jacksonville, FL, in 1888 and during the aftermath of the Johnstown, PA flood in 1889 (Leighow 1997).

Roswell Park, a physician and surgeon during the late 19th century, helped disseminate the principles of antisepsis during surgical procedures in the United States. Park used the findings of English scientist Joseph Lister to advocate for the use of antiseptic techniques and appropriate wound care in the treatment of surgical cases well before such approaches were common in the United States (Gage 1997).

Nicholas J. Pisacano, a physician who practiced in the middle and late 20th century, recognized the need to upgrade the general practitioner's skills as new technologies and treatments were developed. He worked tirelessly to develop and promote the specialty of family practice in the United States (Adams and Moore 1997).

Ernst P. Boas, a physician who practiced in New York City during the first half of the 20th century, was among the first to call for the coordinated, interdisciplinary care of the chronically ill. Prior to his advocacy, the chronically ill often were considered incurable. He believed that the development of new therapeutics and restorative technologies could return people with chronic illnesses to better health and productivity. His work led to the establishment of the Goldwater Memorial Hospital for Chronic Diseases on Welfare Island in New York City (Brickman 1997, 21).

Mary Steichen Calderone, medical director of the Planned Parenthood Federation of America during the 1950s, launched a clinical investigation program to scientifically identify effective contraceptive methods. Hers was one of the first efforts to identify appropriate clinical practice through the use of scientific evidence in a controversial area (Meldrum 1997).

Hospital Standardization and Accreditation

In 1910, Dr. Edward Martin suggested that the surgical area of medical practice become more concerned with patient outcomes. He had been introduced to this concept through discussions with Dr. Ernest Codman, a British physician who believed that hospital practitioners should track their patients for a significant time after treatment to determine whether the end result was positive or negative. Dr. Codman also advocated the use of outcome information to identify practices that led to the best results.

Dr. Martin and others had been concerned about the conditions in US hospitals for some time. Many observers felt that part of the problem was related to the absence of organized medical staffs in hospitals and to lax professional standards. In the early 20th century, hospitals were used primarily by surgeons who required their facilities to treat patients with surgical modalities. Therapies based on medical regimens were not developed until later in the century. It was natural, therefore, for the impetus for improvement in hospital care to come from the surgical community.

In November 1912, the Third Clinical Congress of Surgeons of North America was held. At this meeting, Dr. Franklin Martin made a proposal that eventually led to the formation of the American College of Surgeons (ACS). Dr. Edward Martin made the following resolution (Roberts et al. 1987, 936):

> Be it resolved by the Clinical Congress of Surgeons of North America here assembled, that some system of standardization of hospital equipment and hospital work should be developed to the end that

those institutions having the highest ideals may have proper recognition before the profession, and that those of inferior equipment and standards should be stimulated to raise the quality of their work. In this way, patients will receive the best type of treatment, and the public will have some means of recognizing those institutions devoted to the highest levels of medicine.

Through the proposal and the resolution, the ACS and the hospital improvement movement became intimately tied. Immediately upon formation, however, officers of the college realized how important their work would be. They were forced to reject 60 percent of the fellowship applications during the college's first three years because applicants were unable to provide documentation to support their clinical competence (Roberts et al. 1987, 937). Medical records from many hospitals were so inadequate that they could not supply information about the applicants' practices in the institutions. Because of this situation and many others of which they became aware, college officers petitioned the Carnegie Foundation in 1917 for funding to plan and develop a hospital standardization program.

In 1917, a committee on standards was formed by the college and met to consider the development of a minimum set of standards that US hospitals would have to meet if they wanted approval from the ACS. On December 20, 1917, the ACS formally established the Hospital Standardization Program and published a formal set of hospital standards called *The Minimum Standard.*

During 1918 and part of 1919, the ACS undertook review of hospitals across the United States and Canada as a field trial to see whether *The Minimum Standard* would be effective as a measurement tool. In total, 692 hospitals were surveyed, of which only 89 met the standard entirely. Some of the most prestigious institutions in the United States failed to meet the standard. Brief and clear in its delineation of what was believed to promote good hospital-based patient care in 1918, *The Minimum Standard* (cited in ACS 1930, 3) stated:

1. That physicians and surgeons privileged to practice in the hospital be organized as a definite group or staff. Such organization has nothing to do with the question as to whether the hospital is "open" or "closed," nor need it affect the various existing types of staff organization. The word staff is here defined as the group of doctors who practice in the hospital inclusive of all groups such as the "regular staff," the "visiting staff," and the "associate staff."

2. That membership upon the staff be restricted to physicians and surgeons who are (a) full graduates of medicine in good standing and legally licensed to practice in their respective states or provinces; (b) competent in their respective fields; and (c) worthy in character and in matters of professional ethics; that in this latter connection the practice of the division of fees, under any guise whatever, be prohibited.

3. That the staff initiate and, with the approval of the governing board of the hospital, adopt rules, regulations, and policies governing the professional work of the hospital; that these rules, regulations, and policies specifically provide: (a) that staff meetings be held at least once each month (In large hospitals, the departments may choose to meet separately); and (b) that the staff review and analyze at regular intervals their clinical experience in the various departments of the hospital, such as medicine, surgery, obstetrics, and the other specialties; the clinical records of patients, free and pay, to be the basis of such review and analysis.

4. That accurate and complete records be written for all patients and filed in an accessible manner in the hospital—a complete case record being one which includes identification data; complaint; personal and family history; history of present illness; physical examination; special examinations, such as consultations, clinical laboratory, x-ray, and other examinations; provisional or working diagnosis; medical or surgical treatment; gross and microscopic pathological findings; progress notes; final diagnosis; condition on discharge; follow-up; and, in case of death, autopsy findings.

5. That diagnostic and therapeutic facilities under competent supervision be available for the study, diagnosis, and treatment of patients, these to include, at least (a) a clinical laboratory providing chemical, bacteriological, serological, and pathological services; (b) an x-ray department providing radiographic and fluoroscopic services.

The adoption of *The Minimum Standard* marked the beginning of the accreditation process for healthcare organizations. A similar process is still followed today. (For more information, see chapter 15 of this textbook.) Basically, the process is based on the development of reasonable quality standards and a survey of the organization's performance on the standards. The accreditation program is voluntary, and healthcare organizations request participation to improve patient care (Roberts et al. 1987).

The ACS continued to examine and approve hospitals for three decades. By 1950, however, the number of hospitals being surveyed every year had grown unmanageable, and the college could no longer afford to administer the program alone. After considerable discussion and organizing activity, four professional associations from the United States and Canada—the American Medical Association (AMA), the American College of Physicians (ACP), the American Hospital Association (AHA), and the Canadian Medical Association (CMA)—decided to join the ACS to develop the Joint Commission on Accreditation of Hospitals. The new accrediting agency was formally incorporated in 1952 and began accreditation activities in 1953. It continued its activities almost 50 years later as the Joint Commission on Accreditation of Healthcare Organizations (JCAHO) before renaming itself the Joint Commission in 2007.

PI and Modern Healthcare

Until World War II, most healthcare was still provided in the home. Quality in healthcare services was considered a byproduct of appropriate medical practice and oversight by physicians. The positive and negative effects of other factors and the contributions of other healthcare workers were not given much consideration.

In the 1950s, the number of hospitals grew to support developments in diagnostic, therapeutic, and surgical technology and pharmacology. Fueled by an expanding economy, the Hill-Burton Act of 1946 funded extensive hospital construction. A renewed insurance industry helped pay for the new healthcare services provided to groups of individual beneficiaries.

During this period, the Hospital Standardization Program was replaced by the Joint Commission on Accreditation of Hospitals (JCAH) (1952). A whole new set of standards covered every aspect of hospital care. The intent was to ensure that the care provided to patients in accredited hospitals would be of the highest quality.

The construction of new facilities and the growth of the medical insurance industry, however, did not guarantee access to services. As new treatments and "miracle" drugs such as antibiotics were developed, healthcare services became more and more costly. Many Americans, particularly the poor and the elderly, could not afford to buy healthcare insurance or to pay for the services themselves.

Medicare and Medicaid Programs

The idea of federal funding for healthcare services goes back to the 1930s, the Great Depression, and Franklin Roosevelt's New Deal. Harry Truman also supported a universal healthcare program in the late 1940s. But it was not until the 1960s and the presidency of Lyndon Johnson that the federal government developed a program to pay for the healthcare services provided to the poor and the elderly (AHA 1999).

In 1965, the United States Congress passed Public Law 89-97, an amendment to the Social Security Act of 1935. Title XVIII of Public Law 89-97 established health insurance for the aged and the disabled. This program soon became known as Medicare. Title XIX of Public Law 89-97 provided grants to states for establishing medical assistance programs for the poor. The Title XIX program became known as Medicaid. The objective of the programs was to ensure access to healthcare for citizens who could not afford to pay for it themselves. The Great Society, as the geopolitics of the United States was called in the 1960s, marshaled billions of federal tax dollars to fund care for millions of Americans.

During the 1970s, attempts were made to further standardize and improve the clinical services provided by physicians and hospitals. Under the authority of Medicare officials, hospital audits of physicians' medical records were mandated to identify physicians with substandard practice patterns or excessive patient care costs. Local peer review organizations (PROs), usually sponsored by local medical societies, reviewed the findings at each local institution and developed recommendations for physician continuing education. Such retrospective **quality assurance (QA)** efforts were only partially successful and had little effect on the mounting cost to the government of the Medicare and Medicaid programs. As a result, utilization review (UR) programs were mandated to justify hospital admissions. The concept and practice of UR survives today (see chapter 7). Institutions must still provide payers a rationale for the level of services provided to be reimbursed.

The changes that most significantly improved patient outcomes in the 1970s involved the development and use of sophisticated medical technology and pharmaceuticals. The overall benefits of modern healthcare were evident in increased life spans and better medical outcomes. Americans had come to expect the best and the newest medical care available as a personal right not to be taken away.

By 1980, however, it was obvious that healthcare spending in the United States would consume more and more economic resources if left unchecked. The Medicare and Medicaid programs were on their way to becoming the most expensive government programs in US history. At the same time, healthcare experts also began to understand that increased spending and technological advances did not automatically guarantee quality healthcare.

In the early 1980s, a new nationwide system was developed to standardize reimbursement for hospital services provided to Medicare and Medicaid beneficiaries. Until 1983,

Medicare and Medicaid reimbursement was based on a **retrospective payment system.** In a retrospective payment system, providers are paid for the services they provided to a patient in the past. Retrospective payment is also called fee-for-service payment. The patient goes to the doctor, the doctor cares for the patient, the doctor assigns charges and submits a bill to a payer, and the doctor is reimbursed for his or her charges. The problem with this system is that there is no incentive for the doctor to hold down costs. If the doctor provides more services, then he or she bills more and gets paid more. So, this type of arrangement did not help rein in ever-increasing healthcare costs.

To slow the growth in cost of federal healthcare programs, a prospective payment system was developed. In a prospective payment system, providers receive a fixed, predetermined payment for the services they provide. The reimbursement amounts are determined annually by the Centers for Medicare and Medicaid Services (CMS), and billing of carriers and patients cannot exceed these assigned amounts. Because the amount of reimbursement is fixed and often lower than what the provider would otherwise charge, providers are theoretically motivated to use only those services absolutely necessary to the patient's care. In this way, costs could supposedly be controlled and unnecessary services avoided. However, by the first decade of the 21st century, this system became less and less capable of controlling costs due to a variety of factors, none of which are currently completely understood, and healthcare costs continue to be one of the fastest-growing segments of the gross domestic product as well as one of the most contentious subjects of the US political arena.

In the Medicare and Medicaid prospective payment system, reimbursement for hospital inpatient services has long been based on diagnosis-related groups (DRGs). This system assumes that similar diseases and treatments consume similar amounts of resources and therefore have similar total costs, at least on a regional, if not national, basis. Every hospital inpatient has been assigned to an appropriate DRG on the basis of his or her diagnosis since 1984. Since that time, reimbursement levels for each DRG are updated annually and adjusted for the geographic location of the healthcare facility. For federal fiscal year 2009, however, CMS undertook major revision of the DRG structure to create groups that reflect the medical severity of the patient's condition (MS-DRGs) by recognizing conditions that by their concurrent occurrence with the reason for admission significantly inflate the use of resources and the overall costs of the provision of care.

The Healthcare Common Procedure Coding System (HCPCS) was developed in the early 1980s. HCPCS codes are used to report the healthcare services provided to Medicare and Medicaid beneficiaries treated in ambulatory settings. HCPCS initially included three separate levels of codes: (level I) Current Procedural Terminology (CPT®) codes, (level II) national codes, and (level III) local codes. The level III local codes were eliminated by CMS in 2003 (CMS 2008).

A prospective payment system for hospital outpatient and ambulatory surgery services provided to Medicare and Medicaid beneficiaries was implemented in 2001. This system is based on ambulatory payment classification (APC) groups. The APCs are generated on the basis of the HCPCS CPT codes assigned for services such as outpatient diagnostic procedures and outpatient radiology procedures. A similar system has been implemented for the reimbursement of professional fees. This resource-based relative value scale (RBRVS) system takes into consideration the level of services provided by the physician in terms of time spent with the patient, complexity of physical exam and information gathering, and the diagnostic and procedural actions performed to arrive at the reimbursement amount.

US hospitals and physicians provide billions of dollars worth of care to Medicare and Medicaid patients every year. The implementation of prospective payment systems has made it necessary for healthcare organizations to devise ways to control costs without endangering safe and effective patient care. It is necessary to recognize, however, that there are limits to the amount of dollars that can be extracted from the system by these methods.

The issue of linking payment of services to quality and performance has continued to evolve and has led to the development of value-based purchasing or pay-for-performance systems. **Value-based purchasing** is seen primarily in the public sector and is a "system in which purchasers hold providers of healthcare accountable for both the costs of healthcare and its quality" (Casto and Layman 2011, 264). In the private sector, pay-for-performance programs are more common and base provider payments on performance and incentives.

Managed Care Revolution

The growth of managed care in the United States also has had a tremendous impact on healthcare providers. *Managed care* is a broad term used to describe several types of managed healthcare plans. Health maintenance organizations (HMOs) are one of the most familiar types of managed care. Members of an HMO (or their employers) pay a set premium and are entitled to a specific range of healthcare services. HMOs control costs by requiring beneficiaries to seek services from a preapproved list of providers, by limiting access to specialists and expensive diagnostic and treatment procedures, and by requiring preauthorization for inpatient hospitalization and surgery.

Other types of managed care include preferred provider organizations (PPOs) and point-of-service (POS) plans. These types of managed care plans negotiate discounted rates with specific hospitals, physicians, and other healthcare providers. Many also restrict access to specialists and require preauthorization for surgery and other hospital services. In PPOs, enrollees are required to seek care from a limited list of providers who have agreed in advance to accept a discounted payment for their services. Enrollees in POS plans pay for a greater portion of their healthcare expenses when they choose to seek treatment from providers who do not participate in their plan.

Together, the Medicare and Medicaid programs and the managed care insurance industry have virtually eliminated fee-for-service reimbursement arrangements. At the same time, healthcare consumers are demanding more services and greater quality. Hospitals and physicians now find that they have no choice but to become more efficient and effective if they are to stay in business. Programs that promote **efficiency** and **effectiveness** have become the only way for providers to add value to the services they provide and ensure their financial viability.

Total Quality Management in Healthcare

In the 1980s, leaders in the healthcare industry began to take notice of a theory from general industry called **total quality management (TQM)**. The concept of TQM was developed by W. Edwards Deming in the early 1950s as an alternative to authoritarian, top-down management philosophies. Philip Crosby and J.M. Juran each further adapted TQM and developed similar approaches. TQM mobilizes individuals directly involved in a work process to examine and improve the process with the goal of achieving a better product or outcome. It does not matter what the product or outcome might be. TQM is firmly based in the statistical analysis of objective data gathered from observation of the process being examined. The data are then carefully analyzed to identify the steps in the process that lead to a less-than-ideal product or outcome. Once the problematic steps in the process have been identified, individuals or teams can make recommendations for changing the process to get a better product or outcome. Key to Deming's philosophy is the concept that problematic processes, not people, cause inferior products and outcomes.

TQM revolutionized industrial production in Japan during the post–World War II period. When Japanese automobiles took over much of the US car market in the late 20th century, American manufacturers began to take notice of TQM. They recognized that Deming's management philosophy might help them create more efficient and effective manufacturing processes.

Avedis Donabedian (1966) was one of the first theorists to recognize that the TQM philosophy could be applied to healthcare services. Beginning in 1966, Donabedian advocated the assessment of healthcare from four perspectives: **structure, process,** outcome, and **cost.** Only in the 1990s, however, were his approaches widely adopted. As the concept of TQM (or continuous quality improvement [CQI], as it became known in the US healthcare system) was integrated into the healthcare industry's quest for improvement, the industry began using Donabedian's four perspectives to identify processes of providing care that could be improved. Using the team approach from Deming and his emphasis on objective data gathering to describe a process clearly, members of the industry began a self-examination that focused very specifically on the processes of care, rather than on the individuals who provided it. Many improvements were made for the nation's recipients of care in all types of healthcare organizations using this variant of Deming's TQM.

By the end of the 1990s, however, some individuals involved in the improvement of quality in healthcare had made a significant realization: Quality in healthcare was tied very closely to the performance of individuals in the healthcare organization. Unlike the products of manufacturing firms that utilized machinery to shape raw materials into physical products, the products of healthcare organizations were the services provided to patients by healthcare professionals who defined processes of practice. The performance of the professionals in healthcare processes often determined the quality of the services. Quality improvement initiatives in healthcare organizations were renamed *performance improvement* initiatives, at least in those organizations affected by the JCAHO's PI standards. Quality improvement was refocused to examine the performance of the people in the organization, rewarding those who obtained good outcomes or costs, and requiring those working in the healthcare industry to become more accountable for their patient or client outcomes.

Federal agencies began to emphasize quality improvement in the programs they sponsored during this time as well. The approach by federal Medicare and Medicaid programs retained the quality improvement terminology but focused largely on the same kinds of process issues. Today, contracted healthcare examiners—once called PROs and now called quality improvement organizations (QIOs)—retrospectively examine the care provided to beneficiaries and compare it with comparable providers' performance in different regions of the country.

This comparison of providers' performance is facilitated by the collection and submission of mandated data sets by the Joint Commission and CMS, called **core measures,** on the most common diagnoses such as pneumonia, congestive heart failure, or myocardial infarction. The core measures define the practices used in managing a health condition that achieve the best outcomes, often on the basis of research identifying the best practices and methodologies used across the country. Analysis of the core measure data allows providers to examine where their performance on various characteristics of care does not measure up to what the general community is accomplishing. Thereby, they can identify aspects of their services that can be improved.

Also in the first decade of the 21st century, some important changes in the philosophy of the Joint Commission have evolved. Most important, a new emphasis on patient safety has arisen in response to an analysis revealing that hundreds of thousands of patients die in hospitals every year from mistakes or miscommunication involving the care they are receiving. In particular, mistakes occurring in medication administration and provision of surgical procedures have been highlighted. In response, Joint Commission (2011) developed a set of National Patient Safety Goals (NPSGs) that all institutions participating in accreditation must promote and train their staffs providing care to adhere to. Since 2003, the Joint Commission has revised and fine-tuned the original set of NPSGs, moving some of them into the formal accreditation standards (see chapter 10). Finally, the Joint Commission has undertaken radical restructuring of the survey processes used to examine hospitals for accreditation, emphasizing foremost the processes by which nurses and other allied healthcare professionals provide care at the bedside rather than emphasizing the development of policy and procedure and retrospective review of records.

In parallel with these changes in the philosophy of the Joint Commission, the federal government has sponsored more and more research into the issues inherent in the US healthcare delivery system through its Agency for Healthcare Research and Quality (http://www.ahrq.gov/consumer). In the private sector, organizations such as the National Quality Forum have brought together a variety of stakeholders, including researchers, providers, consumer advocates, payers, and accreditors, to develop quality measures for use across most healthcare organizations (http://www.qualityforum.org). The IOM has used its funding from a variety of sources to examine the areas in which the system is failing the American people and to make recommendations on systematic improvement (http://www.iom.edu). Since its inception, the IOM has published hundreds of reports on different healthcare topics.

In particular, the student of healthcare quality improvement might want to read *Crossing the Quality Chasm: A New Health System for the 21st Century* (IOM 2001). After acknowledging that the current system is overly complex and inequitable with respect to various socioeconomic groups, the IOM cites six core requirements necessary to focus US healthcare delivery in the 21st century: Care should be "safe, effective, patient-centered, timely, efficient, and equitable." At the same time, the IOM (2001) proposed a set of 10 rules or general principles to inform efforts in redesigning the healthcare system:

- Care is based on continuous healing relationships. Patients should receive care whenever they need it and in many forms, for example, over the Internet, by telephone, and by other means in addition to in-person visits.

- Care is customized according to patient needs and values.

- The patient is the source of control, being given the necessary information and opportunity to exercise the degree of control they choose over healthcare decisions that affect them.

- Knowledge is shared and information flows freely.

- Decision making is evidence-based. Patients should receive care based on the best available scientific knowledge. Care should not vary from clinician to clinician or from place to place.

- Safety is a system [priority]. . . . Reducing risk and ensuring safety require greater attention to systems that help prevent and mitigate error.

- Transparency is necessary. . . . Information describing the system's performance on safety, evidence-based practice, and patient satisfaction [should be readily available].

- [Patient] needs are anticipated.

- Waste is continuously decreased.

- Cooperation among clinicians is a priority.

Following publication of *Crossing the Quality Chasm* and heightened dialogue by accrediting and licensing agencies regarding some of its recommendations, renewed emphasis has been placed on the issues it and others raised regarding safety of care, patient centricity of care, the scientific basis for care, and the transparency of the outcomes of care. In 2008, the IOM published *Knowing What Works in Health Care: A Roadmap for the Nation* to further elucidate how the science, on which healthcare is increasingly based, could be more certainly promulgated to providers and consumers in the nation as a whole. It makes recommendations for a national clinical effectiveness assessment program "with authority, overarching responsibility, sustained resources, and adequate capacity to ensure production of credible, unbiased information about what is known and not known about clinical effectiveness." It goes on to make specific recommendations regarding how the assessment should be undertaken:

- Set priorities for, fund, and manage systematic reviews of clinical effectiveness and related topics.

- Develop a common language and standards for conducting systematic reviews of the evidence and for generating clinical guidelines and recommendations.

- Provide a forum for addressing conflicting guidelines and recommendations.

- Prepare an annual [summary] report to Congress (IOM 2008).

Many of these dialogues have taken place alongside political discussions, debates, and demonstration projects about healthcare reform in the face of burgeoning healthcare costs in the first decade of the 21st century and the projected financial inadequacies of the Medicare and Medicaid programs taking effect as the century progresses. Many of the political figures of this period have assumed that they have an adequate understanding of the complexities of US healthcare delivery to formulate plans to solve the issues. Few undertook a solid attempt at doing so at the federal level, however, until those of the last two years of the decade. Prior to that, those charged with administration of the Medicare and Medicaid programs put forward little in the way of reform, except to require the development of more specific data sets: MS-DRGs; the International Classification of Diseases, tenth revision, Clinical Modification (ICD-10-CM); and the Procedural Classification System (ICD-10-PCS). MS-DRGs are now implemented, but the latter two are scheduled for final implementation October 1, 2013. There is a tremendous amount of systems development and education that must be accomplished before then by all payers, providers, and ICD data users. Managed care programs have proliferated, but little is really known about their effectiveness or their patients' satisfaction with them. Stand by also for the assessments of mandated insurance reform and participation by employers and the populace in the state of Massachusetts and, as well, the mandated participation by employers and the populace in "healthcare coverage" of a noninsurance type undertaken by the City and County of San Francisco in California.

After many years of debate, at the very end of the first decade of the 21st century, the US Congress managed to pass three sets of legislation that could have large positive impacts on the quality of care in the healthcare system as a whole. The American Recovery and Reinvestment Act, the Health Information Technology for Economic and Clinical Health (HITECH) Act, and the Patient Protection and Affordable Care Act all have provisions designed to improve the quality of a patient's healthcare: the Recovery Act by focusing funding on the expansion of the healthcare workforce; the HITECH Act by stimulating investment in the information systems infrastructure of professional practices, clinics, and hospitals; and the Affordable Care Act by mandating increased quality measure reporting by payers and providers at all levels of care, by implementing penalties for poor care in terms of reimbursement, and by improving access for the millions of Americans who, prior to the act's implementation, had nowhere to turn but the nation's emergency departments. New quality measure reporting would establish a quality measurement program for Medicaid and require long-term care and hospice facilities to submit data on their quality of care for the first time. Unfortunately, at the time of publication of this text, the Affordable Care Act has become mired in the deep political divide among conservatives, liberals, and independents in this country. The final outcome of this revolutionary but complicated solution will not be known until well after the 2012 election results are evident. In particular, the federal mandate contained therein for as many citizens as possible to participate in some kind of healthcare coverage for payment of received services makes it likely that the debate will continue until the publication of the sixth edition of this text.

Why Care about PI?

An individual working in the US healthcare industry today hears many terms that reflect the long-term development of quality improvement philosophy, including *quality assurance*, *quality improvement*, *quality management*, and *performance improvement*. The differences in meaning are subtle, reflecting the time and place of their origins, as well as the individuals and philosophies that generated them. But they are all, in reality, focused on one thing: helping people with challenged health return to healthier, more productive lives and doing so by the most efficient and effective means possible. It is an evolving mission and one that is always seeking a better way.

Healthcare professionals must be concerned with PI. There is a long tradition of seeking improvement in the healthcare industry. Today, PI is the key to ensuring high-quality care, and a PI philosophy pervades leading healthcare organizations. To contribute to personal and organizational success, one must commit to participate in PI. Today's patients increasingly are choosing their professional and institutional providers on the basis of quality. Furthermore, most contemporary payers prefer to negotiate with organizations that provide high-quality, yet cost-effective, services. Today's healthcare organizations must be able to back up their espousal of quality with reliable, objective data. Government-sponsored and commercial health plans, employers, and consumers are all now asking for more information on the quality of the healthcare services they receive and pay for. Additionally, a focus on quality is the key to meeting regulatory, licensure, and accreditation requirements. Demonstrating quality and improving performance are the definitive keys to success in the healthcare industry's mission to provide high-quality care.

Summary

Quality and PI in healthcare have a long tradition in the United States. With the examination and licensure of physicians, the standardization of hospitals, and the adoption over time of a philosophy of continuous quality improvement, the healthcare industry has committed itself to improving the health of its customers in the most efficient and effective ways possible. Along the way, the government has tried to stimulate the processes of improvement in the industry through innovative payment and review programs. Improvement initiatives at the end of the 20th century concentrated on refining improvement methodologies and making improvement processes more scientific. Indeed, improvement initiatives have become one of the most important functions that healthcare organizations perform today to thrive in the healthcare marketplace. However, the answer to the mandate for quality healthcare at a viable cost to all constituencies still largely eludes the nation, and much in the way of political and social dialogue must continue in order to meet the mandate in the 21st century.

References

Adams, D.P., and A.L. Moore. 1997. Nicholas J. Pisacano. In *Doctors, Nurses, and Medical Practitioners: A Bio-Bibliographical Sourcebook.* Edited by Magner, L.N., 222–226. Westport, CT: Greenwood Press.

American College of Surgeons. 1930. *Manual of Hospital Standardization and Hospital Standardization Report.* Chicago: American College of Surgeons.

American Hospital Association. 1999. *100 Faces of Health Care.* Chicago: Health Forum.

Bowditch, N.I. 1972. *History of the Massachusetts General Hospital.* Boston: Arno Press and New York Times.

Brickman, J.P. 1997. Ernst P. Boas. In *Doctors, Nurses, and Medical Practitioners: A Bio-Bibliographical Sourcebook.* Edited by Magner, L.N., 19–24. Westport, CT: Greenwood Press.

Bullough, V.L. 1997. Robert Latou Dickinson. In *Doctors, Nurses, and Medical Practitioners: A Bio-Bibliographical Sourcebook.* Edited by Magner, L.N., 75–78. Westport, CT: Greenwood Press.

Casto, A., and E. Layman. 2011. *Principles of Healthcare Reimbursement*, 3rd ed. Chicago: AHIMA Press.

Centers for Medicare and Medicaid Services. 2008. HCPCS: General information. http://www.cms.hhs.gov/MedHCPCSGenInfo/.

Donabedian, A. 1966. Evaluating the quality of medical care. *Milbank Quarterly* 44:166–203.

Flexner, A. 1910. *Medical Education in the United States and Canada, Bulletin Number Four* (The Flexner Report). New York: The Carnegie Foundation for the Advancement of Teaching. http://www.carnegiefoundation.org/files/elibrary/flexner_report.pdf.

Gage, A. 1997. Roswell Park. In *Doctors, Nurses, and Medical Practitioners: A Bio-Bibliographical Sourcebook*. Edited by Magner, L.N., 204–208. Westport, CT: Greenwood Press.

Haller, J.S. 1981. *American Medicine in Transition 1840–1910*. Chicago: University of Illinois Press.

Hill, P.E. 1997. Maude E. Callen. In *Doctors, Nurses, and Medical Practitioners: A Bio-Bibliographical Sourcebook*. Edited by Magner, L.N., 49–54. Westport, CT: Greenwood Press.

Hill-Burton Act of 1946. 42 USC 6.

Institute of Medicine. 2001. *Crossing the Quality Chasm: A New Health System for the 21st Century*. Washington, DC: National Academy Press.

Institute of Medicine. 2008. *Knowing What Works in Health Care: A Roadmap for the Nation*. Washington, DC: National Academy Press.

Joint Commission. 2011. Facts about the National Patient Safety Goals. http://www.jointcommission.org/facts_about_the_national_patient_safety_goals/.

Joint Commission on Accreditation of Hospitals. 1952. *Standards of Hospital Accreditation*. Oakbrook Terrace, IL: JCAHO.

Kalisch, P.A., and B.J. Kalisch. 1995. *The Advance of American Nursing*. Philadelphia: J.B. Lippincott Company.

Leighow, S.R. 1997. Lavinia Lloyd Dock. In *Doctors, Nurses, and Medical Practitioners: A Bio-Bibliographical Sourcebook*. Edited by Magner, L.N., 79–85. Westport, CT: Greenwood Press.

Medicaid. 1965. Public Law 89-97, Title XIX.

Medicare. 1965. Public Law 89-97, Title XVIII.

Meldrum, M. 1997. Mary Steichen Calderone. In *Doctors, Nurses, and Medical Practitioners: A Bio-Bibliographical Sourcebook*. Edited by Magner, L.N., 43–48. Westport, CT: Greenwood Press.

Morton, T.G. 1973. *The History of the Pennsylvania Hospital*. New York: Arno Press.

Roberts, J.S., J.G. Coate, and R. Redman. 1987. A history of the Joint Commission on Accreditation of Hospitals. *JAMA* 256(7):936–940.

Trent, J.C. 1977. An early New Jersey medical license. Chapter X in *Legacies in Law and Medicine*. Edited by Burns, C.R., 90–92. New York: Science History Publications.

Resources

Agency for Healthcare Research and Quality. http://www.ahrq.gov.

Crosby, P.B. 1980. *Quality Is Free*. New York: Mentor Books.

Crosby, P.B. 1984. *Quality without Tears*. New York: Plume Books.

Deming, W.E. 1986. *Out of the Crisis*. Cambridge, MA: MIT Press. First published in 1982 as *Quality, Productivity, and Competitive Position*.

Donabedian, A. 1980. *The Definition of Quality and Approaches to Its Management*. Volume 1: *Explorations in Quality Assessment and Monitoring*. Ann Arbor, MI: Health Administration Press.

Donabedian, A. 1988. The quality of care: How can it be assessed? *JAMA* 260(12):1743–1748.

HR 4157. 2006. International Classification of Diseases, tenth revision, Procedural Classification System (ICD-10-PCS).

Juran, J.M. 1945. *Management of Inspection and Quality Control*. New York: Harper & Brothers.

Juran, J.M. 1951. *Quality Control Handbook*. New York: McGraw-Hill.

Juran, J.M. 1964. *Managerial Breakthrough*. New York: McGraw-Hill.

Juran, J.M. 1967. *Management of Quality Control*. New York: Joseph M. Juran.

Juran, J.M. 1970. *Quality Planning and Analysis*. New York: McGraw-Hill.

Juran, J.M. 1980. *Upper Management and Quality*. New York: Joseph M. Juran.

Juran, J.M. 1988. *Juran on Planning for Quality*. New York: Free Press.

Silin, C.I. 1977. A state medical board examination in 1816. In *Legacies in Law and Medicine*. Edited by Burns, C.R., 93–106. New York: Science History Publications.

Walton, M. 1986. *The Deming Management Method*. New York: Perigee Books.

Walton, M. 1990. *Deming Management at Work*. New York: G. P. Putnam and Sons.

Part I
A Performance Improvement Model

Chapter 1
Defining a Performance Improvement Model

Learning Objectives

- To explain the cyclical nature of performance improvement activities
- To introduce terminology and standards common to performance improvement activities
- To distinguish between organization-wide performance improvement activities and team-based performance improvement activities
- To outline the organization-wide performance improvement cycle
- To outline the team-based performance improvement cycle

Key Terms

Continuous monitoring
Leadership
Opportunity for improvement
Performance improvement (PI) team
Process redesign
QI toolbox techniques

Background and Significance

Efforts to ensure the quality of the healthcare services provided in the United States have been in place for more than 30 years. Through the years, these efforts have had many different names: quality assurance (QA), total quality management (TQM), quality improvement (QI), continuous quality improvement (CQI), quality management (QM), and performance improvement (PI). Each of these terms represents a quality and PI model or methodology that healthcare organizations have used with varying degrees of success. Many books and articles have been written on the subject, and new models and terminology will likely be developed in the future.

A new professional entering the healthcare field will probably work for many organizations over his or her career and participate in many quality and PI projects. He or she will learn to use specific quality and PI models and techniques as needed. With experience, healthcare professionals will develop the skills necessary to customize the models to specific organizations and healthcare services.

The goal of this chapter is to provide a general overview of quality and PI as it is applied in healthcare organizations. The chapter describes a generic PI model, defines commonly used PI terms, and explains the basic philosophy of continuous performance improvement.

PI as a Cyclical Process

Various healthcare organizations, including accreditation bodies, groups of clinical professionals, quality management professionals, healthcare providers, and government regulatory and policy-making entities, all have unique perspectives on quality in healthcare. Many have developed their own methodologies for quality and PI. Most PI models applied in healthcare today share one structural characteristic: They are cyclical in nature.

The cyclical model is based on the assumptions that PI activities will take place continually and that services, processes, and outcomes can always be improved. Quality should not be treated as a goal that is accomplished and then forgotten. Rather, it should be an ongoing mission that guides everyday operations.

Accreditation and licensing agencies expect hospitals and other healthcare facilities to strive for the highest quality of care possible at all times. Healthcare leaders and their boards of directors are responsible for the quality of the organizations' services. Many large healthcare organizations employ experts in quality management who are responsible for organizing PI activities and reporting results to the leadership and the boards of directors. At the same time, however, all employees are expected to have a basic understanding of PI principles and participate in PI activities.

The general PI model presented in this textbook includes two interrelated cycles. The cycle illustrated in figure 1.1 represents the organization's ongoing performance-monitoring function. The cycle illustrated in figure 1.2 represents the activities of individual PI teams working on specific PI projects. Together, the two cycles make up the healthcare PI model (figure 1.3).

Monitoring Performance through Data Collection

Performance monitoring is data driven. Monitoring performance based on internal and external data is the foundation of all PI activities. Each healthcare organization must identify and prioritize which processes and outcomes (in other words, which types of data) are important to monitor on the basis of its mission and the scope of care and services it provides. A logical starting point in identifying areas in which to monitor performance

Figure 1.1.   Organization-wide PI process

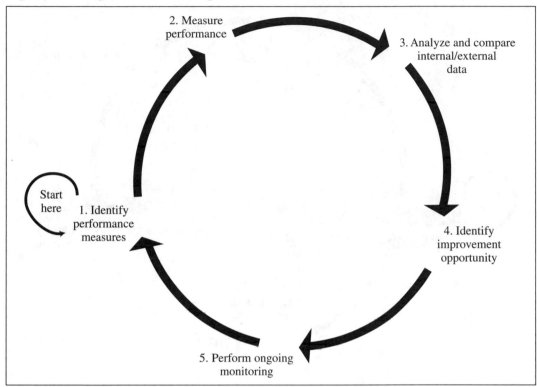

Figure 1.2.   Team-based PI process

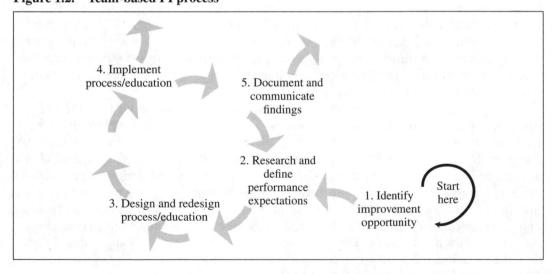

Figure 1.3.   PI model

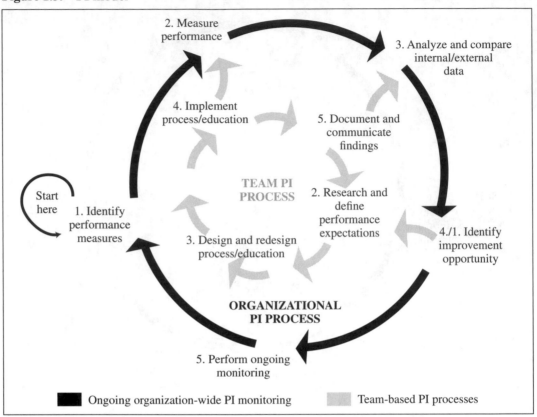

includes those that perform important organizational functions (addressed in part II of this text), particularly those that are high risk, high volume, or problem prone. Outcomes of care, customer feedback, and the requirements of regulatory agencies are additional areas that organizations consider when prioritizing performance monitors. Once the scope and focus of performance monitoring are determined, the leaders define the data collection requirements for each performance measure.

As shown in figure 1.1, monitoring performance depends on the identification of performance measures for each service, process, or outcome deemed important to track. Performance measure is "a quantitative tool (for example, a rate, ratio, index, percentage) that provides an indication of an organization's performance in relation to a specified process or outcome" (Joint Commission 2011). Monitoring selected performance measures can help an organization determine process stability or identify improvement opportunities. Specific criteria are used to define the organization's performance measures. Components of a good performance measure include a documented numerator statement, a denominator statement, and a description of the population to which the measure is applicable. In addition, the measurement period; baseline goal; data collection method; and frequency of data collection, analysis, and reporting must be identified.

One important outcome that hospitals are required to continuously monitor is the monthly delinquent health record rate. The criteria used to establish this performance measure include:

$$\frac{\text{Number of incomplete health records that exceed the}}{\text{medical-staff–established time frame for chart completion}}$$

$$\text{Average monthly discharges}$$

The populations included in this performance measure are the medical staff and inpatient health records. Tracking this outcome allows the hospital to continuously monitor its rate or percentage of delinquent health records. (See figure 1.1.) If the health record delinquency rate exceeds the hospital's established performance standards (an internal comparison) or nationally established performance standards (external comparison), an **opportunity for improvement** has been identified. Following this, a team-based PI process may be initiated. (See figure 1.2.)

When an organization compares its current performance with its own internal historical data, or uses data from similar external organizations across the country, it establishes a *benchmark*, also known as a standard of performance or best practice, for a particular process or outcome. Establishing a benchmark for each monitored performance measure assists the healthcare organization in setting performance baselines, describing process performance or stability, and identifying areas for more focused data collection. The Joint Commission (until 2007, known as the Joint Commission on Accreditation of Healthcare Organizations) is one available external resource that can be used to establish the performance measure of the average monthly health record delinquency rate for a hospital. The Joint Commission will cite the healthcare organization with a requirement for improvement if the total average health record delinquency rate exceeds 50 percent of the average monthly discharges in any one quarter. Hospitals commonly set the benchmark for their health record delinquency rate at less than 50 percent.

Once a benchmark for each performance measure is determined, analyzing data collection results becomes more meaningful. Results that fall outside the established benchmark often trigger further study or more focused data collection on a performance measure. When variation is discovered through **continuous monitoring,** or when unexpected events suggest performance problems, members of the organization may decide that there is an opportunity for improvement. The opportunity may involve changing a process or an outcome to better meet customer feedback, needs, or expectations.

An example of the PI model used as an improvement opportunity identified from ongoing data collection at Community Hospital of the West is shown in figure 1.4. The hospital administration had previously identified the employee turnover rate as an important performance measure to monitor and had collected a number of years of historical internal data on this performance measure. Additionally, it researched external comparison data from other hospitals in the community and throughout the state and determined that the best-practice rate for employee turnover in its area should be 5 percent. Accordingly, the administration set its employee turnover rate benchmark at less than 5 percent.

Figure 1.4.   Community Hospital of the West employee turnover rate

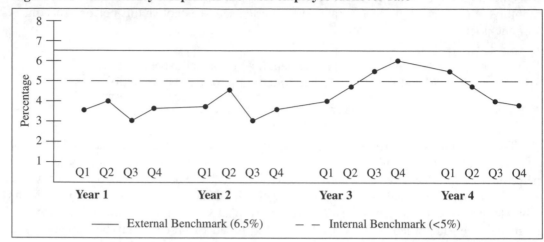

During the third year, the employee turnover rate began to steadily increase from 3 percent to 6 percent. After receiving third-quarter data that showed a continued increase in turnover, the Performance Improvement and Patient Safety Council recommended further data analysis by job class. The findings from this analysis showed a pattern in employee turnover within nursing. Exit survey data received from nursing staff were also studied, with reasons for leaving linked to salary and benefits. The council immediately recommended that the human resources department research community salary and benefits packages offered to nurses. The results of the research revealed that Community Hospital of the West's salary and benefits package had not remained competitive, and nursing personnel were being recruited by hospitals with more attractive benefits packages. Once Community Hospital of the West redesigned, implemented, and advertised its benefits package for nurses, the turnover rate decreased to below the established benchmark. Figure 1.5 shows how the PI model was applied in this situation.

It has been a common practice in many healthcare organizations and is now a Joint Commission requirement to appoint a **leadership** group to oversee organization-wide PI activities. This leadership group (sometimes named the Performance Improvement and Patient Safety Council or quality council) is responsible for defining the organization's PI program. Establishment of a PI program includes the following steps:

1.   Define and implement the organization-wide PI model.

2.   Establish a staff education plan to train employees in PI.

3.   Prioritize and define PI measures.

4.   Define data collection and reporting responsibilities.

5.   Appoint PI teams when process variation exceeds established benchmarks.

6.   Maintain a process of reporting significant findings and corrective actions to the board of directors and other stakeholders.

Part III of this text covers PI leadership responsibilities in greater detail.

Figure 1.5.   Community Hospital of the West PI model

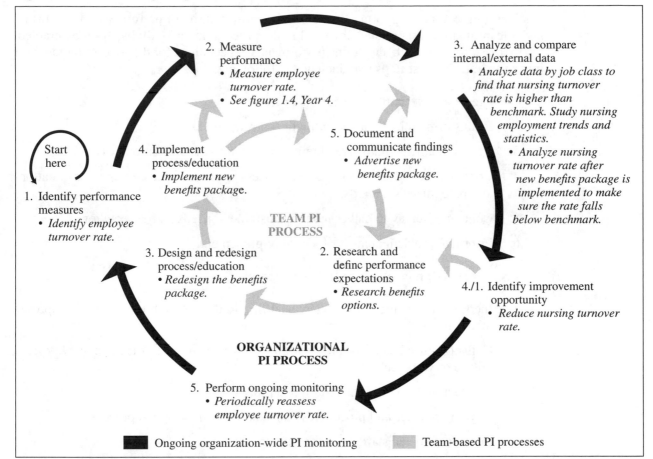

Who identifies opportunities for improvement? Participation depends primarily on leadership's commitment to establishing a culture of continuous improvement. Ideally, PI opportunities should be identified by those closest to care or service processes.

There is a wide spectrum of PI mind-sets in healthcare organizations. In some organizations, employees may not feel free to offer suggestions for improvement. Managers who have a traditional style of management may believe that only managers should direct change and thus might feel threatened by PI processes. In such situations, managers assume responsibility for identifying opportunities for improvement.

Once an improvement opportunity has been identified, the leadership group can respond in a variety of ways. When the improvement opportunity is believed to be the result of a lack of knowledge or experience, an educational program may be recommended. When the improvement opportunity is the result of inefficiency or ineffectiveness in a work process, the leadership group may convene a **performance improvement (PI) team** to examine the process. (The relationship between organization-wide performance monitoring and team-based PI processes is illustrated in figure 1.3.)

Team-Based PI Processes

Once an improvement opportunity has been identified through performance monitoring, and a team that consists of staff involved in the process under study has been assembled, the first task is to research and define performance expectations for the process targeted for improvement. The first steps may include the following:

1. Create a flow chart of the current process.

2. Brainstorm problem areas within the current process.

3. Research any regulatory requirements related to the current process.

4. Compare the organization's current process with performance standards or nationally recognized standards.

5. Conduct a survey to gather input on customers' needs and expectations.

6. Prioritize problem areas for focused improvement.

Process redesign involves the following steps:

1. Incorporate findings or changes identified in the research phase of the improvement process.

2. Collect focused data from the prioritized problem areas to further clarify process failure or variation.

3. Create a flow chart of the redesigned process.

4. Develop policies and procedures that support the redesigned process.

5. Educate involved staff about the new process.

PI teams can use a variety of tools to accomplish their goals. This textbook calls these quality improvement tools collected from traditional quality improvement practice and theory **QI toolbox techniques.** The tools make it easier to gather and analyze information, and they help team members stay focused on PI activities and move the process along efficiently. Several chapters in part I of this textbook, and all of the chapters in part II, introduce at least one technique from the QI toolbox.

After implementing a new process, the team continues to measure performance against customers' expectations and established performance standards. The team may need to redesign the process or product if measurements indicate that there is room for further improvement. When measurement data indicate that the improvement is effective, ongoing monitoring of the process is resumed (as in figure 1.1). The team documents and communicates its findings to the leadership group and other interested parties in the organization. Results also may be communicated to interested groups in the community.

The team is usually disbanded at this point in the cycle, and routine organizational monitoring of the performance measures is resumed. If another opportunity for improvement arises, the team-based improvement process may be reinstituted.

Summary

PI in healthcare is a cyclical process. Healthcare professionals are expected to continually look for opportunities to improve the quality of processes, services, and outcomes. Many PI methodologies can be applied in healthcare organizations. Most methodologies, however, follow a model of continuous performance monitoring, ongoing identification of improvement opportunities, and team-based improvement processes.

Reference

Joint Commission. 2011. Performance measurement. http://www.jointcommission.org/performance_measurement.aspx.

Resources

Kelly, D.L. 2011. *Applying Quality Management in Healthcare, Third Edition: A System's Approach.* Chicago: Health Administration Press.

McLaughlin, C.P., and A.D. Kaluzny. 2006. *Continuous Quality Improvement in Health Care: Theory, Implementations, and Applications*, 3rd ed. Sudbury, MA: Jones & Bartlett Learning.

Ransom, S.B., S.J. Maulik, and D.B. Nash. 2008. *The Healthcare Quality Book: Vision, Strategy and Tools*, 2nd ed. Chicago: Health Administration Press.

Chapter 2
Identifying Improvement Opportunities Based on Performance Measurement

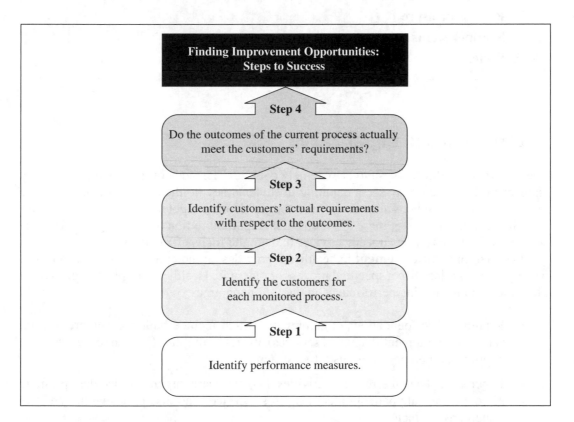

Learning Objectives

- To explain the principal aspects of healthcare that are targeted for performance measurement

- To describe the significance of outcomes and proactive risk reduction in performance improvement methodology

- To explain how brainstorming and the nominal group technique can be used in performance improvement activities

Key Terms

Affinity diagrams
Benchmarking
Brainstorming
Nominal group technique
Outcome measure
Outcomes
Performance measurement
Performance measures
Process measure
Sentinel events
Systems

Background and Significance

The American healthcare system is extremely complex. The idea of improving even a tiny element of the system may seem daunting to students new to the concept of performance improvement (PI). Where does the process begin? How are potential areas for improvement identified? To answer these questions, it is important to first develop a general understanding of the areas of healthcare services that are the focus of PI efforts.

Performance measurement in healthcare provides an indication of an organization's performance in relation to a specified process or outcome. Healthcare PI philosophies most often focus on measuring performance in the following areas:

- **Systems:** The foundations of caregiving, which include buildings (environmental services), equipment (technical services), professional staff (human resources), and appropriate policies (administrative systems)

- **Processes:** The interrelated activities in healthcare organizations that promote effective and safe patient outcomes across services and disciplines within an integrated environment

- **Outcomes:** The final results of care, treatment, and services in terms of the patient's expectations, needs, and quality of life, which may be positive and appropriate or negative and diminishing

Most PI projects address the organization's performance in at least one of these areas.

Continuous Improvement Builds on Continuous Monitoring: Steps to Success

To discover which systems, processes, or outcomes need to be improved, a healthcare organization must first find out what is and what is not working with respect to the needs and expectations of its customers (for example, results of customer satisfaction surveys and customer complaints). (See the discussion of performance measurement and monitoring in chapter 1.) Most improvement methodologies recognize that the organization must identify and continuously monitor the important organizational and patient-focused functions that they perform, with special emphasis on high-volume, high-risk, and problem-prone outcomes. (See figure 2.1 for an illustration of the process.)

Figure 2.1.   Process of identifying improvement opportunities

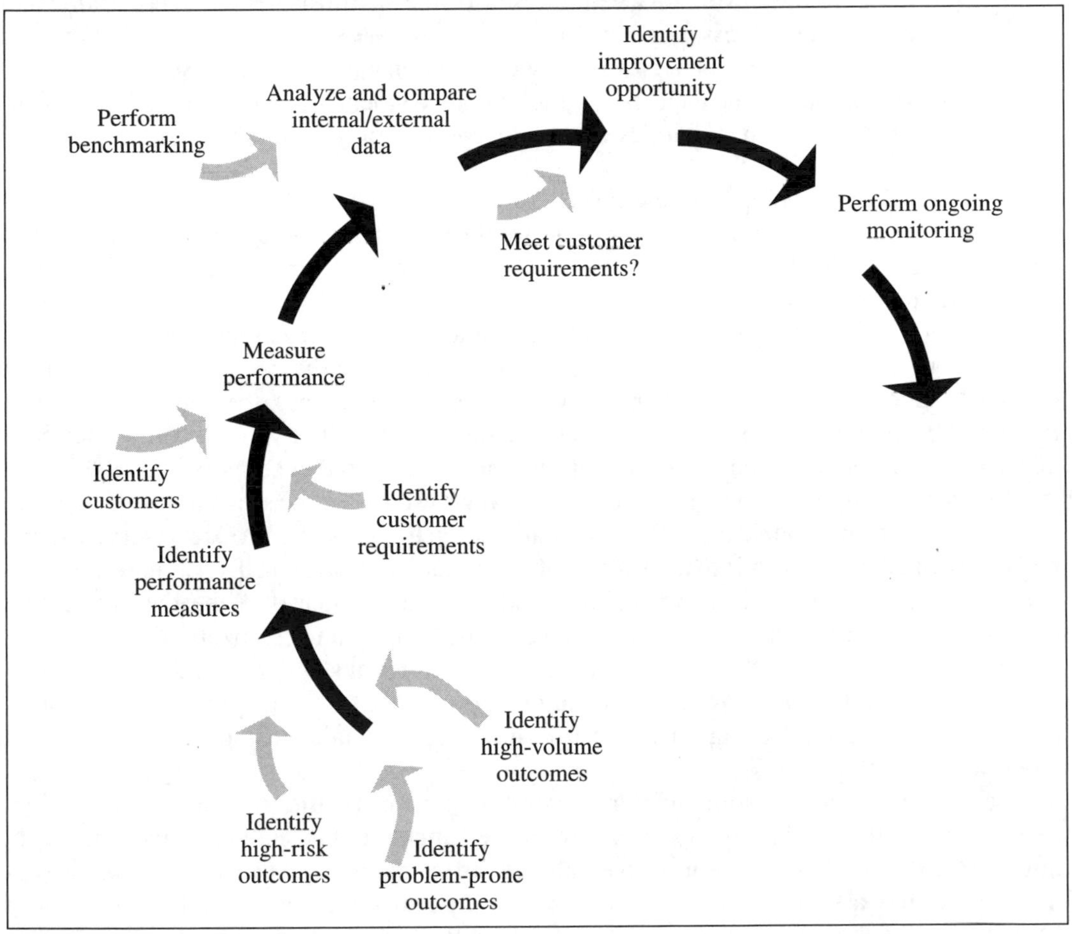

Step 1: Identify Performance Measures

Performance measures include process measures and outcome measures:

- A **process measure** focuses on a way of delivering services that leads to a certain outcome. A scientific or experiential basis must exist for believing that the process, when executed appropriately as designed, will increase the probability of achieving a desired outcome. Examples of process measures are percentage of antibiotics administered immediately prior to open reduction internal fixation (ORIF) surgeries or percentage of deliveries accomplished by cesarean section. These procedure measures might be monitored irrespective of the specific patient outcomes if the medical staff were attempting to move staff practice to a model more widely demonstrated to be more effective in the scientific literature and in the community in which the medical staff was based.

- An **outcome measure** indicates the result of the performance (or nonperformance) of a function or process. For example, an outcome measure may be the effect of care, treatment, or services on a customer, such as an unanticipated adverse event or, as in the example above, the incidence of postoperative wound infections occurring in ORIF procedures in which antibiotics were and were not utilized (Joint Commission 2011a).

Many facilities develop measurable criteria to determine whether customer care, treatment, or services produce desirable or undesirable outcomes. The organization must then develop a data collection process or tool within the facility to track information on customer care, treatment, and services.

In addition, the processes, end products, and outcomes of every organizational unit may affect other organizational units. This means that in addition to the patients, the members of the organization may be one another's customers. For each process, the end products must first be identified, including those received by patient customers as well as other members of the organization. (See the discussion of internal and external customers in chapter 6.)

Benchmarking is another means of identifying systems, processes, and outcomes for improvement. **Benchmarking** is the systematic comparison of the products, services, and outcomes of one organization with those of a similar organization. Benchmarking comparisons also can be made using regional and national standards if the data collection processes are similar. This process of benchmarking against an organization's established norm, which may be based on best practice, state or national standards, or some combination of these thresholds, helps the organization determine whether its processes fall within the acceptable standard deviations of the norm. Items that fall outside the norm may be appropriate for PI projects.

Lastly, organizations sometimes receive dramatic information about the ineffectiveness of a care process through a sentinel event. **Sentinel events** usually involve significant injury to or the death of a patient or an employee through avoidable causes. The Joint Commission defines a sentinel event as an unexpected occurrence involving death or serious physical or psychological injury, or the risk thereof. Serious injury specifically includes loss of limb or function (Joint Commission 2011b). The event is called "sentinel" because it should sound an alarm that requires immediate attention. The phrase "or risk thereof" describes any process variation for which a recurrence would carry significant chance of an adverse reaction. Examples of reviewable sentinel events include a patient suicide in a setting where the patient received 24-hour care, infant abduction or discharge to the wrong family, rape, hemolytic transfusion reaction involving administration of blood or blood products having major group incompatibilities, or surgery on the wrong patient or wrong body part. Such problem-prone outcomes get the organization's attention very quickly. An analysis of the causes of a sentinel event usually allows the organization to make significant improvements in a process. The Joint Commission (2011c) issues a notification called "Sentinel Event Alert" with information related to sentinel events and outcomes. This information outlines risk reduction strategies for many common sentinel events based on root-cause analysis from different organizations. Review of this information allows the organization to measure its own performance against the performance of other organizations. (See chapter 10.)

The most important performance measures are those identified as strategically important to the organization's overall mission. Some organizations use the criteria of high or low volume, high risk, and problem prone to identify the performance measures that should receive the most scrutiny:

- Processes related to high- or low-volume outcomes affect numerous customers. High-volume processes increase the risk of incidents through the sheer number of processes performed. Low-volume processes increase the risk because they may be performed infrequently or be unfamiliar to staff, creating the opportunity for increased errors or patient safety risks.

- Processes related to problem-prone or high-risk outcomes can result in patient injury or negative outcomes that might open the organization to malpractice suits or other legal actions. Either of these process outcomes increases the long-term cost to the patient or the community due to increased length of stay required for additional procedures or costly malpractice fees.

The processes and outcomes related to strategically important services and to the organization's overall mission become the organization's performance measures—those measures by which the performance of the organization and its work units will be monitored by internal and external customers.

Step 2: Identify the Customers for Each Monitored Process

The question to be answered in this step is, who receives the outcomes or end products? The list must be exhaustive and should include internal and external customers (as described in chapter 6). Steps 2 through 4 are initiated when a performance measure shows undesirable trends or outcomes requiring the formation of a PI team.

Step 3: Identify Customers' Actual Requirements with Respect to the Outcomes

Actual requirements must be identified from the customers' perspective. The objective is to identify the factors that the organization's internal and external customers value most (as described in chapter 6).

Step 4: Do the Outcomes of the Current Processes Actually Meet the Customers' Requirements?

When the outcomes of current processes *do* actually meet the customers' requirements, the organization should continue ongoing monitoring of the processes. When the outcomes *do not* meet customers' requirements, a PI team should be formed to examine the processes in greater detail. (See chapter 3.) Alternatively, the organization should develop an educational program to fine-tune staff members' ability to execute the processes effectively.

Real-Life Examples

Some ways that healthcare work units have identified improvement opportunities using the techniques introduced in this chapter are discussed in the following paragraphs.

Registration for Day Surgery

At one hospital, data from customer satisfaction surveys indicated an increase in patient complaints about having to come to the facility two and three times for preoperative testing. The PI team assigned to explore the problem identified the following performance measures, customers, and customers' requirements and determined whether the customers' requirements were met:

Step 1:   *Performance measures?*

Registration information provided and surgery scheduled by physician's office

Preoperative workup completed by day of surgery

Step 2:   *Customers for monitored process?*

Patient and patient's family

Physician and office staff

Surgery staff

Registration staff

Step 3:   *Customers' requirements?*

One-time communication of registration information

Preoperative workup completed prior to day of surgery and coordinated in one visit

Step 4:   *Customers' requirements met?*

Patient satisfaction surveys showed only 76 percent satisfaction with same-day surgery registration and preoperative workup processes.

Registration staff and physician's office staff were hearing complaints from patients that the registration process was cumbersome and not user-friendly.

Duplicate data collection occurred between physician's office registration and same-day surgery registration.

The data collection process indicated patient dissatisfaction with services. Several problems were clearly identified that could lead to an improved outcome for patients through a PI process with a combined team approach.

Business Office and Health Information Management Department

In another hospital, the number of accounts waiting to be billed had increased over the past six months. The business office and health information management (HIM) department decided to look at the timeliness, appropriateness, and effectiveness of their information-processing procedures. A PI team assigned to examine the process developed the following information:

Step 1: *Performance measures?*

Patient insurance and benefits information received at time of registration

Health record documentation complete at time of discharge

Clinical codes assigned and transmitted within 72 hours of patient discharge

Unbilled accounts less than $1 million

Step 2: *Customers for monitored process?*

Patients

Physicians and other clinical staff

Business office staff

HIM staff

Administration

Third-party payers

Step 3: *Customers' requirements?*

Unbilled accounts continuously below $1 million

Health record delinquency rate less than 50 percent

HIM health record completion standards met

Business office benefits verification standards met

Step 4: *Customers' requirements met?*

Unbilled accounts greater than $3 million

Health record delinquency rate greater than 50 percent

HIM backlogs in all chart completion areas

Business office verifying benefits at admission only 48 percent of time

QI Toolbox Techniques

The most common toolbox techniques that PI teams use to determine performance measures, identify customers, identify customers' requirements, and identify whether customers' requirements are met include brainstorming, affinity diagrams, and the nominal group technique.

Brainstorming

Brainstorming can be conducted in a structured or an unstructured way. In *structured* brainstorming, the leader solicits input from team members by going around the table or room. Each team member comments on the issue in turn or passes until the next round. This process continues until participants have no new ideas to suggest or until the time period set in the meeting's agenda has elapsed. In *unstructured* brainstorming, members of the team offer ideas as they come to mind. Some members may have no ideas to offer, and others may contribute a number of ideas. In either method of brainstorming, several general rules are followed:

- Everyone agrees on the issue to be brainstormed.
- All ideas are written down on a white board or flip chart in the team member's own words.
- Ideas are never criticized or discussed during the brainstorming period.
- The process is limited in the time allotted—5 to 15 minutes at most.

Affinity Diagrams

Affinity diagrams are used to organize and prioritize ideas after the initial brainstorming session. This type of diagram is useful when the team generates a large amount of information. The team members agree on the primary categories or groupings from the brainstorming session, and then secondary ideas are listed under each primary category. This process allows the team to tackle a large problem in a more manageable way (Tague 2004). (See figure 2.2 for an example.) Adhesive notes work well for this process. They are easily transferred from one category or grouping to another as team members work to group or rate ideas.

Nominal Group Technique

The **nominal group technique** gives each member of the team an opportunity to select the most important ideas from the affinity diagram. This technique allows groups to narrow the focus of discussion or to make decisions without getting involved in extended, circular discussions during which the more vocal members dominate. All of the ideas obtained during an earlier brainstorming session are written in a place where everyone can see them. Teams usually use white boards or flip charts for this purpose.

Next, team members vote on the various issues or ideas to determine which should be considered first. The facilitator writes the numeral "1" by the idea that each team member chooses as most important. This process continues until all of the team members have ranked all of the issues or ideas on a numerical scale. For example, if five issues were listed, each team member would rank them from 1 to 5, with 1 being the most important and 5 being the least important. Then the facilitator adds up the rankings for each issue. The issue with the lowest sum is selected as the team's choice for most important. The team will work on this issue first, followed by the other four issues in ranked order.

Figure 2.2.   Example of an affinity diagram

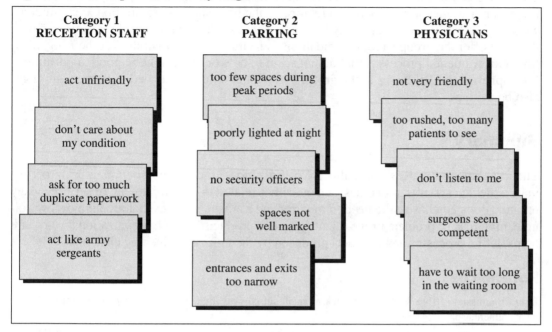

Another way to vote is to use adhesive dots in various colors. Each team member chooses a color, and the members affix their dots to the five issues they think are most important. The issue that has the most dots is the most important. This method works well because members can be influenced by other members' placement of votes, thus allowing consensus to begin to develop during the voting process.

Case Study

Students should watch the movies *The Doctor*, with William Hurt, and *Patch Adams*, with Robin Williams, or any current television program that occurs in a healthcare setting. Students should brainstorm positive and negative healthcare performance issues shown in the film or program. Then they should create an affinity diagram by writing the brainstormed issues on adhesive notes and grouping similar performance issues together on a white board or flip chart. In group settings, the nominal group technique could be used to prioritize the most important performance issues identified from the film or program for action by a team.

Project Application

Students should brainstorm issues or opportunities for improvement that they have observed in their academic environment, general community, work settings, or personal activities.

The issues can be educational processes such as course sequencing, professional practice issues, or customer service issues in relation to the bookstore or registration area. Students working in a healthcare setting may have issues that student teams could work on, and then they can offer the group's recommendations to healthcare administrators at their organization. Governmental processes that do not seem to be working might be good opportunities for improvement. Processes at the grocery store or at church that need improvement might also be evident.

Summary

The most important areas for healthcare organizations to consider when measuring performance include systems, processes, and outcomes related to care, treatment, or service. Many organizations emphasize the need to monitor and evaluate services that are high or low volume, high risk, or problem prone. Identifying end products for each organizational work unit helps define processes and products produced by the unit and valued by customers.

References

Joint Commission. 2011a. Performance measurement. http://www.jointcommission.org/performance_measurement.aspx.

Joint Commission. 2011b. Sentinel event. http://www.jointcommission.org/sentinel_event.aspx.

Joint Commission. 2011c. Sentinel event alert. http://www.jointcommission.org/sentinel_event.aspx.

Tague, N. 2004. *The Quality Toolbox*, 2nd ed. Milwaukee, WI: ASQ Quality Press.

Resources

Abdelhak, M., E. Jacobs, S. Grostick, and M.A. Hanken. 2007. *Health Information: Management of a Strategic Resource*, 3rd ed. Philadelphia: W. B. Saunders.

Agency for Healthcare Research and Quality. http://www.ahrq.gov/consumer/.

Albright, J.M., R.J. Panzer, E.R. Black, R.A. Mays, and C.M. Lush-Ehrmann. 1993. Reporting tools for clinical quality improvement. *Clinical Performance Quality in Health Care* 1(4):227–232.

Donabedian, A. 1988. The quality of care: How can it be assessed? *JAMA* 260(12):1743–1748.

LaTour, K., and S. Eichenwald, eds. 2010. *Health Information Management: Concepts, Principles, and Practice*, 3rd ed. Chicago: AHIMA.

Chapter 3
Using Teamwork in Performance Improvement

Learning Objectives

- To identify the effective use of teams in performance improvement activities

- To enumerate the differences between the roles of the leader and the members in performance improvement teams

- To describe the contributions that team charters, team roles, ground rules, listening, and questioning can make to improve the effectiveness of performance improvement teams

Key Terms

Action plan
Agenda
Blitz team
Cross-functional
Functional
Ground rules
Mission statement
Performance improvement council
Team charter
Team facilitator
Team leader
Team member
Team recorder or **scribe**
Timekeeper
Values statement
Vision statement

Background and Significance

Performance improvement (PI) teams involve a number of people working over long periods of time. They are expensive in terms of both time and money. Therefore, PI teams should be considered an organizational resource to be used appropriately and prudently.

The early quality improvement philosophies of Deming, Juran, and Crosby were based on team processes. Therefore, when quality improvement methodologies were first applied to healthcare organizations, it was assumed that PI activities were best accomplished by PI teams. Experience with PI processes in healthcare settings, however, has shown that PI teams are not always required.

Today, when an improvement opportunity is identified, the organization's leadership or PI council can initiate one of three approaches:

- Establish a blitz team

- Disseminate information or develop an educational training program

- Develop a functional or cross-functional PI team

Sometimes the leaders of an organization may decide that they already have all the facts they need about an improvement opportunity and that the changes required are "quick fixes." In such cases, they may decide to establish a blitz team. A **Blitz team** does not spend a lot of time gathering data and reengineering processes. These teams are usually composed of individuals from a similar group who are very familiar with the processes or end products that need improvement (Caldwell 1998). For example, the members of the health information management (HIM) department may want to increase response time to chart sign-off. The HIM department may plan several ways to make charts more available for all other staff, or they may create a more conducive environment for privacy during documentation. The blitz team constructs relatively simple fixes that improve work processes without going through the whole PI process and without the need to involve other departments. Thus, an improvement can be implemented without a major investment of time, personnel, and resources.

Some improvement opportunities involve only the dissemination of information or better individual training. Again, this approach to implementing an improvement can be accomplished without expending large amounts of resources.

However, when the improvement opportunity is complex or involves multiple departments or multiple work units within a department, the team-based approach should be considered. A PI team is instituted to research, plan, and implement the improvement. PI teams may be **functional** or **cross-functional.** A functional team involves staff from a single department or service area, while a cross-functional team involves more than one department, service area, or discipline. For example, a multidisciplinary or cross-functional team may be needed to address a shortage of blood or blood products in a hospital that cares for emergency, surgical, and obstetrics patients, any of whom may need blood at any time during their hospital stay. Individuals from all areas, including the laboratory, administration, surgery, obstetrics, and the emergency room, may need to help set priorities and explain the particular needs of their own areas.

This chapter discusses the composition of PI teams and the roles of individual members. It explores the purpose of team charters, mission statements, and vision statements; ground rules for meetings; and the skills needed to develop effective teams.

Effective Teams and Team Composition

Effective team function is crucial to the success of PI programs in healthcare organizations. An organization's leaders can take a variety of initiatives to help teams function more effectively. There appears to be one major issue, however, that, more than any other, predicts the likelihood of team effectiveness in the PI realm: the organization's expectations.

Some consultants believe that every team needs development, and consequently, many use team-building exercises as a matter of course. The single most important way for an organization to achieve effective teams is to make team problem solving and team PI part of the organizational culture. From the moment an individual is hired to work within a healthcare organization, the message should be overtly communicated by the organization that the individual is expected to participate in team projects and that this is part of everyone's job description. By making team participation part of the organizational culture, no individual employee will think that he or she is exempt from cooperating in team approaches to organizational issues.

That is not to say that there will not be individuals on a team who are uncooperative or have their own agendas. Individuals who are not team players can be directed into positive team production, however, with knowledgeable and experienced PI teams.

When convening a cross-functional PI team is appropriate, the leadership of the organization must determine the composition of the team. The PI team should be made up of individuals close to the process to be improved, because they are best qualified to accomplish the process review. This may mean that some teams will include more staff than managers. Questions that should be asked to identify individual team members include the following:

- Which departments or disciplines are involved in the process?

- Who are the customers of the process? In other words, who will receive the product or service that the process produces?

- Who supplies the process? That is, who provides (supplies) a product or service that begins the process to be improved?

Applying this line of questioning to the multidisciplinary team addressing the hospital's blood supply shortage, the departments and disciplines identified in the process included the laboratory, administration, surgery, obstetrics, and emergency departments. Some of the disciplines and departments identified on the team are the customers of the process, for example, the patient care areas and the patients requiring the blood products. The suppliers of the process, in this instance, are the laboratory and administration areas, both of which are responsible for coordinating the availability of blood products to the hospital's patient care areas.

Limitations on the number of people who can participate on a team and other factors sometimes mean that all of the people involved in a process to be improved cannot participate directly on the PI team. When this happens, the team must make provisions to contact the other individuals affected by the improvement initiative. Because their perspectives and information are of critical importance, the team must develop some means for obtaining their input.

It is important to keep teams small and manageable. The general rule of thumb is that teams should be made up of 8 to 10 members. Once the team has been formed, the team members should determine which individuals, departments, and disciplines are key players in the process. Then they can bring other individuals, departments, and disciplines into the process on an ad hoc basis.

Team Roles

After the team has been selected, a **team leader** should be chosen. Having a leader is necessary to get the team organized. The organization's leaders may select the team leader, or the team itself may select its own leader.

The team leader should be someone whom the team respects as well as someone who is organized and will take the initiative to see the team through the process. This person should also know or understand the PI process and clearly understand the process to be improved. The team leader is primarily responsible for championing the effectiveness of the process in meeting customers' needs. He or she is also responsible for the *content* of the team's work and for the following specific activities:

- Preparing for and scheduling meetings (standard meeting day, time, and location)
- Sending out announcements of meetings, other necessary materials, and team assignment reminders
- Conducting meetings (the importance of following an agenda is discussed later in the "QI Toolbox Technique" section of this chapter)
- Focusing the group's attention on the task at hand
- Ensuring group participation and asking for facts, opinions, and suggestions
- Providing expertise in the organization's PI methodology, tools, and techniques
- Coordinating data collection
- Assigning tasks
- Facilitating implementation of action plan items
- Critiquing the meetings

- Serving as the primary spokesperson and presenter for the team

- Keeping attendance records

- Contacting absent members personally to review the results of the meeting and provide any materials that were distributed during the meeting

The PI team also may want to identify a **team facilitator.** The facilitator should be someone who knows the PI process well and has facilitated such a team in the past. The facilitator also may be required to train the team in the PI process and quality improvement (QI) tools. The facilitator also is required to understand the process to be improved. The facilitator is primarily responsible for ensuring that an effective PI process occurs. The responsibilities of the team facilitator include the following:

- Serving as advisor and consultant to the team

- Acting as a neutral, nonvoting member

- Suggesting alternative PI methods and procedures to keep the team on target and moving forward

- Managing group dynamics, resolving conflict, and modeling compromise

- Acting as coach and motivator for the team

- Assisting in consensus building when necessary

- Recognizing team and individual achievements

Some teams combine the roles of the leader and the facilitator and assign one person to both functions.

The role of the **team member** includes the following functions:

- Participating in decision making and plan development for the team

- Identifying opportunities for improvement

- Gathering, prioritizing, and analyzing data

- Sharing knowledge, information, and data that pertain to the process under study

The role of **team recorder** (or **scribe**) is vital to the team's success. This team member keeps minutes of the team's work during the meetings, including any documentation required by the organization. The recorder performs the following functions:

- Recording information on a flip chart for the group

- Creating appropriate charts and diagrams

- Assisting with notices and supplies for meetings

- Distributing notices and other documentation to team members in a timely manner along with scheduled meeting times

- Developing meeting minutes within the facility policy timeline and utilizing a reporting format that assigns duties with time frames

- Producing an agenda for new meetings with assignments for team members from the previous meeting

Finally, teams may assign someone to be a **timekeeper.** The timekeeper helps the team manage its time and notifies the team during meetings of time remaining on each agenda item in an effort to keep the team moving forward on its PI project.

Team Charters

In many healthcare organizations, the initiation of a PI team begins with the ongoing data review of performance measures identified by the **performance improvement council** or leadership as important performance markers to monitor. The PI council generally makes a recommendation for the implementation of a PI team when a performance measure shows a negative or downward trend in the performance of a process or outcome. This can then be formalized with a **team charter.**

Team charters explain those issue(s) the team was initiated to address, describe the team's goal or vision, and list the initial members of the team and their respective departments. Team charters are helpful because they keep the team's objective in focus. Usually, team charters also identify any mitigating factors that may limit the PI process, such as financial limitations, full-time employee restrictions, or time constraints. They keep the organization focused on the opportunity for improvement and the team focused on its mission. See figure 3.1 for an example of a team charter.

Mission, Vision, and Values Statements

Healthcare organizations may use a **mission statement,** a **vision statement,** and a **values statement** at many different levels. The corporation as a whole may have a mission and vision statement, as may the separate divisions of the corporation. Departments within facilities may also have mission and vision statements.

To be effective, mission, vision, and values statements should be developed in concert with the organization's overall goals as developed in the organization's strategic plan. The statements should reflect the mission and vision of the overall organization as well as the goals of the individual PI team. The mission statement identifies the PI team, what it does, and whom it serves. For instance, the mission of the health information PI team is to provide quick, accurate billing to all clients and third-party payers in an honest, efficient, and user-friendly manner. The vision statement for the team may be "better service to all," and its values may be honesty, efficiency, and user friendliness.

After the team has been assembled and the leader has been chosen, the team should establish its mission. Developing a mission statement can help both the team and the larger

Figure 3.1.   Example of a team charter

PERFORMANCE IMPROVEMENT TEAM CHARTER (Page 1 of 2)		
Team Name *Clinical Laboratory Services*		**Date Submitted to Performance Improvement Council** *February 15th*

Statement of the Problem, Issue, or Concern to Be Addressed by the PIT

Safety issues or other problems concerning the hospital labs increased 207% over a one-year time frame.

Statement of the Goals, Objective, and Desired End State

Identify specific problem areas within laboratory services, conduct a baseline study to assess each area, analyze results, develop an action plan, implement improvements, and evaluate results.

Proposed Team Members		
Name	Title	Department
Roger Jones	*Chief Clinical Officer*	*Administration*
Jill Andrews	*Lab Manager*	*Laboratory*
Ben Carlson, M.D.	*Emergency Physician*	*E.R.*
Sandy Johnson	*Director of Clinical Ser.*	*Administration*
Kathy Smith, R.N.	*Director of Nursing*	*Nursing*
John Rasmussen	*Lab tech*	*Laboratory*
Sue Hol	*Lab tech*	*Laboratory*
Pam Richards	*Coordinator*	*Quality Management*

Project Resources		
Planned Start Date *February 20th*	Planned Completion Date *June 1st*	Planned Frequency of Meetings *weekly*
Administrative/PIC Support Needed (if any)		Estimated Cost of Team's Work *$1000.00*

(Continued on next page)

Figure 3.1.   *(Continued)*

PERFORMANCE IMPROVEMENT TEAM CHARTER (Page 2 of 2)

**What Important Organizational or Patient Care Functions Will the Project Measure or Improve?
(Check all that apply.)**

☐ Ethics Rights, Responsibilities

☑ Provision of Care, Treatment, and Services

☑ Improving Organizational Performance

☐ Leadership

☑ Management of the Environment of Care

☐ Management of Information

☑ Management of Human Resources

☐ Surveillance, Prevention, and Control of Infection

☐ Medication Management

Project Benefits
How Will the Project Support the Mission/Values and/or Achieve the Organization's Strategic Goals?

☐ Improved Patient Outcomes

☑ Cost Savings

☑ Improved Service

☐ Time Savings

☐ Other _____

_____

How?   *reduce safety violations in the laboratory and rework*

_____

_____

_____

_____ *Jill Andrews* _____   _____ *Feb. 15th* _____

Signature of Applicant   Date

To Be Completed by Performance Improvement Council

Comments

_____

_____

Performance Improvement Council Recommendations _____

_____

_____

_____   _____
Signature   Date

organization identify the goals and purpose of the PI initiative. The team's mission statement should answer the following questions:

- What process is to be improved?
- For whom is the process performed?
- What products does the process produce?
- What is not working with the current process?
- How well must the process function?

(See the example in figure 3.2.)

The team should also articulate its vision for the process. A vision statement describes what the organization or PI team initiative will look like or be in the future, or it describes some milestone the organization or PI team will reach in the future. (See the example in figure 3.3.)

The team's vision of the way a process should function may not be validated by existing data and observations of the process. In such cases, disharmony between the vision and reality becomes apparent. And because humans have a natural tendency to resolve disharmony, the team has an opportunity to improve the process. The more clearly the group maintains its focus on "what should be" and acknowledges "what is," the more focused it will be on implementing its vision of the desired outcome.

Quite often, organizations give up their vision because of the large gap between their vision and the current reality. Some organizations focus on their vision and ignore the way things are, or they believe the current situation is better than it really is. In either case, the natural tendency for resolution or change is dissipated.

The team that focuses on "what should be" while at the same time maintaining an accurate description of the current state of the process takes a powerful step toward creating the results it envisions. When the PI team focuses clearly and consistently on its mission and vision, it naturally and almost effortlessly senses what still needs to be done. New processes present themselves, and the group becomes increasingly aware of additional opportunities for continuing improvement.

Figure 3.2.   Sample mission statement

> Evaluate the HIM lab in regard to accessibility, resources,
> library access, Internet access, quality of equipment, and adequacy of equipment
> while maintaining 95 percent HIM student satisfaction with these services.

Figure 3.3.   Sample vision statement

> The HIM lab provides access to a variety of application software resources,
> library knowledge bases, and the Internet.
> A convenient, comfortable work environment exists.

Ground Rules for Meetings Led by the Facilitator

Establishing ground rules for meetings helps a team maintain a level of discipline. **Ground rules** include a discussion of attendance, time management, participation, communication, decision making, documentation, room arrangements, and cleanup. The ground rules will not be the same for every team, as each team should decide how it wants to proceed. But the ground rules should be well known to everyone on the team, and everyone should have participated in their development. Most teams that use ground rules allow for periodic review and revision of those rules, particularly when team membership changes. New members must be brought up to speed on the ground rules when they begin coming to team meetings. (See figure 3.4.)

The attendance discussion should establish who will schedule meetings, arrange for a meeting room, and notify members. The ground rules also should cover the team's expectations regarding absences, including whether team members can be removed for absenteeism and whether substitutes can attend meetings.

Cancellation of meetings should be discussed in the ground rules, as well as how the team will address issues of tardiness. This discussion also should include how the time

Figure 3.4.   Sample meeting ground rules worksheet

Ground Rules Worksheet

1. Every individual has a viewpoint that is valuable, every individual can make a unique contribution, and every individual can speak freely.

2. All team members must listen attentively and respectfully without interrupting. Only one person should speak at a time.

3. All team members must be willing to accept responsibility for assignments and complete any assigned tasks between meetings.

4. The organizational positions/levels of team members will not be recognized during team meetings. Every member of the team is an equal participant.

5. Solutions must be created with resources that are currently available. Money and additional staff are not considered issues.

6. _____

7. _____

8. _____

9. _____

10. _____

---

allotted to agenda items will be monitored. For example, will the team assign a timekeeper at the start of each meeting?

Discussion of team member participation should include the team's expectations regarding advance preparation. The team should have a plan for encouraging all members to make equal contributions, determining how activities will be monitored to ensure productive meetings, deciding how assignments and expectations for their completion will be made, and deciding how ad hoc members will be invited and prepared for their input.

Communication ground rules are imperative for team effectiveness, particularly regarding how candid members may be and whether information discussed in the team process must remain confidential. PI data are considered confidential in most facilities and may be legally protected from reproduction or use outside the facility or agency.

The team needs to clearly define how information will be managed and protected during the project. The team also should decide what will happen when discussions get off track, how interruptions or side conversations will be handled, what listening skills are expected, how differences of opinion and conflict among members will be expressed and resolved, and how creativity will be encouraged and negative thinking discouraged. Finally, the team must decide whether consensus or majority decisions will be taken on issues that require a vote.

Other questions that may require discussion include the following:

- Will there be meeting breaks, and if so, how will they be handled?

- Who is responsible for setup and cleanup of the meeting room?

- Does the team require information technology support? If so, who will coordinate it?

- How, when, and why should administration be involved?

- How will department managers be notified of the need for department employees to participate on a team?

- Is overtime necessary for this team to complete its assignment?

Problem-Solving Techniques, Listening, and Questioning

Encouraging team productivity can be a major issue in many organizations. This is an outgrowth of the common management styles that most organizations exhibit. Organizations tend to gravitate to one of two management styles. One style is inclusive: All viewpoints are considered with respect to their potential contribution to solving the PI issue at hand. The other style is exclusive: Its goal is to get to a result as quickly as possible. Each style has positive and negative aspects. People who operate by the inclusive style can get mired in details and discussion and achieve results only after extensive processing. People who operate by the exclusive style can fail to perceive important details in their rush to implement a solution. A combination of the two styles is more effective than either style alone. Each style can be employed at appropriate points in the development of a team process.

The management style employed will depend on the maturity of the team and its effectiveness. To improve team effectiveness in PI, the cyclical PI methodology was developed to give teams a structure to follow in problem solving. QI toolbox techniques were developed to give teams an easy way to organize and analyze data, and the concept of facilitation was developed to help move teams along.

Another area that is extremely important in the development of good team interaction and functioning is the ability to listen and question. PI team members need to be able to do both, and team leaders may need to work with team members to develop this skill. Commonly, in human communication in organizations, individuals tend to be either active communicators or passive listeners. Active communicators can quickly dominate a team meeting. They are accustomed to expressing themselves and being heard. Sometimes their listening skills are eclipsed by their own volubility. These team members may need to be reoriented to practice listening more often, allowing the quieter individuals on the team an opportunity to express their perspectives. Similarly, the quieter members may have become accustomed to listening to other people and not voicing their opinions. They may have to be reoriented to contribute, sharing their knowledge and expertise with the group so that important details are not ignored.

Often, too, in human communication in organizations, individuals become invested in their own perspectives and ways of seeing and interpreting situations. This can happen with both active communicators and passive listeners. The active communicators often react by trying to persuade everyone else on the team of the justness of their perspectives. The passive listeners may say nothing but internally retain their commitment to their own perspectives. Neither of these tactics moves the team toward resolving the problem it was convened to solve. Team members may have to be reoriented to listen carefully to others' perspectives and to seek a common understanding of those perspectives using questioning techniques.

The power of the question lies in the fact that it compels an answer. When the right questions are asked, the information, experience, reactions, perspectives, and attitudes that they prompt provide important answers. Not asking questions may result in only one perspective, which may or may not reflect the reality of various situations. One individual can never know as much about an opportunity for improvement as the collective members of the team. Trying to make decisions without sufficient information decreases the likelihood that a new solution will solve the problem. So it is important for PI team members to use effective questioning techniques.

When using questioning methods, team members should maintain a positive attitude about the importance of asking rather than telling and remember that each person's unique experience, background, and training allows him or her to contribute unique information. It is also important to recognize that there is more than one type of questioning. Different styles of questioning can be used to gather different types of information. Note the types of questions shown in figure 3.5 and the purposes of each.

Figure 3.5.   Types of questions and their purposes

Type	Purpose	Examples
Factual	To get information To open discussion	*How* and all of the *W* questions: *what, where, why, when,* and *who*
Explanatory	To find reasons and explanations To broaden discussion To develop additional information	In what way would this help solve the problem? What aspects of this issue should be considered? Just how would this action be done?
Justifying	To challenge old ideas To develop new ideas To find reasons and proof	Why do you think so? How do you know? What evidence do you have?
Leading	To introduce a new idea To advance a suggestion	Should we consider this idea as a possible solution? Would this idea be a feasible alternative?
Hypothetical	To develop new ideas To suggest another, possibly unpopular opinion To change the course of discussion	What would happen if we did it this way? Would it be feasible for us to do this the way company X does it?
Alternative	To choose an alternative To obtain agreement	Which of these solutions is better? Does this solution represent our choice in preference to other alternative solutions?
Coordinating	To develop consensus To obtain agreement To take action	Can we conclude that this is the next step we should take? Is there general agreement on this plan?
Direction of Questions		
Overhead: directed to the group	To open discussion To introduce a new phase To give everyone a chance to comment	How shall we begin? What shall we consider next? What else might be important?
Direct: addressed to a specific individual	To call on an individual for specific information To get an inactive individual involved in the discussion	George, what are your suggestions? Gracie, have you had any experience in this area?
Relay: referred back to another individual or to the group	To help the leader avoid giving his or her own opinion To get others involved in the discussion To call on someone who knows the answer	Would someone like to comment on Peter's question? Mary, how would you answer Paul's question?
Reverse: referred back to the individual who asked the question	To help the leader avoid giving his or her own opinion To encourage the questioner to think for himself or herself To bring out opinions	Well, Bing, how about giving us your opinion first? Heddie, tell us first what your own experience has been in this area?

Source: Burns 1960. Reprinted with permission.

People Issues

Finally, in discussing the effectiveness of PI teams, we must specifically recognize the effects that individuals have on PI processes. In reality, all of the team-development techniques are intended to help teams function *through* the people issues and become effective teams. Effective teams typically succeed in the following objectives:

- Establishing goals cooperatively, with all members who have perspectives on the issues contributing.

- Communicating in a two-way mode, with all members participating. Members who do not spontaneously communicate are encouraged and held responsible for doing so.

- Valuing open expression of both ideas and feelings as important perspectives on organizational issues.

- Distributing leadership and responsibility among all team members, with each member responsible for tasks that make important contributions to team accomplishments.

- Distributing power among all team members. Power is distributed on the basis of information, ability, and contribution to team activities, not on the basis of a team member's place in the formal organizational structure.

- Matching decision-making techniques to the type of decision-making situation. Important decisions are usually made through consensus, meaning that the group as a whole agrees on the appropriate course of action.

- Viewing periodic controversy and conflict among team members as a positive aspect of team growth and understanding in working through the processes the team has been initiated to improve.

- Focusing on the issues that the team has been organized to address and keeping at the heart of its work the mission, vision, and values of both the overall organization and the PI team.

- Making sure that the team's PI efforts and management of project design or tools are cost conscious.

Even those new to the team concept generally can see the importance of these factors. However, in real situations there may be conflict between individuals' roles in the formal organizational structure and their roles in maintaining an effective team structure. Formal organizational roles often require authority for various functions and responsibilities. Effective teams share authority for team performance. Therefore, when individuals are new to the team concept or team approaches to problem solving, they will have to get reoriented; for some, this reorientation is difficult.

Most individuals coming to a PI team for the first time are unfamiliar with the data collection and analysis aspects of team functioning. Some may not want to be involved with such detailed activities and may not have the mathematical skill necessary to perform these activities with ease. The team may have to spend some time helping such individuals accomplish their team tasks in specific areas.

Many individuals in healthcare, particularly clinicians, managers, and administrators, are comfortable with decision making. However, effective teams make decisions as groups, often by consensus, acknowledging perspectives of all participants. For many, giving up the right to make individual decisions is difficult. The team or the leadership of the PI initiative may have to help such persons learn a new, team-oriented decision-making style.

Conversely, people sometimes come to a team with little or no management experience. These individuals make few decisions in their work outside of day-to-day job procedures. Dealing with PI issues without carrying out someone else's orders may be difficult for these people. Some team members may resist being empowered because they come from a culture where employees complain rather than look for solutions to a problem. Encouraging such individuals to participate and mentoring them through the process can help them develop some new skills.

Real-Life Examples

Three examples of the effectiveness of PI teams follow. The first example focuses on the triage process in a small metropolitan hospital. The second example explores HIM and business office department processes. The third example considers safety issues in a hospital laboratory.

Continuum of Care Team

Customer satisfaction surveys indicated that the triage process in the emergency department of a small metropolitan hospital was inadequate. Communication was fragmented, precertification was not taking place in a timely manner, intake-processing time had increased, the main patient waiting area was not private, and referral volume was increasing.

To address these problems, a PI team was chartered. The team charter included the following:

- Team leader: Emergency department intake coordinator

- Team members: Representatives from the business office, HIM, administration, utilization review, and finance

- Ad hoc members: Representatives from regulatory affairs, reception, nursing, and case management, and an emergency department physician

- Team mission statement: Evaluate the emergency department's clinical assessment process regarding patient privacy, data collection, and staff communication, while maintaining 95 percent patient and employee satisfaction with this process

- Team vision statement: Design a centralized clinical assessment center to facilitate patient privacy, data collection, and staff communication

HIM and Business Office Services

An organization's HIM department was experiencing an increase in physician chart delinquencies, delays in diagnosis and procedure coding, and delays in processing requests for patient information. In addition, the business office was experiencing delays in the billing process due to incomplete insurance information and an increase in accounts payable due to the chart completion problems occurring in the HIM department.

To address these issues, a PI team was formed. The team was composed of the following individuals:

- Team leader: HIM consultant

- Team members: Representatives from the HIM department, the business office, registration, and administration, and the physician chairman of the HIM committee

- Team mission statement: Evaluate the physician chart completion and admission interview processes and their impact on coding, billing, release of information, and accounts payable, while providing support to organization-wide management of information, financial viability, and the billing and collection process

- Team vision statement: Achieve timely physician chart completion and a detailed admission interview, which will lead to timely and effective coding and billing of patient information

The HIM department's vision was to "contribute and provide support to the effective organization-wide management of information." The business office's vision statement was to "give support to organization-wide financial viability and provide accurate and timely exchange of financial information that allows for an efficient and effective billing and collection process."

This team made a recommendation to the HIM committee to change the physician chart completion policy from 30 days after discharge to 7 days after discharge. This change improved the coding turnaround time and processing of requests for patient information, which in turn improved the billing cycle. An additional process change was to have a business office representative interview patients upon admission. This eventually improved the accuracy of financial information needed for billing and collection.

Clinical Laboratory Services

Safety issues and other problems concerning the laboratory department at one hospital increased 207 percent over a period of one year. The objectives of the PI team were to identify specific problem areas within laboratory services, conduct a baseline survey to assess each area, analyze the survey results, develop an **action plan,** implement improvements, and evaluate the results of the changes. The team charter was made up of the following:

- Team leader: Chief of pathology

- Team members: The laboratory manager, an emergency department physician, the director of nursing, and a laboratory technician

- Team mission statement: Identify, analyze, and implement changes to improve safety issues and other problem areas within the laboratory department

- Team vision statement: Provide reliable, timely diagnostic services for the clinical staff

The survey indicated that inappropriate techniques for specimen collection were being used, and the reference laboratory was slow to return results to the organization. Team recommendations included education and training on specimen collection and a change in the contract reference laboratory used by the organization.

QI Toolbox Technique

For a meeting to be effective, the team must operate with a common purpose and specific goal. Communication of the meeting's common purpose and specific goal is usually accomplished by establishing an **agenda.** An agenda is a list of the tasks to be accomplished during a meeting. Using an agenda ensures that every team member knows which items will be discussed or worked on. The agenda should be sent to all team members before the meeting. This allows them to prepare to discuss specific agenda items. The agenda also should indicate how long the team will spend on each item. (See the sample agenda in figure 3.6.) Setting time frames for agenda items helps the team leader keep the group focused on the process and moving forward.

Standard agendas begin with a review and approval of the last meeting's minutes. Once this has been accomplished, the PI team should review the agenda for the current meeting and approve the time frames that have been set. This allows the individual team members to have input on how long a certain agenda item should be discussed.

Figure 3.6.   Sample agenda

AGENDA	
Date: January 15 **Time:** 10:00 a.m.	**Team:** Registration Process **Place:** Conference Room B
Time Allotted:	**Item:**
5 minutes	1. Review and approve minutes from last meeting
5 minutes	2. Review agenda and time frames
15 minutes	3. PI step: Registration process discussion on how the computer system affects the registration process
15 minutes	4. PI step: Registration process discussion on what happens now when the computer system is "down"
15 minutes	5. Brainstorm possible ideas to improve the computer system
10 minutes	6. Process (evaluate) meeting
10 minutes	7. Plan next steps, assign team members' duties, and set agenda for next meeting

As a closing item of business, many teams find it helpful to evaluate the effectiveness of the meeting. Asking the following questions may be helpful:

- Did the team accomplish what it set out to accomplish during the meeting?
- Is the PI process moving forward?
- Does the team need to ask additional people to sit in on the process meetings?
- Did members participate appropriately, listen effectively to other members' suggestions, and stay focused on the agenda?

Finally, the next meeting's agenda and team member assignments should be agreed upon and tied to the current meeting's evaluation process and minutes. In other words, the next meeting should be structured based on the accomplishments of the current meeting.

Case Study

"Well, why does it have to take so darn long?" the nurse shouted into the telephone receiver. "We've got to be able to order tests for our patients! They can't wait until next Christmas for their meds!" She slammed the receiver onto its cradle and turned to the rest of the staff collected at the nursing station. "The patient in room 436 was transferred here from ICU two hours ago, and I still can't enter any orders. How do those idiots in Admitting think we're supposed to get our work done? I will never understand why it has to take so long to get a patient transferred in that darn system."

"That witch!" exclaimed the admissions clerk to her supervisor as she hung up the phone. "If someone would let us know once in a while what they're doing with patients in this place, maybe we could do our jobs! Evidently, they transferred Mr. Campbell to 436 from ICU hours ago!"

The clerk walked over to the report printer. A long, wide ribbon of paper hung from it onto the floor, where it curled in a short pile. She yanked at the hanging pages and ripped them along a perforation. Then she sat down at a desk and began sorting the half-sheet messages from the hospital network communication system into different piles. When she was finished, she began entering the status and location changes for each of the patients into the patient accounting and order-entry system.

"But instead of giving us a call and telling us that the patient's been transferred, they'd rather wait 'til a couple of hours later when the patient doesn't have his meds and then call up and rag on us like it was *our* fault!" She entered "Campbell, Roy" from one of the half-sheets, and the patient's location data appeared on the screen. She keyed "4-3-6" in the location field and pressed "Enter."

Western States University Hospital employees have been dealing with this conflict for two years, ever since management purchased a new patient accounting and order-entry system from ABC Company. Previously, clinicians used XYZ software to look up patient histories, laboratory reports, and other diagnostic data for both inpatients and outpatients.

The software had also provided departments with information about the current location of the patient so that they would know where to send the final paper-based reports of blood tests, x-rays, and other diagnostic reports. But the nursing staff had never been very careful about transferring or discharging patients in the XYZ system. It was one of those tasks that was secondary to the other patient-oriented duties they had to perform in their hectic schedules.

Western States University Hospital is the principal tertiary care hospital in a community of 200,000, and patients are referred to it from all over the state. The census never dips below 70 percent. As a result, the nursing units are almost always full, and the patients have high acuity levels.

The admitting and patient accounting departments had been requesting a new information system for many years when administration finally agreed to invest in the ABC system. The new system allows them to tie order-entry functions to the geographic location of the patient in the hospital. Thus, the system provides more accurate information to help lab and other diagnostic testing personnel, such as ECG and x-ray, locate patients when tests are ordered. This feature also ensures that a patient's account is charged the correct room rate, which was never the case when they were using the XYZ system. Nursing staff never seemed to get changes in room location entered into the system in a timely fashion. And *everyone* knew that the census from the XYZ system was never accurate.

The managers of the admitting and patient accounting departments had stood their ground when the new work procedures were developed around the ABC system. They were adamant that nursing was *not* going to be in charge of patient census management. It had been obvious for years that nursing could not take it seriously. The admitting department staff would be making all patient-location changes in the system, and the system would generate an accurate daily inpatient census. They had information system (IS) programmers add a short utility in XYZ so that whenever a patient was discharged or transferred in the XYZ census management application, the admitting department printer would print a notification message. Throughout the day, the admitting clerks would enter the messages into the ABC system. If, for some reason, they were not notified, they had the authority to go into the system and change the dates and times of the discharge or transfer so that the accounting files would be correct and the patients' bills would reflect correct charges. One additional characteristic of the ABC system, however, was that orders on a patient could only be entered from the nursing unit on which the system currently had the patient located.

Case Study Questions

1. In your opinion, is there an opportunity for improvement in this system? Why or why not?

2. If there is room for improvement, is a PI team appropriate in this context?

3. From your knowledge of hospital organizational structure, who should be on the PI team? What departments should be represented? What staff positions would you include? What is your rationale for including each individual?

Student Project Application

Students should form teams of two to four members. Each team should select a process or service to evaluate for improvement opportunities. Then, each team should develop a mission statement and a vision statement for its process. This will help the team identify its goals and purposes for the PI process and clarify what it is trying to accomplish. Mission and vision statements can be written on newsprint flip-chart paper. The statements should be displayed on the wall so that the students can share their initial mission and vision statements and introduce their proposed projects.

Summary

PI teams often undertake improvement activities in healthcare organizations. The team process allows the members to represent the varied perspectives of departments and other entities in the organization. At a minimum, a team should include a leader and several members. Team charters, mission and vision statements, and meeting agendas help keep the team focused on its activities. Team members also may need to learn effective listening and questioning techniques and to accept responsibility for participating in collaborative problem solving and other team activities.

References

Burns, R.K. 1960. *The Questioning Techniques*. Chicago: Industrial Relations Center, University of Chicago.

Caldwell, C., ed. 1998. *Handbook for Managing Change in Health Care*. Milwaukee, WI: ASQ Quality Press.

Resources

Adams, T., J.A. Means, and M. Spivey. 2007. *The Project Meeting Facilitator: Facilitation Skills to Make the Most of Project Meetings*. San Francisco: Jossey-Bass.

Blanchard, K., A. Randolph, and P. Graizer. 2005. *Go Team! Take Your Team to the Next Level*. San Francisco: Berrett-Kochler Publishers.

DeMarco, T., and T.R. Lister. 2000. *Peopleware: Productive Projects and Teams*, 2nd ed. New York: Dorset House Publishing.

Fast Company Magazine. 2001. *What Makes Teams Work: The Teamwork Syllabus* (eBook). New York: Gruner + Jahr USA Publishing.

Johns, M.L. 2007. *Creating, Coaching and Managing High-Powered Work Teams*. Chicago: Lulu Press.

Katzenbach, J.R., and D.K. Smith. 2001. *The Discipline of Teams: A Mindbook-Workbook for Delivering Small Group Performance*. New York: John Wiley & Sons.

Katzenbach, J.R., and D.K. Smith. 2003. *The Wisdom of Teams: Creating the High-Performance Organization*. New York: Harper Collins Publishers.

Leeds, D. 2000. *Smart Questions: The Essential Strategy for Successful Managers*. New York: Berkley Publishing Group.

Lencioni, P.M. 2002. *The Five Dysfunctions of a Team: A Leadership Fable*. San Francisco: Jossey-Bass.

Lencioni, P.M. 2005. *Overcoming the Five Dysfunctions of a Team: A Field Guide for Leaders, Managers, and Facilitators*. San Francisco: Jossey-Bass.

Chapter 4
Aggregating and Analyzing Performance Improvement Data

Learning Objectives

- To differentiate between internal and external benchmark comparisons
- To identify common healthcare data collection tools
- To introduce the concept of data aggregation in support of data analysis
- To describe the various data types
- To recognize the correct graphic presentation for a specific data type
- To design graphic displays for a given set of data
- To analyze the data for changes in performance displayed in graphic form

Key Terms

Absolute frequency
Bar graph
Check sheet
Continuous data
Control chart
Discrete or **count data**
Histogram
Likert scale
Line chart
Mean (*M*)
Median
Nominal data

Ordinal data
Pareto chart
Pie chart
Pivot table
Relative frequency
Sampling
Standard deviation (*SD*)

Background and Significance

After the performance improvement (PI) team has administered its survey or collected data by abstracting them from other sources, it is ready to aggregate and analyze the data. Other sources of data may include health records, organization-wide incident reports, and annual employee performance evaluations and staff competency results. Abstracted data and survey results can provide invaluable information about a process and thereby point the team in a specific direction for improvement. Internal and external data comparisons, also known as benchmarking, can provide additional information about why and how well the process works—or does not work—in meeting the customers' expectations.

It is best to conduct an internal data comparison with data collected over a period of time. Collecting data over a three- to six-month time frame, for example, establishes an internal baseline for benchmark purposes. To establish the baseline, the organization averages all collected data. This internal baseline becomes the organization's benchmark to maintain or improve upon when external benchmark comparisons are not available.

Comparing an organization's performance with the performance of other organizations that provide the same types of services is known as external benchmarking. The other organizations need not be in the same region of the country, but they should be comparable in terms of size and patient mix. The use of external benchmarks can be instructive when comparisons are made with an organization doing an outstanding job with a process similar to the process on which the PI team is focusing. For example, if the national standard for the average number of adverse drug reactions were X, then comparing an organization's number with the national average would give the team information about the effectiveness of the organization's medication program. The Joint Commission (2011a) Core Measure data are another external benchmark that permits rigorous comparison of the actual results of care across hospitals.

In figure 4.1, note the comparison of Western States University Hospital's physician specialty lengths of stay. This report allows the organization to do both internal and external comparisons. Internal comparisons can be performed on the mean length of stay observed (Mean LOS Obs) between specialties of practice. For instance, note the difference in mean length of stay between the Family Practice Service and the General Internal Medicine Service. External benchmarking also can be performed by comparing the mean length of stay observed and the mean length of stay expected (Mean LOS Exp). Note also the major differences in standard deviation for length of stay (*SD* LOS Obs) between the two services.

Figure 4.1. LOS summary by attesting physician specialty

Physician Specialty	Cases	Mean LOS (Obs)	SD LOS (Obs)	Mean LOS (Exp)	LOS Index	Savings Opp (Days)	% 30 Day Readmit	% With Comps	% Deaths (Obs)	% Deaths (Exp)	% Early Deaths
Cardiology	1	6.00	—	6.36	0.94	0	0	0	0	0.75	0
Endocrinology	1	3.00	—	3.93	0.76	−1	0	0	0	0.83	0
Family Practice	17	8.47	11.44	6.26	1.35	38	11.76	0	0	4.27	0
Infectious Disease	4	4.00	2.94	4.35	0.92	−1	0	0	0	1.13	0
General Internal Medicine	34	3.82	3.00	4.89	0.78	−36	0	0	5.88	4.39	2.94
Nephrology	3	3.67	0.58	4.99	0.73	−4	0	0	0	4.03	0
Neo/Perinatal Medicine	1	4.00	—	3.69	1.08	0	100.00	0	0	0.92	0
Prev/Occ Med	6	4.83	4.83	6.37	0.76	−9	16.67	0	33.33	16.57	16.67
General Pediatrics	7	3.43	2.15	3.55	0.97	−1	0	0	0	0.18	0
Pulmonary/Crit Care	2	17.50	21.92	14.65	1.19	6	0	0	50.00	61.46	50.00
General Diag/Interv Radiology	1	1.00	—	12.02	0.08	−11	0	0	100.00	80.25	100.00
Rheumatology	1	2.00	—	3.40	0.59	−1	0	0	0	0.39	0
Internal Med Heme/Onc	1	3.00	—	3.71	0.81	−1	0	0	0	0.90	0

Legend:

Comps = Complications	Opp = Opportunity
Crit = Critical	Prev = Preventive
Diag = Diagnostic	Readmit = Readmission
Exp = Expected	SD = Standard deviation
Heme = Hematology	
Interv = Interventional	
LOS = Length of stay	
Med = Medicine	
Neo = Neonatal	
Obs = Observed	
Occ = Occupational	
Onc = Oncology	

Benchmarking on mortality can be performed using the columns "% Deaths (Obs)" and "% Deaths (Exp)." Where might Western States University Hospital want to focus attention on improving hospital lengths of stay?

PI teams can use several tools for data aggregation, analysis, and presentation. These tools are discussed in more detail later in this chapter.

Data Collection Tools

Certain types of data and information need to be accumulated over time to support clinical and management functions. The organization must assess its need for aggregate data and information and define the types of required data and information to support individual care and care delivery, decision making, management and operations, analysis of trends over time, performance comparisons over time within and outside the organization, and PI. The common types of data collection tools used in healthcare organizations include incident reports, safety and infection surveillance reports, employee performance appraisals, staff competency examinations, restraint use logs, adverse drug reaction reports, surveys, diagnosis and procedure indices, case abstracts, and peer review reports. Individually, these tools do not describe the quality of care provided by the healthcare organization. So the data from these reports must be aggregated to provide useful information about the organization's performance in key areas.

To aggregate data, the values of one data element over a set period of time (such as a month or quarter) are added together. These aggregated data are then compared with previous months or quarters to determine if there is a variance from the established benchmark. Chapter 16 discusses the transformation of data into knowledge in more detail, and figure 16.1 shows an example of aggregate data over time between quarters.

Sometimes, the organizational characteristic or parameter about which data are being collected occurs too frequently to measure every occurrence. In this case, those collecting the data might want to use sampling techniques. **Sampling** is the recording of a smaller subset of observations of the characteristic or parameter, making certain, however, that a sufficient number of observations have been made to predict the overall configuration of the data. (See Layman [2009, 2010] for additional reading.) The Joint Commission (2011b) recommends the following sampling methodologies for use in monitoring its requirements:

- For a population size of fewer than 30 cases, sample 100 percent

- For a population size of 30 to 100 cases, sample 30 cases

- For a population size of 101 to 500 cases, sample 50 cases

- For a population size greater than 500 cases, sample 70 cases

Other approaches to sampling methodologies can be found in a standard statistical textbook.

When an organization needs to collect a new data element, a variety of data collection tools can be used. First and also simplest is the check sheet.

Check Sheets

A **check sheet** is used to gather data based on sample observations in order to detect patterns. When preparing to collect data, a team should consider the four *W* questions:

- *Who* will collect the data? For example, using the Joint Commission's Core Measure Set (2011a) for heart failure, determining who will collect the data is vital to data accuracy. More often than not, the individual collecting the heart failure measures will be a clinician with a background in cardiology. A nonclinical person can be trained to look for specific documentation of the measure in the health record, but the complexity of the heart failure data makes a cardiology clinician the best candidate for this type of data collection.

- *What* data will be collected? Here, the Joint Commission Core Measure (2011a) is defined for the organization. The data elements for this core measure include discharge instructions, left ventricular systolic function, treatment with angiotensin-converting enzyme inhibitor (ACEI) or angiotensin receptor blocker (ARB) for left ventricular systolic dysfunction, and adult smoking-cessation counseling.

- *Where* will the data be collected? Most often, data for the heart failure core measure will be abstracted or collected from the individual patient health record. However, some measures may have to be collected from other data sources. Conceivably, there could be core measures that require the abstractor to go to other electronic systems, like those used in the ICU, that might not be printed for the paper-based record.

- *When* will the data be collected? This question is defined by time parameters. The data for the Joint Commission Core Measures are collected on patients for a three-month period (such as July, August, and September) and must be reported to the Joint Commission four months from the end of the last month of the reporting quarter (for reporting on July, August, and September, this is the end of January) (Joint Commission 2011a).

Once the team answers the four *W* questions, it can develop a check sheet to collect the data. (See figure 4.2.) Check sheets make it possible to systematically collect a large volume of data. It is important to make sure that the data are unbiased, accurate, properly recorded, and representative of typical conditions for the process.

Figure 4.2.   Example of a check sheet

Problem	Day			
	1	2	3	TOTAL
A	II	III	II	7
B	I	I	I	3
C	IIII	II	IIII	10
TOTAL	7	6	7	20

A check sheet is a simple, easy-to-understand form used to answer the question, how often are certain events happening? It starts the process of translating opinions into facts. Constructing a check sheet involves the following steps:

1. The PI team determines who is responsible for collecting the data: a clinician, a technician, or another person.

2. The PI team agrees on which event to observe.

3. The team decides on the time period during which the data will be collected. The time period can range from hours to weeks.

4. The team determines the appropriate source from which the data will be collected. This may be health records, charge slips, and so forth.

5. The team designs a form that is clear and easy to use. The team should make sure that every column is clearly labeled and that there is enough space on the form to enter the data.

6. The team collects the data consistently and honestly. Enough time should be allowed for this data-gathering task.

Check sheets can also be used to tally survey responses. (See "Survey Design" in chapter 6.) For example, if a survey included a question that asked for the days of the week on which patients had surgery, the results could be tabulated by using a check sheet that included each day of the week.

Healthcare organizations do not have to develop new data collection methods for every PI project. Organizations must determine what they are already collecting and how those data can be used in future PI measurement processes.

Types of Data

Before a PI team can decide on how to display performance data, it must determine which types of data have been collected. The four data categories are nominal, ordinal, discrete, and continuous.

Nominal data, also called categorical data, include values assigned to name-specific categories. For example, gender can be subdivided into two groups, "male" and "female," or two categories, "1" and "2." Nominal data are usually displayed in bar graphs (figure 4.3) and pie charts (figure 4.4).

Ordinal data, also called ranked data, express the comparative evaluation of various characteristics or entities, and relative assignment of each, to a class according to a set of criteria. Many surveys use a Likert scale to quantify or rank statements. A **Likert scale** allows the respondent to state the degree to which he or she agrees or disagrees with a statement. It typically ranges from 1 to 5. This type of scale allows the PI team to determine how respondents feel about issues. Ordinal or ranked data, like nominal data, are also best displayed in bar graphs and pie charts.

Discrete or **count data** are numerical values that represent whole numbers, for example, the number of children in a family or the number of unbillable patient accounts. Discrete data can be displayed in bar graphs.

Figure 4.3. Example of a bar graph

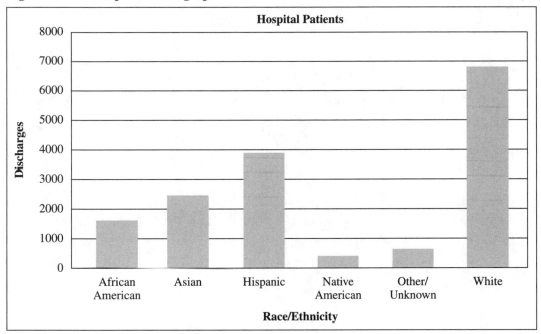

Figure 4.4. Example of a pie chart

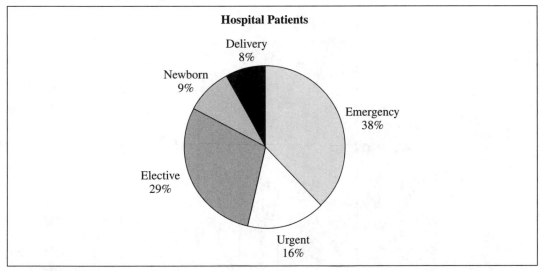

Continuous data assume an infinite number of possible values in measurements that have decimal values as possibilities. Examples of continuous data include weight, blood pressure, and temperature. Continuous data are displayed in histograms (figure 4.5) or line charts (figure 4.6).

Figure 4.5.   Example of a histogram

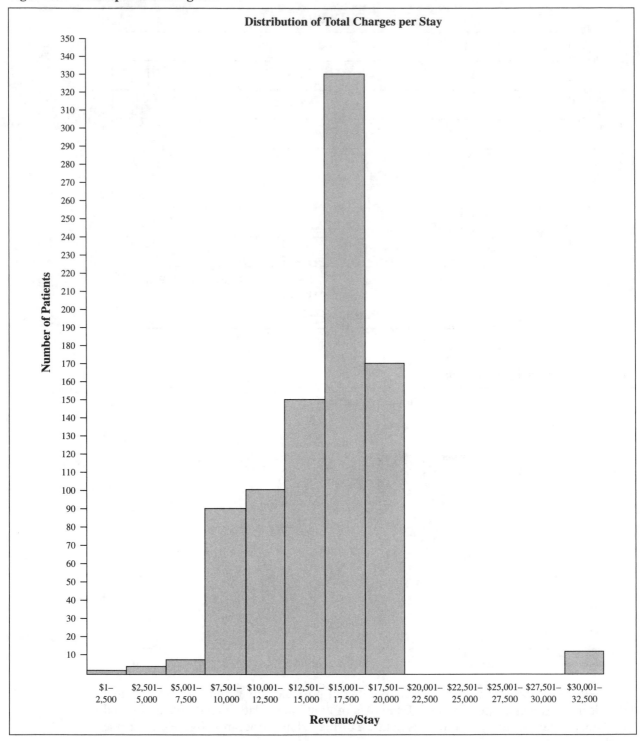

Figure 4.6.   Example of a line chart

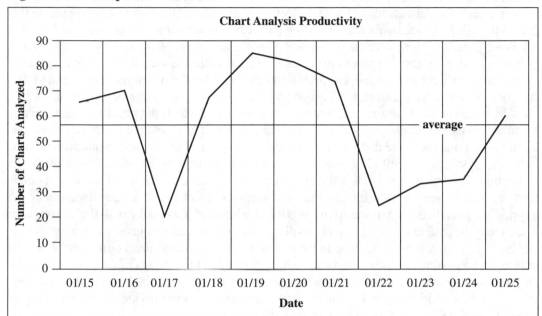

Table 4.1.   Sample data set

Date and Time	Respiration Rate Recorded
Jan. 5, 8:00 a.m.	22/min
Jan. 5, 12:00 noon	25/min
Jan. 5, 4:00 p.m.	25/min
Jan. 5, 8:00 p.m.	22/min
Jan. 5, 12:00 midnight	21/min
Jan. 6, 4:00 a.m.	23/min
Jan. 6, 8:00 a.m.	25/min

Two terms often used in data analysis are **absolute frequency** and **relative frequency.** Absolute frequency refers to the number of times a score or value occurs in the data set. For example, in the data set shown in table 4.1, the frequency of the score or value 25 is 3. Relative frequency is the percentage of the time that the characteristic appears. In the example, the percentage of observations in which the respiration rate was 25 was 3:7, or 42.9 percent—its relative frequency.

Management of Data Sets

Today's healthcare organizations maintain multiple large databases that are used to support various aspects of their operations. Patient management systems record all aspects of patient registration for service, type of service requested, dates and times the service was rendered, rendering providers, clinic or hospital census bed utilized, and so on. Patient financial systems manage the data associated with collecting charges, manifesting a bill, outputting that bill to the UB2004, receiving and recording payments from insurers or patients, and posting all those transactions as necessary to general ledger accounts. More and more often today, one sees clinical systems deployed to capture the information associated with the actual condition of the patient and the clinical provision of service by the provider, deriving such data as blood pressure, temperature, findings on physical examination, probable diagnosis, and the like. Many hospitals have provider order-entry systems in which the provider electronically communicates requirements for care provision to nursing and ancillary services staff, and each system maintains the data details for each of the order transactions. In addition to these principal systems, a multitude of smaller systems are utilized by individual departments or collections of departments in healthcare organizations, such as the radiology management system, the medication-ordering and management systems of the pharmacy department, the myriad of specialized systems used in the clinical laboratories to perform all the various tests used today in patient evaluation, and the diagnosis and procedure encoding system used in health information services to encode the summary diagnoses and procedures performed for billing and research purposes. Therefore, when working out the details of data collection, it is important to identify systems that may be a source of data that can be beneficial to the organization's PI activities and to use the systems' reporting tools to provide often very complex data sets to the PI teams for analysis and interpretation.

The use of data sets for PI purposes must be designed very carefully. First, one must examine the nature of the data to be sure they accurately reflect the subject under investigation. Reliability can be significantly influenced by what the sources of the data set were when the data were created, how carefully data were derived from those original sources, how carefully data were transcribed to paper- or computer-based record systems by users, and how faithfully data were interfaced from one electronic system to another. If data in the set were coded using either a standardized coding system (such as the International Classification of Diseases, ninth revision, Clinical Modifications [ICD-9-CM]) or a homegrown system, nonstandardized code structures specifically built into system tables for a specific organization, the structure of the codes, the conventions of their usage, and their definitions in relationship to the PI team's requirements must be examined carefully prior to use for PI activities. Using data without a clear picture of these aspects may lead a PI team to make inappropriate interpretations. Reporting them externally without examination in satisfaction of core measure or state data reporting activities may lead an organization to be judged inaccurately by the Centers for Medicare and Medicaid Services (CMS) or groups or individuals using that data published on public Web sites.

An example of this type of complexity occurring at Western States University Hospital was the request from an external public health monitoring agency for data regarding the hospital's experience with "severe sepsis." Now, obviously, the cases appropriate for reporting to this agency would have to be retrieved using ICD-9-CM codes assigned at discharge by the health information services staff. However, given the inconsistent usage of the term "sepsis" and its related terms by hospital house staff and attending staff, what is written in the health record could end up being coded as any one of the following ICD-9-CM codes:

038.0–038.9   Septicemia due to a variety of bacterial organisms

790.7   Bacteremia

995.90	Systemic inflammatory response syndrome, unspecified
995.91	Sepsis
995.92	Severe sepsis

Patients may also have expired in any or all of these categories, making the designation "severe" possible for any of them. Using only the cases coded with 995.92 might leave out many other cases relevant to the measure of "sepsis" in the hospital. Depending on the adequacy of the clinical documentation, a patient coded with Bacteremia might also have met the other requirements for severe sepsis (bacterial blood or urinary tract infection as well as some type of organ failure due to the infection) without the word "sepsis" ever occurring in the health record. Therefore, in working up the reported data for a monitoring agency or a PI team, quality management staff must be very careful to work with infection control staff to identify appropriate cases. Such complexities, overlaps, and inconsistencies may be inherent in any data set one attempts to use for PI and quality management purposes in healthcare.

Once the data set to be used by a PI team has been identified, the actual extraction and reporting of specific incidences must be considered carefully. The process of extraction of relevant cases from the entire data set is known as "querying." If a simple case list for one or a few parameters or characteristics of a patient population similar to the sepsis example above is required, the extraction probably will be fairly straightforward. However, if a multilevel query is involved, one that begins by extracting cases exhibiting one relevant characteristic and then creating one or two subsets against other relevant characteristics, the process of the query needs to be planned out carefully. In reality, the multilevel query is more common, so individuals involved in this work usually deal with a fair amount of complexity. An example built on the earlier discussion of sepsis would probably find a multilevel query defining a time period of interest, requesting the ICD-9-CM codes for sepsis to be extracted from the time period, and then perhaps further limiting that set by whether the sepsis was present on admission or developed during hospitalization. The resulting three-level set would probably still require validation by infection control staff against infection control databases.

Statistical Analysis

Methods of statistical analysis that are necessary to the graphic display of data include the mean and standard deviation. Although an in-depth discussion of these techniques can be found in any elementary statistics text (for example, Osborn [2006]), a brief review is provided here before the discussion of graphic display.

The **mean (M)** is also known as the arithmetic average of a distribution of numerical values. The values may be discrete or continuous in nature. If the data are discrete (or count), the mean should be rounded to the nearest whole value; if the data are continuous, whole numbers or numbers with decimal fractions can be reported.

To calculate the mean, the various observed values are first summed or added together. There may be repetitions of specific values, all of which are included. Then, the sum is divided by the number of observations made. For example, 15 observations of a person's systolic blood pressure revealed the following data set:

| 122 | 124 | 116 | 115 | 120 | 128 | 126 | 122 | 121 | 121 | 124 | 120 | 117 | 116 | 121 |

Note there are three 121s and two 122s in the set. All are summed. The sum of those observations is 1,813, which is then divided by the number of observations made (15). This equals 120.866666666666 . . . , which should be rounded to a whole number because systolic blood pressure is commonly expressed as a whole number. The reported mean, or average, systolic measurement is 121.

The **median** usually is derived without calculation. The observed values are placed in ascending or descending order; the value that is in the very middle of the set is taken as the median. There has to be an odd number of observations for there to be a value in the middle. In the following data set, the values are rearranged in ascending order as follows:

115	116	116	117	120	120	121	121	121	122	122	124	124	126	128

Note again that the repeated values are retained. The middle value is 121, as indicated by the arrow. Thus, 121 is the median. If, however, there were an even number of values, the middle would fall between the two values at places 7 and 8 in the row.

115	116	116	117	120	121	121	121	121	122	122	124	124	126

The values in places 7 and 8 are added together and divided by 2: 121 + 121 = 242, which divided by 2 = 121. If the values in places 7 and 8 were 122 and 125, adding them together would equal 247, which divided by 2 would equal 123.5, which should be rounded to 124 because systolic blood pressure is expressed in whole numbers.

It is sometimes better to use a median value in displaying some graphic representations of data, particularly if there is a lot of variation in the observed values or if they are skewed to one side. *Skewing* means that there are a lot of very high or very low values in the observations that distort the calculated mean. Because the median is not calculated, if the data set is greatly distorted by the extreme values, it can help to define a truer picture of the middle of the set.

The **standard deviation (*SD*)** is a more complex analysis technique used in developing control charts for the display of some PI data. (See the discussion of control charts later in this chapter.) The standard deviation is most easily calculated using the statistical analysis feature of a spreadsheet application. To do so, enter and highlight the column of data and select the standard deviation function from the menu bar "fx" button. Alternately, choose a cell to contain the *SD*, type =STDEV(), then record the range inside the parentheses.

Although the *SD* is easily calculated using a spreadsheet application, what this statistic reveals about a data set is more difficult to understand. When a PI team begins observing a continuous measure, the observations are plotted along the X- and Y-axes with very little clustering, or no discernable pattern or trend. The first nine values from the systolic blood pressure data set above can be graphed as in figure 4.7 on an X-Y axis, where the X-axis is the value of the measure and the Y-axis is the absolute frequency of that value in the set.

Here we see 115 with an absolute frequency of 1, 116 with an absolute frequency of 2, 117 with an absolute frequency of 1, and so on. As the measure is observed more and more

Figure 4.7.   Spread of data in initial observations of a continuous measure

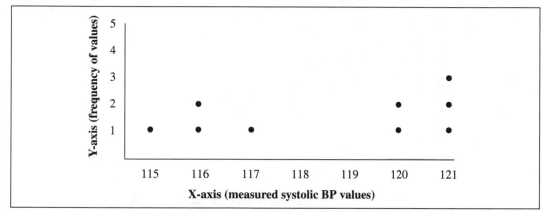

Figure 4.8.   Spread of data in later observations of a continuous measure

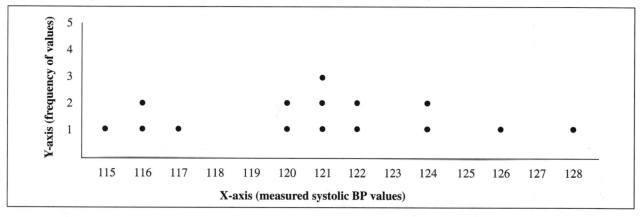

times, however, the observed values begin to congregate more often around the mean, as in figure 4.8.

As the number of observations increases into the hundreds or thousands, a graph similar to figure 4.9 begins to form, the typical bell-shaped curve of what is called a normal distribution. Almost all measures, when graphed, take on this bell-shaped or "normal" appearance as the number of observations increases.

At the center or vertex of the normal distribution is the calculated mean. For the small data set above, 121 was calculated as the mean of the observed blood pressures. Many people know that the commonly accepted "normal" or mean value for systolic blood pressure is 120, so that calculation is relatively close. It has the greatest absolute frequency in this data set as denoted by the apex of the curve residing at that 121 value. As we examine the absolute frequencies of the measured values of the data set to the left and right sides of the mean, we see them decrease until there are no observations below 80 or above 160 in relatively "normally" functioning human beings.

Figure 4.9.   A normal distribution

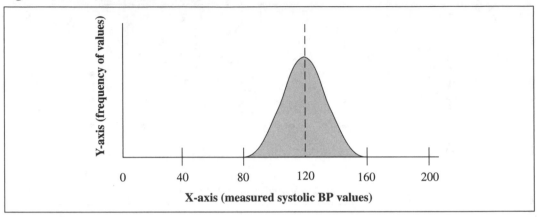

Figure 4.10.   One standard deviation from the mean

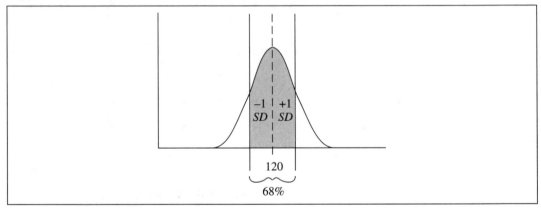

For the purposes of control chart construction, the standard deviation can be defined by the percentage of the frequencies contained beneath various portions of the normal distribution. Approximately 68 percent of the observations occur in the interval under the curve from –1 *SD* from the mean to +1 *SD* from the mean. (See figure 4.10.)

Approximately 95 percent of the observations occur in the interval under the curve from –2 *SD* from the mean to +2 *SD* from the mean. (See figure 4.11.)

Finally, approximately 99 percent of the observations fall in the interval under the curve from –3 *SD* from the mean to +3 *SD* from the mean.

The standard deviation is a useful statistic for PI in healthcare. It helps define the interval in which 95 percent of the observations should be made. Any observation that occurs outside the interval defined by +/–2 *SD* from the mean can be identified as a variant. If many observations fall outside the +/–2 *SD* interval, the process under examination could be "out of control" and contributing negatively to the provision of healthcare services.

Figure 4.11.   Two standard deviations from the mean

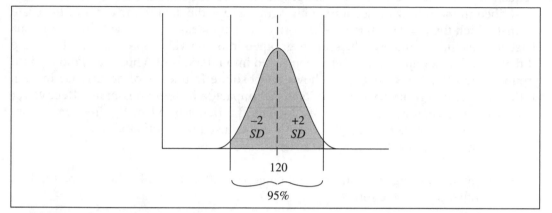

Data Display Tools

The display tools most commonly used in PI activities include bar graphs, histograms, Pareto charts, pie charts, pivot tables, line charts, and control charts.

Once the data have been collected, the PI team should sort the data and identify any significant findings. Charts and graphs of the data make it easier to identify trends and significant relationships. Graphs can be used to compare data sets from different years or over time to visually illustrate a trend in the data or a change in performance. The PI measures reported to a board of directors often highlight variances in data using graphs, tables, or charts (see figure 16.1). For example, in a bar graph, a change in the height of a bar indicates an increase or decrease in the data represented by the bar. The PI team would then have to determine whether this increase or decrease was a significant change in the performance of the related process.

When constructing charts, graphs, and tables, the team must provide explanatory labels and titles. Data display should be simple and accurate. Team members must report all of the data, even when the data appear to have positive or negative implications for the organization. Sometimes what appears to be a negative trend may actually turn out to be a positive trend after the team fully analyzes the data. (See AHIMA [2011] for additional information.)

Bar Graphs

A **bar graph** is used to display discrete categories, such as the gender of respondents or the type of health insurance respondents have. Such categories are shown on the horizontal, or X, axis of the graph. The vertical, or Y, axis shows the number or frequency of responses. The vertical scale always begins with zero. Most spreadsheet software can be used to "draw" a bar graph from a given data set. An example of a bar graph is in figure 4.3.

Histograms

A **histogram** is a bar graph that displays data proportionally. Histograms are used to identify problems or changes in a system or process. They are based on raw data and absolute frequencies, which determine how the graphs will be structured. Unlike a Pareto chart (described in the following section), a histogram keeps the data in the order of the scale against which they were obtained. The horizontal axis measures intervals of continuous data, such as time or money. The scale is grouped into intervals appropriate to the nature of the data. For example, time might be grouped into intervals of 6 hours and money into groups of $5,000. The vertical axis shows the absolute frequency of occurrence in each of the interval categories. Because of its visual impact, a histogram is more effective for displaying data than a check sheet of raw data, particularly when the frequencies are large. A histogram rather than a pie chart should be used for continuous data.

Histograms have the following characteristics:

- They display large amounts of continuous data that are difficult to interpret in lists or other nongraphic forms.

- They show the relative frequency of occurrence of the various data categories indirectly using the height of the bars.

- They show the distribution of the absolute frequencies of the data in the grouped intervals.

The first step in creating a histogram is to gather the data. The data can be collected on check sheets or gathered from department logs or other resources. A histogram should be used in situations in which numerical observations can be collected, for example, cost in dollars for a surgical procedure. Once the data have been gathered, the team can begin to group the data into a series of intervals or categories. A check sheet can be used to count how many times a data point appears in each interval grouping. For example, the cost of a surgical procedure on each patient might be grouped into the following intervals: $0 to $24,999; $25,000 to $49,999; $50,000 to $74,999; and $75,000 to $99,999.

To create the actual histogram, set up the horizontal axis with the interval groupings and the vertical axis with the absolute frequencies, always beginning at zero for both. Each bar should be drawn upward as it relates to the tabulated frequencies from the check sheet.

To analyze a histogram, look for things that seem suspicious or strange. The team should review the various interpretations and write down its observations.

The histogram in figure 4.5 shows data related to the number of patients and their total charges. The horizontal axis lists the revenue per stay by dollar amounts, and the vertical axis shows the interval groupings indicating the number of patients.

Pareto Charts

A **Pareto chart** is a kind of bar graph that uses data to determine priorities in problem solving. Using a Pareto chart can help the PI team focus on problems and their causes and demonstrate which are most responsible for the problem. Follow these steps to construct a Pareto chart:

1. Use a check sheet to collect the required data. Figure 4.12 shows the top 10 major diagnostic categories (MDCs) by total charges. A check sheet is used to collect cases by MDC and to total the hospital charges for that MDC.

Figure 4.12. Example of a Pareto chart

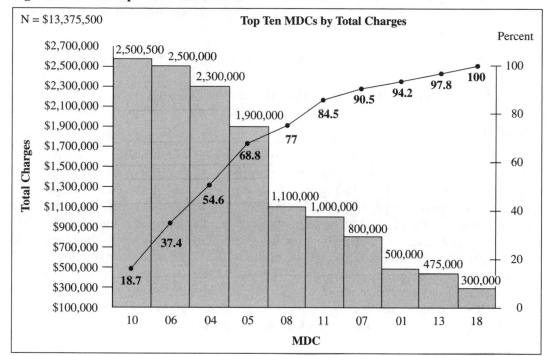

2. Arrange the data in order, from the category with the greatest frequency to the category with the lowest frequency. In the figure, the data are arranged from the MDC with the highest charges to the MDC with the lowest charges.

3. Calculate the totals for each category. Figure 4.12 lists MDC 10 first, with charges totaling approximately $2,500,500; then MDC 06 with charges totaling $2,500,000; MDC 04 with charges of $2,300,000; and so forth to MDC 18, with charges totaling approximately $300,000.

4. Compute the cumulative percentage. This is accomplished by calculating the percentage of the total for each category and then adding the percentage for the greatest frequency to the percentage for the next greatest frequency, and so on. Using the example in figure 4.12, the charges for MDC 10 ($2,500,500) represent 18.7 percent of all charges listed, while the charges for MDC 06 ($2,500,000) represent 18.7 percent of all charges listed. The cumulative percentage is obtained by adding the percentages together—MDC 10's 18.7 percent plus MDC 06's 18.7 percent equals 37.4 percent. This cumulative percentage is then calculated for all categories until 100 percent is obtained.

5. Draw horizontal and vertical axes on graph paper. The horizontal axis is "MDC" and the vertical axis is "Total Charges."

6. Scale the vertical axis for absolute frequency (0 to the total calculated above).

7. Working from left to right, construct a bar for each category, with height indicating the frequency. Start with the category with the largest value and add categories in descending order.

8. Draw a vertical scale on the right side of the graph and add a percentage scale (0 to 100 percent).

9. Plot the cumulative percentage line, as shown in figure 4.12.

Pie Charts

A **pie chart** is used to show the relationship of each part to the whole, in other words, how each part contributes to the total product or process. The 360 degrees of the circle, or pie, represent the total, or 100 percent. The pie is divided into "slices" proportionate to each component's percentage of the whole. To create a pie chart, first determine the percentages for each data element of the total population, and then draw the slice accordingly. Creating pie charts by hand requires the use of a protractor. For example, if a slice represents 45 percent of the whole, multiply the 360 degrees of the circle by .45 to find that 45 percent of the pie equals 162 degrees. Then, using the protractor, mark off 162 degrees on the pie and draw lines to the center to configure the slice. Spreadsheet programs can automatically create pie charts from a given data set (see instructions under "Line Charts"). (See figure 4.4 for an example of a pie chart.)

Pivot Tables

"**Pivot tables** are an excellent Excel tool to summarize data according to categories [as they can be done manually using a check sheet discussed previously]. For example, they may be used to summarize charges according to department, counts of coded data elements, etc. Pivot tables also provide flexibility for the end user or analyst to organize and filter the data in various ways before finalizing the analysis." Table 4.2 "is a small example

Table 4.2.   Example of a pivot table

Count of Dx			
Dx	Female	Male	Grand Total
4242		1	1
4254	2		2
4280	1		1
4290	1		1
5119		1	1
7455	1		1
78341	1		1
7861	1		1
E8780		1	1
Grand Total	7	3	10

Source: AHIMA 2011.

of a pivot table totaling diagnosis codes according to sex" (AHIMA 2011, 10). Microsoft Office (2011) provides detailed instructions on how to create pivot tables in Excel.

Line Charts

A **line chart** is a simple plotted chart of data that shows the progress of a process over time. By analyzing the chart, the PI team can identify trends, shifts, or changes in a process over time. The chart tracks the time frame on the horizontal axis and the measurement (the number of occurrences or the actual measure of a parameter) on the vertical axis. The data are gathered from sources specific to the process that has been evaluated. Each set of data (measurement or number of occurrences and time frame) must be related.

A line chart can be created by going through the following steps:

1. Select a time frame.

2. Identify the data to be tracked.

3. Use a check sheet to collect frequency data or a tally sheet to collect measurement data.

4. Draw the chart and place the measurement or frequency on the vertical axis and the time frame on the horizontal axis.

5. Label the chart with specific details.

6. Plot the data in the sequence they appear.

7. Connect the points to form a relationship line.

8. Take the average of the data points collected.

9. Finally, draw a line parallel with the horizontal axis to represent the average.

To analyze the chart, the team should look for peaks and valleys that indicate there may be a problem with the process.

Periodically redoing the line charts for a process helps the team monitor changes over time. A line chart is a good way to display trends in the data. For example, a line chart could be displayed on a large plastic graph that could be updated each month. When the team evaluates the results, it should look for seasonal peaks and valleys. For example, summer vacation times may show a change in a chart plotting staff productivity. Figure 4.6 provides an example of a line chart.

To create the line chart using Excel for the data displayed in figure 4.6, enter the data points into the spreadsheet. This includes one column for the dates and a second column indicating the number of charts analyzed for the corresponding date. Then high-light the data in both columns with the cursor. Next, select the insert tab in Excel, and then select the type of chart—in this case, a line chart—that you want the program to create. The software will display the chart on the screen. To add the axis labels, use your mouse to click in the chart; the chart tools tab should appear on the menu bar at the top of the screen. Using this tab, select the layout option. Next, locate the axis titles option; select this icon and add the X-axis title ("date") and the Y-axis title ("number of charts analyzed"). To add a chart title, use the chart tools to select the layout icon and then the chart title; use the drop-down menu options to define the location of the title. To add the data values on the chart, select the data labels icon under the chart tools layout option and the values should appear on the chart. The chart can then be copied and pasted into your report (Microsoft Office 2011).

Control Charts

A **control chart** can used to measure key processes over time. Using a control chart focuses attention on any variation in the process and helps the PI team determine whether that variation is normal or a result of special circumstances. Normal variation also may be called *common cause variation*, or the expected variance in a process, because the process will not or cannot be performed in exactly the same manner each and every time. When a special circumstance or unexpected event occurs in the process, this will result in what is called *special cause variation*. It is this special cause variation that the PI team needs to investigate.

The specific statistical calculations used to determine the upper and lower limits of a control chart depend on the type of data collected. The calculations used for statistical process control are the data mean, the median of the range between data points, and the standard deviation. (Refer to discussion of the mean and standard deviation in the section "Statistical Analysis," and see Meisenheimer [1997].) The appearance of the control chart is like turning the classic bell curve on its left tail and running it horizontally left to right as the time on the X-axis goes by. (See figure 4.13.)

The upper and lower control limits are always +/–2 standard deviations from the mean. As each successive month of data is added to the chart, the standard deviations are recalculated and may fluctuate in value. As the process is tightened up and improved over time, the standard deviation should become smaller and smaller as variation is driven out of the process. If the standard deviation expands, the process becomes less controlled, taking on variation and most likely less quality. The latest calculated standard deviation is always used in the current display of the chart. Data points that lie outside the upper or lower control limits may signal special cause variation that should be examined.

Figure 4.13.   Example of a control chart

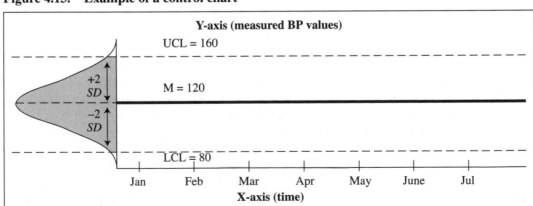

The following list shows the steps in developing a control chart:

1. Determine which process and what data to measure.

2. Collect about 20 observations of the measure.

3. Calculate the mean and standard deviation for the data set. Various spreadsheet software programs can be used to make these calculations. The mean, or average, becomes the centerline for the control chart.

4. Calculate an upper control limit and a lower control limit. The upper control limit is usually represented by a dashed line two standard deviations above the mean, and the lower control limit is usually two standard deviations below the mean.

The resulting control chart becomes the standard against which the team can compare all future data for the process. For example, figure 4.13 displays systolic blood pressure measurements for a patient. The mean is calculated at 120, and the standard deviation is calculated at 20. The upper control limit (UCL) is two standard deviations above the mean, or 160. The lower control limit (LCL) is two standard deviations below the mean, or 80.

Advanced Statistical Analysis

More advanced forms of statistical analysis are sometimes used in PI activities. Examples include analysis of variance (ANOVA), linear regression, and correlation. Information on these methods is available in the resources section for this chapter.

Real-Life Example

Table 4.3 shows a portion of a patient profile for one hospital in the years 2006 and 2011. When the 2006 data are compared with the 2011 data in a bar graph (figure 4.14), we see that the hospital's customer base has experienced an increase in the number of Asian patients. The hospital must look at how this increase affects its processes. For example,

Table 4.3.   Data set for bar graph

Profile of Hospital Patients			
2006		**2011**	
Race/Ethnicity	**Discharges**	**Race/Ethnicity**	**Discharges**
White	6,254	White	6,874
Black	1,859	Black	1,763
Hispanic	4,251	Hispanic	3,954
Native American	254	Native American	301
Asian	1,352	Asian	2,514
Other/Unknown	750	Other/Unknown	594

Figure 4.14.   Bar graph comparison of patient profile data

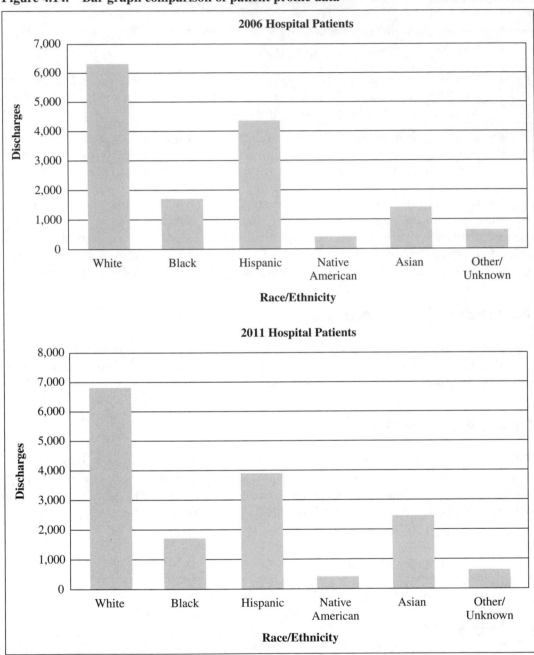

what changes might be required in the dietary area? What staffing changes might be required to accommodate patients who have religious and cultural differences? How will the organization ensure patient rights and safety in the face of language barriers to effective communication?

Table 4.4.   Data set for pie chart

Profile of Hospital Patients			
2006		**2011**	
Admission Type	**Discharges**	**Admission Type**	**Discharges**
Emergency	2,163	Emergency	5,987
Urgent	4,325	Urgent	2,478
Elective	5,784	Elective	4,458
Newborn	1,659	Newborn	1,342
Delivery	1,478	Delivery	1,270

Figure 4.15.   Pie chart comparison of patient profile data

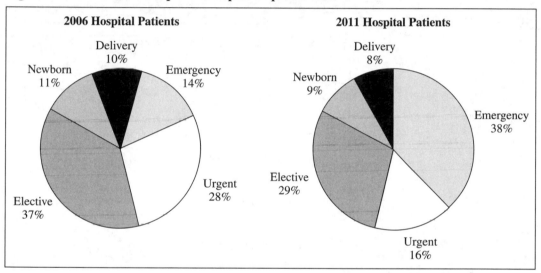

Table 4.4 shows another set of data from the hospital's patient profile. The two pie charts in figure 4.15, which were created from the data, show that over five years, the number of emergency admissions increased by 24 percentage points and the number of urgent admissions decreased by 12 percentage points. This information indicates that either the admissions are being categorized incorrectly or the incidence of trauma is increasing. The facility may need to look at its emergency department capacity and procedures or consider changes to its admission criteria.

Case Study

Students should select three sets of data from table 4.5 and create an appropriate graph to represent those data. They should keep in mind the type of data in the table and choose the best graphic display tool for those data.

Table 4.5. Data set for case study

PROFILE OF HOSPITAL PATIENTS, CALIFORNIA

PAGE 84
HSA 11 – HFPA 933 — LAKEWOOD REGIONAL MED CTR – SOUTH ST
REPORTS

ID# 106190240   SEE VOLUME III FOR LTC

AGE	DISCHARGES MALE	FEMALE	TOTAL	AVER STAY	ADJUSTED TOTAL CHARGES TOTAL $	$/DAY	$/STAY
<29 DAYS	546	502	1,048	1.6	781,716	476	746
29-364 DY	6	5	11	1.9	29,432	1,402	2,676
1- 4 YRS	14	10	24	1.9	74,596	1,622	3,108
5-14 YRS	28	33	61	2.3	280,570	1,990	4,600
15-18 YRS	24	121	145	2.1	641,857	2,077	4,427
19-44 YRS	616	1,672	2,288	3.0	17,251,826	2,528	7,540
45-64 YRS	835	798	1,633	4.9	24,390,763	3,064	14,936
65-69 YRS	291	397	688	5.8	12,545,685	3,159	18,235
70-74 YRS	381	437	818	6.2	15,700,837	3,078	19,194
75-84 YRS	417	700	1,117	6.6	21,994,942	2,998	19,691
85+ YRS	128	278	406	6.4	6,490,931	2,499	15,988
TOTAL	3,286	4,953	8,239	4.4	100,183,155	2,787	12,160

UTILIZATION & CHARGES FOR MOTHERS & BABIES

	DISCHRGS	DAYS	ALOS	ADJUSTED TOTAL CHARGES TOTAL $	$/DAY	$/STAY
NORMAL NEWBRN (1)	910	1,379	1.5	623,095	452	685
DELVRY—VAGINL (2)	853	1,275	1.5	2,594,805	2,035	3,042
DELVRY—C.SECT. (3)	168	490	2.9	1,073,141	2,190	6,388

DEFINITIONS: (1) DRG 391; (2) DRGS 372 THRU 375; (3) DRGS 370 & 371.

MAJOR DIAGNOSTIC CATEGORY	DISCHARGES	%	AVER STAY	ADJUSTED TOTAL CHARGES # TOTAL $	$/DAY	$/STAY
01 NERVOUS SYSTEM	433	5.3	5.4	6,037,289	2,587	13,943
02 EYE	11	0.1	3.1	91,369	2,687	8,306
03 EAR, NOSE, ETC	63	0.8	3.5	494,246	2,247	7,845
04 RESPIR SYSTEM	783	9.5	6.7	14,830,414	2,807	18,941
05 CIRCU SYSTEM	1,728	21.0	5.1	33,469,870	3,788	19,369
06 DIGESTIV SYSTM	598	7.3	5.0	8,158,578	2,723	13,643
07 HEPATO SYSTEM ETC	209	2.5	4.7	3,208,921	3,268	15,343
08 MUSCULOSKEL SYSTEM	656	8.0	5.5	9,884,375	2,760	15,068
09 SKIN, BREAST, ETC	174	2.1	5.3	2,008,206	2,195	11,541
10 ENDOCRIN, NUTRI, ETC	269	5.7	4.8	4,547,948	2,017	9,697
11 KIDNEY/URINARY	257	3.1	4.8	2,713,015	2,222	10,556
12 MALE REPRODUCTV	148	1.8	4.1	1,664,124	2,242	11,244
13 FEMALE REPRODUCTV	132	1.6	3.6	1,311,264	2,738	9,934
14 PREGNCY/CHILDBIRTH	1,104	13.4	1.8	4,058,449	2,092	3,676
15 NEWBORN/NEONATE	1,047	12.7	1.6	781,465	476	746
16 BLOOD, ETC.	35	0.4	4.6	362,063	2,249	10,345
17 MYELOPROLIF, ETC	54	0.7	5.6	731,165	2,413	13,540
18 INFEC & PARASIT	142	1.7	8.5	3,225,324	2,668	22,714
19 MENTAL DISORDERS	23	0.3	3.3	162,376	2,165	7,060
20 ALC/DRUG USE ETC	43	0.5	4.0	398,022	2,341	9,256
21 INJURY/POISON/DRUG	104	1.3	4.1	1,389,320	3,223	13,359
22 BURNS	3	0.0	13.0	68,008	1,744	22,669
23 OTHER FACTORS	14	0.2	4.7	127,105	1,926	9,079
24 MULTI SIG TRAUMA	1	0.0	5.0	14,540	2,908	14,540
25 HIV INFECTIONS	8	0.1	20.3	445,699	2,751	55,712
UNGROUPABLE	0	0.0	.0	0	0	0
TOTAL	8,239	100.0	4.4	100,183,155	2,787	12,160

EXPECTED SOURCE OF PAYMENT	DISCHARGES	%	AVER STAY	ADJUSTED TOTAL CHARGES TOTAL $	$/DAY	$/STAY
MEDICARE	2,862	34.7	6.5	52,618,588	2,836	18,385
MEDI-CAL	1,836	22.3	3.2	12,966,166	2,194	7,062
INSURANCE CO	812	9.9	3.0	6,189,201	2,512	7,622
HMO/PHP	2,020	24.5	3.3	21,706,087	3,269	10,746
BLUE X/SHIELD	31	0.4	3.2	291,884	2,919	9,416
SELF PAY	423	5.1	2.9	3,139,734	2,551	7,423
MED INDIGENT	0	0.0	0.0	0	0	0
OTHER GOVMT	0	0.0	3.3	32,663	3,266	10,888
WORKERS COMP	251	3.0	4.1	3,236,576	3,124	12,895
OTHER	0	0.0	0.0	0	0	0
NONGOVMT	0	0.0	0.0	0	0	0
NO CHARGE	0	0.0	0.0	0	0	0
TITLE V	1	0.0	1.0	2,256	2,256	2,256
UNKNOWN	0	0.0	0.0	0	0	0
TOTAL	8,239	100.0	4.4	100,183,155	2,787	12,160

PERCENTILES OF $/STAY

10TH	50TH	90TH
3,462	8,682	27,240
1,413	5,497	13,293
4,905	13,088	40,052
4,218	10,712	48,831
3,160	7,335	22,872
3,976	8,740	27,930
4,153	11,050	26,487
3,096	7,001	19,284
2,533	5,973	17,435
2,999	8,177	18,577
5,793	9,014	19,010
5,587	8,815	14,482
2,214	3,101	8,245
438	567	1,177
3,632	6,887	26,568
2,517	8,806	29,828
4,442	13,583	52,218
2,886	5,201	15,823
1,990	3,381	22,500
2,733	5,074	17,604
886	6,684	25,358

RACE/ETHNICITY	DISCHARGES	%	STAY
WHITE	5,235	63.5	4.8
BLACK	772	9.4	4.3
HISPANIC	1,597	19.4	3.1
NATIVE AMER	98	1.2	3.8
ASIAN	482	5.9	3.8
OTHER & UNKNOWN	55	0.7	3.3

ADMISSION SOURCE	DISCHARGES	%	STAY
ROUTINE	3,585	43.5	4.2
EMERGENCY ROOM	3,299	40.0	5.2
HOME HEALTH SVC	0	0.0	3.0
SHRT TERM ACUTE HOS	117	1.4	4.5
SNF/ICF	167	2.0	8.4
OTHER FACILITY	38	0.5	4.7
NEWBORN	1,032	12.5	1.6
OTHER & UNKNOWN	0	0.0	0

DISPOSITION	DISCHARGES	%	STAY
ROUTINE	6,710	81.4	3.6
SHRT TERM ACUTE HOS	318	3.9	3.6
OTHER FACILITY	187	2.3	7.8
HOME HLTH SRVC	277	3.4	9.1
SNF/ICF	417	5.1	10.2
DIED	245	3.0	8.2
LEFT AGNST MED ADV	85	1.0	2.9
OTHER & UNKNOWN	0	0.0	.0

ADMISSION TYPE	DISCHARGES	%	STAY
EMERGENCY	606	7.4	7.2
URGENT	4,704	57.1	5.2
ELECTIVE	868	10.5	4.3
NEWBORN	1,032	12.5	1.6
DELIVERY	1,022	12.4	1.7
OTHER & UNKNOWN	7	0.1	1.7

EXCLUDES DISCHARGES WHERE TOTAL CHARGES WERE REPORTED AS UNKNOWN

Project Application

Using the data collected from their quality improvement projects, students should select data to be displayed and determine the best graphic presentation. They should use a spreadsheet software program to design graphs for their projects.

Summary

It is important for PI teams to learn to use data analysis tools and data aggregation techniques. Making improvement decisions based on actual experience is much better than making decisions based on intuition or gut feelings. Graphs help translate data into meaningful information by allowing the team to clearly see the magnitude of changes, and graphic depictions of process outcomes are also easier to track over time. The most commonly used graphic tools include bar graphs, pie charts, Pareto charts, histograms, pivot tables, line charts, and control charts.

References

AHIMA. 2011. *Health Data Analysis Toolkit*. Chicago: AHIMA. Web only.

Joint Commission. 2011a. http://www.jointcommission.org/performance_measurement.aspx.

Joint Commission. 2011b. *Hospital Accreditation Standards*. Oakbrook Terrace, IL: Joint Commission Resources.

Layman, E. 2009. Data collection: Sampling. Chapter 10 in *Health Informatics Research Methods: Principles and Practice*. Edited by Layman, E., and V. Watzlaf. Chicago: AHIMA.

Layman, E. 2010. Research methods: Data collection methods. Chapter 16 in *Health Information Management: Concepts, Principles, and Practice*, 3rd ed. Edited by LaTour, K., and S. Eichenwald-Maki. Chicago: AHIMA.

Meisenheimer, C.G., ed. 1997. *Improving Quality: A Guide to Effective Programs*, 2nd ed. Gaithersburg, MD: Aspen Publishers.

Microsoft Office. 2011. Excel help and how-to. http://office.microsoft.com/en-us/excel-help/.

Osborn, C. 2006. *Statistical Applications for Health Information Management*, 2nd ed. Gaithersburg, MD: Aspen Publishers.

Resources

Lighter, D., and D.C. Fair. 2004. *Principles and Methods of Quality Management in Health Care*, 2nd ed. Gaithersburg, MD: Aspen Publishers.

McLaughlin, C.P., and A.D. Kaluzny. 2006. *Continuous Quality Improvement in Health Care: Theory, Implementation, and Applications*, 3rd ed. Gaithersburg, MD: Aspen Publishers.

National Center for Health Statistics (NCHS) and the Centers for Medicare and Medicaid Services (CMS). International Classification of Diseases, Ninth Revision, Clinical Modification (ICD-9-CM). http://www.cdc.gov/nchs/about/otheract/icd9/abticd9.htm.

Chapter 5
Communicating Performance Improvement Activities and Recommendations

Learning Objectives

- To apply communication tools such as minutes, quarterly reports, and storyboards in performance improvement processes
- To recognize the key elements in a storyboard and critique a storyboard layout

Key Terms

Storyboard
Storytelling

Background and Significance

The effective communication of information about the activities of performance improvement (PI) teams is vital to the PI process in healthcare organizations. All PI activities should be reported using the committee or meeting structure defined by the healthcare organization. This structure may include medical staff standing committees, PI team workgroups, or department meetings. The hospital committee structure and organizational flow of information are further defined and discussed in chapter 14.

The Performance Improvement and Patient Safety Council is an example of a standing committee in most healthcare organizations that is responsible for coordinating and reporting PI and safety activities. This council receives committee reports of PI activities and, in turn, reports significant findings to the leaders of the organization—typically, the executive committee and board of directors.

Figure 5.1.   **Flow of information from chartered PI teams to the Performance Improvement and Patient Safety Council**

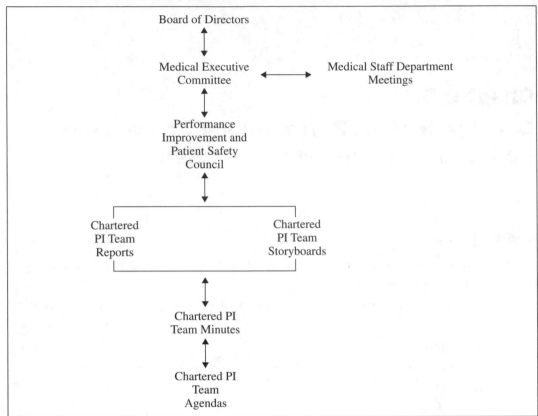

Evidence of PI activity is also required by various regulatory and accreditation agencies. Such organizations require that PI activities take place within every healthcare organization, and they look for PI compliance during the survey process.

Common methods of communicating PI activities include minutes, quarterly reports, and storytelling. This chapter focuses on these three basic communication tools. Figure 5.1 shows the flow of information from the chartered PI teams to the Performance Improvement and Patient Safety Council, regardless of the reporting method.

Minutes

It is important that the PI committee or team keep track of its progress and activities. Documentation of these activities is often recorded in the form of minutes.

Organizations should select the methods they will use to set agendas for their meetings and allocate meeting times for action items and discussions. (Information on setting agendas can be found in chapter 3.) The responsibility for distributing the agendas for upcoming meetings and the minutes from past meetings should be discussed and assigned. The role of recorder, or secretary, should be assigned to an individual trained in the process of recording minutes.

Many different formats can be used to record the minutes of meetings. One that is particularly helpful for PI documentation is the CRAF method. CRAF stands for the following categories of recordable information:

- *C*onclusions of group discussion
- *R*ecommendations made by the committee or team
- *A*ctions that the committee, team, or individual members decide to take
- *F*ollow-up activity (See figure 5.2 for an example.)

By using the CRAF format, the recorder can avoid getting distracted from the discussion. The format allows the recorder to focus only on necessary documentation.

The *conclusions* section of the minutes should document the results of the discussion and any decisions the group makes about future actions. The recorder should be sure to clarify the conclusions at the end of a discussion if there is any ambiguity.

The *recommendations* section of the minutes should capture the team's plan for putting its decision into effect, with justification points if necessary. The approach to solving the problem at hand should be listed as a recommendation.

The recorder then documents the *actions* planned for the different process steps. In figure 5.2, the actions section documents who was assigned to accomplish which activities during the next work period. Activities between meetings might include gathering data, talking with people involved in and responsible for the process being examined, or doing a literature search.

The *follow-up* section documents whether the actions were accomplished and whether the group is ready to make decisions and recommendations for future activities. Assessing and documenting progress ensures that the PI team is following the process plan appropriately and conducting sufficient analysis of previous actions.

Reports

In addition to documenting meeting activities, the committee or team must provide regular reports to the organization's Performance Improvement and Patient Safety Council. The frequency of reporting is usually based on the committee or team meeting schedule. At a minimum, quarterly reports should be submitted to the council. The quarterly report is based on the documented meeting minutes and should include information about PI activities, such as summaries of data collection, conclusions, and recommendations. (See the sample reporting form in figure 5.3.)

Figure 5.2.   Sample minutes from a PI meeting

Committee Name: HIM Laboratory	**Approval:**	
Attendance/Name and Title: HIM 3320 Class		
Date: January 15	**Beginning/Ending Time:** 10:05 a.m.–11:20 a.m.	
Recorder: John Smith		
Leader: Sue Jones		
Facilitator: Kathy Anderson		

Conclusions	Recommendations	Actions	Follow-up
Reviewed and finalized customer survey tool.	Additions/changes to customer survey: • Add "WSU" and class name to survey title. • Add A, B, C, . . . to question responses on survey (all questions as applicable). • Add "on average" to question #2 on survey x2. • Change question #5 wording on survey from "do you have knowledge" to "are you aware." • Add to question #6, "If not applicable to you, circle NA." • Change under question #6 "CPU" to "computer." • Add "NA" column for each response in #6. • Add month and year (1/00) to last page of survey—bottom left corner to indicate design date.	Terry to update survey per team recommendations by 1/20. Request HIM department secretary to copy survey once changes have been made.	Consensus reached on survey tool questions and administration of same

Figure 5.2. *(Continued)*

Conclusions	Recommendations	Actions	Follow-up
Administer survey next week during Stats class and HIM 3010 classes.		Lori and Terry to administer survey to Stats class next week. Michelle to administer survey to HIM 3010 class next week.	
Tabulate results of survey during meeting next week.	Break out in teams, compile data, decide on best QI tool(s) to use in presenting data and which software applications to use.		
Individual teamwork completed on outputs (i.e., identifying customer requirements, possible measure[s] for each requirement, and flowcharting the process)	Break out in teams and assign leader, facilitator, and recorder per each team. Document and report all meeting decisions/actions.	Teamwork completed on following outputs: • Transcription • Chart analysis • Lab/resource accessibility	Assignment complete Team roles practiced
Additional assignments given in preparation for next week's meeting: • Read handout "Developing an Information Management Plan." • Be prepared to discuss the Joint Commission IM standards, which one is related to HIM Laboratory.			
Evaluate meeting. Trouble with amount of time allotted per each agenda item Adjourn			

Figure 5.3. Example of a quarterly report

Committee Name:	HIM Laboratory
Leader:	Sue Jones
Facilitator:	Kathy Anderson
Date:	January 15

Opportunity Statement	Student complaints have been received about the quality of resources and technology available in the HIM Laboratory.
Mission	Evaluate the HIM lab in regard to accessibility, resources, library access, Internet access, quality of equipment, and adequacy of equipment for HIM students.
Vision	The HIM lab provides access to a variety of application software resources, library knowledge bases, and the Internet. A convenient, comfortable work environment exists.
Performance Measure	Survey student satisfaction with HIM Laboratory.
Sample	All HIM and HIT students
Summary of Progress to Date	Survey will be administered to the students during the next week. Data will be tabulated and recommendations will be made. PI team should wrap up its activities by the end of February.
Conclusions	Not applicable at this time
Recommendations	In progress

Reported To: _____   Date: _____

Signature: _____   Date: _____

Storytelling

Storytelling is another effective method of reporting PI activities by chartered teams. Storytelling has always been a powerful method of teaching and learning, and a storyboard or computer-based presentation helps teams explain their work to those who may not be familiar with the PI process. The purpose of creating storyboards or presentations is to summarize an entire PI project in a graphic format. The team uses words, pictures, and graphs to tell the story of the project in a fashion that permits listeners to grasp the team's thought process and to understand its specific applications of PI tools. Storyboards and presentations also demonstrate a growing knowledge of customer needs and the understanding of gathered statistical data. Electronic presentation software has significantly streamlined storytelling because such software provides standard formatting and key symbols to display the PI tools. However, healthcare organizations often use the storyboard because it provides the organization with a valuable teaching tool for its customers and staff. In addition, prominent display of the storyboard recognizes the accomplishments and participation of the organization's staff and employees. Storyboards are actually more effective than computer-based presentations because they show a snapshot of the entire PI team process to date without requiring someone to explain it, as is usually necessary with the computer-based presentation. They force the storytelling to be far more succinct and focused. And when posted in a public place, they are available to a wider audience than are the presentations.

Who started PI storytelling? In the early 1980s, Kaoru Ishikawa called attention to the importance of relaying the PI process in a structured manner to support learning and organization-wide PI (Ishikawa 1986). Since the technique was introduced, elaborate rules outlining the process have been developed. Leaders in continuous quality improvement and total quality management continue to emphasize the importance of these rules.

Who benefits from PI storytelling? Actually, very few people do not benefit from learning in a clear, concise manner how a PI effort proceeded. Examples of how individuals can benefit from the storytelling process include the following:

- Team accomplishments are documented over an extended period of time in an organized and succinct way.

- Presentations are focused, and the presenter gains practice in sharing the pride that comes from working on PI projects.

- Team members crystallize their thinking about the process of improvement.

- Teamwork is tracked in a focused manner, thus facilitating communication while reducing the accumulation of paper.

- Team members receive the public recognition that they are due and learn how they might contribute more in the future.

- Members of other groups or departments learn how to think in new ways about their work and improve the systems that they manage. Questioning one another helps create clearer awareness of how much people can learn from their associates.

- The professional staff can clearly see the impact of their role in improving overall patient care. They also learn how they can actively participate in PI work themselves.

- The board of directors can learn a great deal about the organization by studying the application and effect of PI processes on outcomes. It also can better meet its responsibility of ensuring that the organization provides high-quality patient care.

- The administrative team can prepare itself to lead and teach the process of management and improvement throughout the organization. In addition, it can recognize the contributions of the staff and encourage everyone to do just a little bit more. It also can provide regular opportunities to celebrate gains made in the continuing PI journey.

- Storytelling provides an outstanding forum for introducing new employees to PI and what it is all about.

- Guests, suppliers, and others can learn about PI without placing a significant additional burden on the PI team.

- The dominant culture of the organization becomes one of continuous improvement, and everyone in the organization learns to make improvements in everything they do.

There are several key elements to successful storytelling, including:

- Organization
- Structure
- Timeliness
- Frequency
- Connection
- Celebration
- Feedback

To create effective storyboards, keep the following rules in mind:

- Map the board in advance with labels for each section.
- Prepare clean boards for group presentation and display.
- Keep detailed information in a team record binder for reference.
- Plan the presentation to fit the size of the storyboard (36 × 48 inches is standard) and the general size of the panels.
- Use large fonts (24 point or greater) so that people can read the boards from a distance.
- Be creative with the use of color and other visual enhancements.

Every entity of the healthcare organization will benefit from the storytelling process. By following these basic rules for storyboard development, healthcare organizations can communicate PI activities to the entire organization and recognize individual contributions to the process. The basic storyboard layout is illustrated in figure 5.4.

Once a PI project is complete, the organization may decide to communicate the outcome to its communities of interest, such as patients, medical staff, or employers in the region. Organizations that have improved their services often want to market this fact.

Figure 5.4.   Sample storyboard layout

Storyboard Title		
• Opportunity statement (mission/vision) • Team members • Customers • Relevant dimension of performance	• Key team activities in process steps • Flow charts • Cause-and-effect (fishbone) diagram • Benchmarks	• Data gathered and analyzed (baseline and during PI activities) • Gantt chart • Future plans and goals

Several approaches can be used to communicate information on PIs. For example, some large healthcare corporations routinely present performance data on their Web sites to show customers and other stakeholders how they are progressing with important performance measures.

Many healthcare organizations also publish information about care quality initiatives in their annual reports. Such reports are an excellent vehicle for communicating performance information, emphasizing an organization's mission within its community, and communicating ongoing efforts to provide the community with the best healthcare possible.

In some segments of the healthcare industry, such as long-term care, report cards provide consumers and other stakeholders with information on the performance of individual facilities. Report cards usually present data on an organization's performance with respect to a preestablished set of criteria relevant to the organization's service segment. The Department of Health and Human Services publishes report cards for every licensed long-term care facility in the country (HHS 2011). The report cards show how each facility performed with respect to meeting the state's established licensing criteria.

Real-Life Example

The storyboard in figure 5.5 shows a student project. The PI project examined services at the campus student health center. Students were concerned about customer satisfaction in terms of hours of operation, quality of care, and confidentiality. So the student PI team developed mission and vision statements and identified both the center's customers and those customers' requirements. Then the group surveyed students, faculty, and staff to assess customer satisfaction with the center.

Case Study

Using the following criteria, students should critique the storyboard shown in figure 5.5.

Case Study Questions

1. Is the storyboard pleasing to look at, and is the text easy to read?

2. Is the storyboard set up logically?

3. Is each of the PI steps taken into account?

4. Are the steps in the process easy to read and understand?

5. Are all of the elements of a good mission statement present?

6. Are all of the elements of a good vision statement present?

7. Does the storyboard identify the external and internal customers of the process? (See the discussion of internal and external customers in chapter 6.)

Figure 5.5.   Example of a student team's storyboard presentation

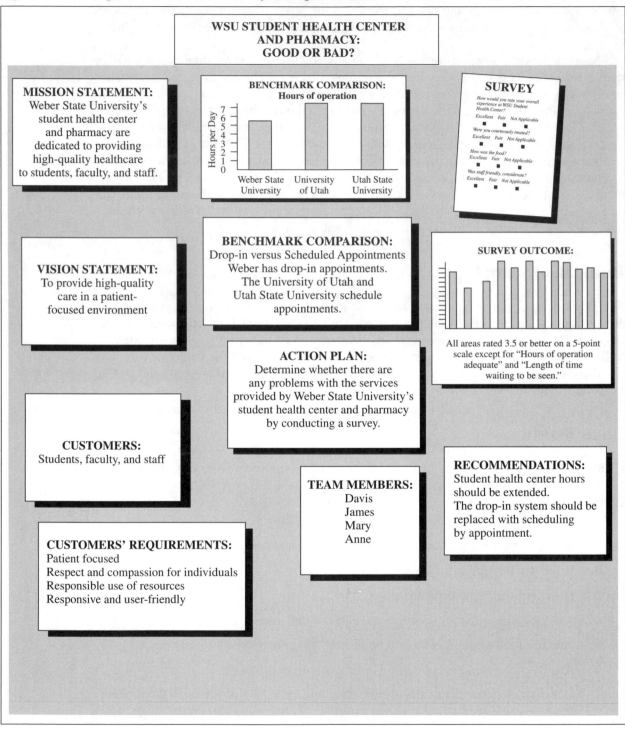

8. Does the storyboard identify the customers' requirements? If so, how? If not, why not?

9. Does the storyboard display the team's improvement process findings?

10. Are the team's recommendations based on the data the team collected? Are the recommendations sound? Are there other recommendations that the team did not identify?

Project Application

Students should develop a storyboard or electronic presentation for their projects. The presentation or storyboard should include each of the steps in the PI process as well as the students' findings and recommendations. Electronic presentations should include no more information than a storyboard would include.

Summary

Communication among the various constituencies involved in healthcare PI activities is of paramount importance. Team members must keep the organization's leadership or Performance Improvement and Patient Safety Council informed of their progress. The team also must track its activities carefully so that it stays focused on the issues for which it was convened. The use of meeting minutes facilitates this communication and tracking. When the team has completed its work, it must communicate its activities to the whole organization to inform everyone of changes in work processes and to allow the people not involved in the project to see how the team arrived at its conclusions. Storyboards or electronic presentations are effective vehicles for this internal communication. Sometimes the organization may want to communicate PI information to external stakeholders. Annual reports, information on Web sites, and report cards are tools that facilitate external communication.

References

Department of Health and Human Services. 2011. Nursing home compare. http://www.medicare.gov/nhcompare/home.asp.

Ishikawa, K. 1986. *Guide to Quality Control*. Milwaukee, WI: ASQ Quality Press.

Resources

Bemowski, K., and B. Stratton, eds. 1999. *101 Good Ideas: How to Improve Just about Any Process*. Milwaukee, WI: ASQ Quality Press.

Denning, S. 2000. *The Springboard: How Storytelling Ignites Action in Knowledge-Era Organizations*. Woburn, MA: Butterworth-Heinemann.

Denning, S. 2005. *The Leader's Guide to Storytelling: Mastering the Art and Discipline of Business Narrative*. San Francisco: Jossey-Bass.

Drennan, D., and S. Pennington. 1999. *12 Ladders to World Class Performance*. London: Kogan Page Ltd.

McLaughlin, C.P., and A.D. Kaluzny. 2006. *Continuous Quality Improvement in Health Care: Theory, Implementation, and Applications*, 3rd ed. Gaithersburg, MD: Aspen Publishers.

Meisenheimer, C.G., ed. 1997. *Improving Quality: A Guide to Effective Programs*, 2nd ed. Gaithersburg, MD: Aspen Publishers.

Part II
Continuous Monitoring and Improvement Functions

Chapter 6
Measuring Customer Satisfaction

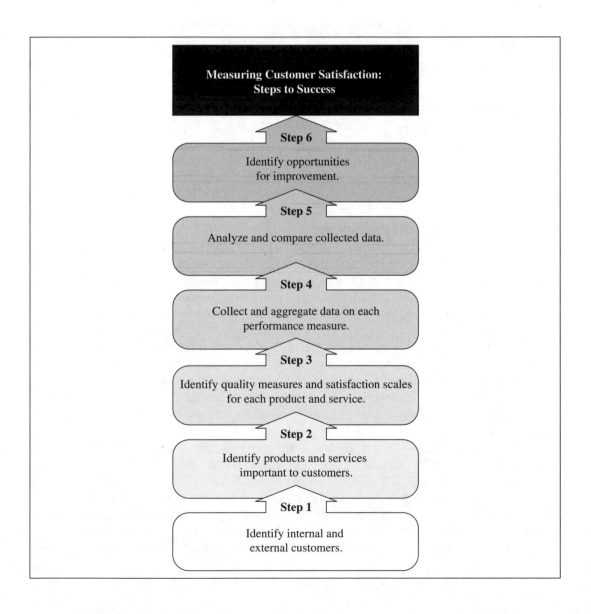

Measuring Customer Satisfaction:
Steps to Success

Step 6
Identify opportunities
for improvement.

Step 5
Analyze and compare collected data.

Step 4
Collect and aggregate data on each
performance measure.

Step 3
Identify quality measures and satisfaction scales
for each product and service.

Step 2
Identify products and services
important to customers.

Step 1
Identify internal and
external customers.

Learning Objectives

- To identify the differences between internal and external customers
- To outline the reasons customers' perspectives are important to the performance improvement process
- To describe the differences between surveys and interviews
- To outline the characteristics that make surveys and interviews effective
- To critique a survey or interview format

Key Terms

Customers
Direct observation
Expectations
External customers
Internal customers
Interviews
Survey tools

Background and Significance

As discussed in chapter 1, researching and defining performance expectations includes an investigation of what the customers of an organizational process expect from that process. Because there are many types of organizational processes, there are also many types of customers. Their **expectations** must be identified and incorporated into the design or redesign of an effective process.

Customers receive a product or service as a result of an organizational process. Just as we can identify the customers of a dress shop or an auto dealership, we can also identify the customers of a healthcare process. For example, when a nurse inserts a catheter into an artery to administer medication, the patient is receiving a service from the nurse. Similarly, when a pharmacist dispenses a medication to a patient, the patient is receiving a product from the pharmacist.

Identifying the patient, client, or long-term care resident as a customer should seem fairly straightforward. But customers can be identified for all kinds of healthcare processes. The families and friends of patients are the customers of volunteer services when they ask for a patient's room number. Emergency care physicians are the customers of central supply services when they request sterile suturing trays to close a patient's laceration. Surgeons are the customers of the pathology laboratory when they request frozen-section examination of tissue in the operating room during resection of a breast lesion.

Types of Customers

Customers can be placed in one of two categories: **internal customers** or **external customers.** Within the healthcare organization setting, internal customers are individuals within the organization who receive products or services from an organizational unit or department. In the preceding examples, surgeons are the internal customers of the pathology laboratory, and emergency care physicians are the internal customers of central supply services.

External customers are individuals from outside the organization who receive products or services from within the organization. In the preceding examples, patients, family members of patients, and friends of patients are external customers.

In determining the customers of a process, however, the organizational frame of reference also must be taken into consideration. Sometimes the frame of reference modifies the customer type, as is graphically displayed in figure 6.1. Figure 6.2 graphically displays an overhead view of figure 6.1. The large oval is Western States University Hospital as a whole organization. Patients are external customers because their frame of reference comes totally from outside the organization. When we think of the organization as a whole, surgeons, on the other hand, are identified as internal customers because they are members of an organizational unit—the medical staff.

Figure 6.1.   Examples of the internal and external customers of a pathology laboratory

External customers:
Patients

Internal customers:
Surgeons

Organization level

External customers:
Patients and surgeons

Internal customers:
Pathologists

Department or unit level

Figure 6.2.   Patients as external customers and physicians as internal customers of Western States University Hospital

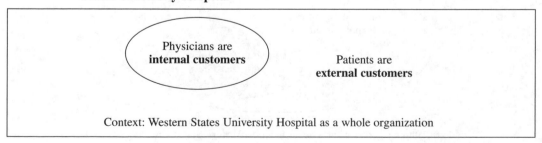

Physicians are
internal customers

Patients are
external customers

Context: Western States University Hospital as a whole organization

Now, if the frame of reference is at the departmental level, as depicted in figure 6.3, the surgeons would be identified as the external customers of pathology lab processes and the pathologists would be identified as the internal customers of the laboratory technicians who process the specimens.

It is important to recognize that internal and external customers must be identified in relation to the organizational process under consideration. Each process has a unique set of customers whose needs and expectations must be recognized.

The opinions of internal and external customers regarding the effectiveness of a health-care process should be of primary importance to healthcare organizations. No one is a better judge of products and services than the customer. Additionally, a dissatisfied customer is said to tell 10 times as many people about a negative experience than the satisfied customer is to relate a positive experience.

There are several ways for an organization to obtain information about its customers' perceptions of its products and services. With internal customers, the organization can simply ask them. Many internal customers never get the opportunity to express their expectations in a positive context. Often, the only time a department representative hears about the expectations of internal customers is when a process has been mismanaged or has resulted in a negative outcome. Giving internal customers the opportunity to vocalize their expectations increases their overall satisfaction.

With external customers, particularly patients, identifying expectations about service quality is more complicated. Patients' expectations are multifaceted and often based on the condition for which the patient is being treated. Assessments of patient expectations must be undertaken judiciously.

Administrative subjects, such as parking, hours of operation, room decor, and so forth, can be assessed using an anonymous patient satisfaction survey. Clinical subject matter pertaining to the patient's condition and medical and nursing treatment, however, may need to be assessed from the viewpoint of the clinicians involved in the patient's care and the outcomes achieved through that care. (See chapter 8.)

Patient expectations about subjective topics, such as pain management, are completely different from one patient to the next. Another highly subjective area that influences a patient's satisfaction is the patient's return to an acceptable quality of life after treatment.

Figure 6.3.   Surgeons as external customers and pathologists as internal customers of Western States University Hospital

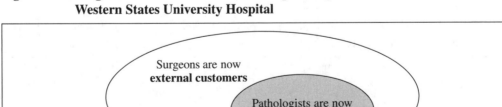

One of the most important factors that influences patients' assessments of their care is how they are treated by caregivers (Atlantic Information Services 1995, 5–6).

Because of this inherent complexity, assessment of patient satisfaction might best be performed by multidisciplinary teams using carefully tailored assessment tools. Nationally recognized vendors offer patient satisfaction surveys. (See table 6.1.) Most of these surveys

Table 6.1. Vendors of patient satisfaction surveys

Vendor Name/ Contact Information	Product Description
NRC Picker http://www.nrcpicker.com	• Affords the only worldwide patient-experience benchmark database with the longest continuous measurement record • Champion of the Eight Dimensions of Patient-Centered Care • Developed Qualisys, state-of-the-art technology that seamlessly automates reporting for measurement and improvement • Offers exclusive source for Picker Institute surveys, educational products, and resources • Assists hundreds of providers with public reporting of performance measures
Deyta, Inc. 7400 New LaGrange Rd. Suite 200 Louisville, KY 40222 http://www.deyta.com	• Developed Factual Foresight application to manage data collection and analysis • Audits employee satisfaction; provides data for compliance and accreditation • Offers consulting services to aid in survey design • Maintains processing center for mailing, collection, scanning, comment typing, coding, and reporting • Offers online access to internal and external benchmarking information
Press Ganey Associates 404 Columbia Place South Bend, IN 46601 http://www.pressganey.com	• Specializes in patient satisfaction measurement via direct mail surveys • Produces quarterly reports that detail hospital-wide performance and compare individual units, noting satisfaction trends and national benchmarking statistics for HCAHPS compliance • Offers online access to completed surveys • Produces special annual reports that contain detailed demographic analyses of individual hospital data and national comparative data
SullivanLuallin, Inc. 3760 Fourth Avenue, Suite 1 San Diego, CA 92103 http://www.sullivan-luallin.com	• Specializes exclusively in ambulatory care performance improvement • Produces standard and customized patient satisfaction surveys • Produces Web-based surveys of internal physicians, managers, and staff members • Produces patient assessments to provide feedback from the patient's view • Provides coaching consultations for human resources improvement

(Continued on next page)

Table 6.1. *(Continued)*

Vendor Name/ Contact Information	Product Description
RAND Health Communications 1776 Main St. Santa Monica, CA 90407 http://www.rand.org/health	• Provides quality assessment instruments in the areas of CAHPS, evidence-based practice, inpatient and ambulatory patient satisfaction, appropriateness of treatment, chronic illness management, and nursing home outcomes • Taps global satisfaction as well as six important aspects of patient satisfaction: technical quality, interpersonal manner, communication, financial considerations, time spent with doctor, and accessibility
Professional Research Consultants, Inc. 11326 P Street Omaha, NE 68137 http://www.prconline.com	• Uses proven methodology for patient satisfaction telephone interviewing • Incorporates patient satisfaction and expectation assessments with outcomes research (not health assessment outcomes) • Provides statistically valid measurement of perceptions of "quality" with open-ended response capabilities
California Institute for Health Systems Performance 1215 K Street Sacramento, CA 95814	• Conducts PEP-C III patient satisfaction survey for selected hospitals in California • Allows hospitals to compare their performance on key dimensions with other participating institutions • Uses Web-based analysis and reporting tools that allow hospitals immediate access to results and flexibility in conducting data analyses

Source: Adapted from Atlantic Information Services 1995, 5–6.

Also see: HCAHPS Approved Vendor List. http://www.hcahpsonline.org/app_vendor.aspx.

also provide healthcare organizations with important benchmarking feedback, which measures their customers' satisfaction against that of other, similar organizations.

Monitoring and Improving Customer Satisfaction: Steps to Success

To monitor and improve customer satisfaction, an organization must know:

- Exactly who its customers are
- What its customers want and value
- What improvements could be made to better meet its customers' needs

Step 1: Identify Internal and External Customers

Assessing whether a process meets the expectations of its customers is difficult when some customers have not yet been identified. To identify customers, the performance improve-

Figure 6.4.   Monitoring and improving customer satisfaction

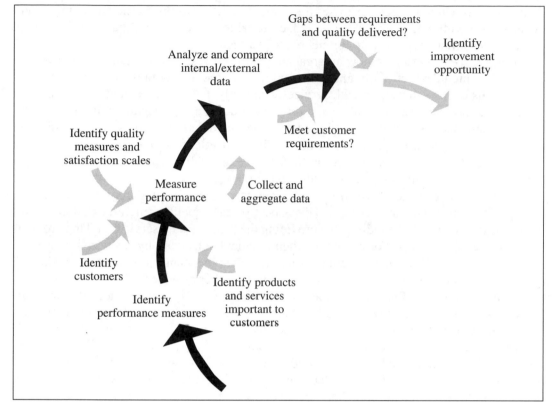

ment (PI) team should list everyone who comes in contact with the process and takes away a product or a service. (See figure 6.4.)

Step 2: Identify Products and Services Important to Customers

The PI team should develop a list of the products and services used by internal and external customers. However, not every product is tangible—it is not always seen and evaluated as an object in the environment. Commonly, tangible products include such things as facilities, equipment, and appearance of personnel. But a more intangible product would be information that is collected in a database. It is used by many customers, but only rarely would that database be printed out on paper in its tangible form.

Outcomes of care are not necessarily tangible, either. To report outcomes of care, the recipient of the care service needs some established means of describing the outcome, or clinical staff may have to use healthcare monitoring instruments to determine improvements in the patient's condition. For example, heart-monitoring equipment might need to be used to determine if a drug has had the appropriate effect on a patient's arrhythmia.

Another aspect of quality that customers may emphasize in their evaluations of healthcare performance is reliability. *Reliability* is the level at which an organization can provide an offered product or service when requested and as advertised. For example, one hospital in the western United States advertises that patients visiting its emergency department will receive care within 15 minutes. To be judged reliable by customers, that 15-minute goal must be met when they show up for emergency services.

Responsiveness refers to how an organizational staff responds to unanticipated service needs. This includes staff willingness to continuously monitor both the customer's condition and his or her satisfaction with services. Currently, pain management is an important function, as noted by various public and private entities. Pain management is a continuous process; patients' pain must be monitored, and their medication dosages must be adjusted, when necessary, to keep pain within their individual tolerance levels. Customers judge responsiveness to pain management on the basis of the staff's willingness to go the extra distance to attend to this often continually changing need.

The healthcare PI term *assurance* describes the knowledge and courtesy of the staff that provide the goods and services. This aspect of care quality generates customer trust and confidence in both the individuals providing the products and services and the products and services themselves. For example, when a patient selects a physician, assurance is a key consideration. If the new patient does not trust the physician's judgment, he or she will probably question the outcome of all visits or find another provider.

Empathy can be defined here as the staff's willingness to relate to customers during the provider-customer relationship as fellow human beings who have feelings and emotions. This can be a particularly important aspect in healthcare settings because when people are ill, they frequently have emotional reactions to the illness. When major illness strikes, or when fragile individuals such as children or the elderly are involved, the emotional response can be intense. Healthcare customers expect that staff and providers will understand these kinds of feelings and help them cope with these trying situations.

Features are the aspects of healthcare services that distinguish one organization from another or that add particular value in the customer's evaluation of an organization. For example, an organization may be renowned in its community for providing exceptionally successful heart disease treatment with few negative outcomes, while employing the latest in diagnostic imaging and therapeutic modalities; or an organization may have upgraded its service by adding a number of new birthing centers at its facility.

Finally, *perceived quality* is also an important aspect of healthcare service. This consists of the organization's reputation for the quality of its services and consumer reaction to these services and products based on their experiences with the organization.

It may or may not be important to look at the quality of a healthcare product or service from all of these aspects. In the process of planning the PI activities for a period of time, leadership must be willing to prioritize the impact of the possible projects on the organization's performance, the number and scope of projects that realistically can be undertaken given available resources, and the criticality of making the improvement at this particular time. Once the process or service is identified for improvement, the PI team must determine which aspects are relevant to the process or service under examination and then complete the cycle of measurement and improvement, as necessary, regarding each aspect.

Step 3: Identify Quality Measures and Satisfaction Scales for Each Product and Service

For each quality aspect of a product or service, performance measures must be identified. For example, if a PI team was assessing a patient's experience at a physician's office for a medical appointment, waiting time would be a relevant performance measure. After the team identified waiting time as a performance measure, it would need to develop a satisfaction scale. The PI team would need to decide whether to measure waiting time in seconds, minutes, or hours.

For Medicare participants, the Agency for Healthcare Research and Quality (AHRQ) has developed a patient satisfaction tool called the Hospital Consumer Assessment of Healthcare Providers and Systems (HCAHPS), the data and outcomes of which are now required to be submitted to the Centers for Medicare and Medicaid Services (CMS) (AHRQ 2008). The questionnaire is mailed to a sample of discharged hospital patients who, after completing it, return it to a vendor for aggregation and analysis of results. The vendor then reports the results to CMS. The areas of focus on the survey include:

- Quality of interactions with nurses in terms of courtesy and respect
- Quality of nurses' ability to listen to the patient
- Ability of nurses to explain relevant aspects of care to the patient
- Call button response times and attitudes
- Quality of interactions with physicians in terms of courtesy and respect
- Quality of physicians' ability to listen to the patient
- Ability of physicians to explain relevant aspects of care to the patient
- Cleanliness and quietness of the care environment
- Quality of assistance with ambulation and elimination activities
- Sufficiency and attentiveness of staff to pain medication
- Education of patient about medications administered in hospital
- Planning for post-discharge assistance and continuing care
- Overall rating of the hospital (Hospital Consumer Assessment of Healthcare Providers and Systems 2011)

Step 4: Collect and Aggregate Data on Each Performance Measure

Next, the PI team should determine the best methods for collecting data on each performance measure being assessed. In assessments of customer satisfaction, the principal methods of data collection are **survey tools, interviews,** and **direct observation.**

The construction of an effective survey tool requires a significant investment of time. (See the discussion of survey tools later in this chapter.) Interviews are often easier to use than survey tools because they consist of a series of open-ended questions. However, it is easier to aggregate data from a survey than information from an interview because surveys usually are composed of structured responses. The responses to interview questions, on the other hand, must be analyzed to identify common themes and perceptions.

The healthcare organization's institutional review board (IRB) should preapprove the use of any data-gathering tool. IRB approval is mandated by federal regulations on the use of human subjects in biomedical and health services research. Although policies and procedures vary across organizations, PI teams using such data-gathering methodologies should recognize their responsibility to obtain IRB approval to maintain the highest research standards respecting their human subjects. If the organization has no IRB, then either the quality council or the committee involved in the approval of PI projects should review the use of all tools. A statement such as, "Your completion and return of this survey implies your consent to use your feedback for quality improvement purposes" should be prominent in the survey introduction so that respondents are aware that their responses will be used individually and collectively. If patient or client responses will be identified as specifically belonging to them by name or associated to information gathered from their health records, organizations may want to include approvals from privacy officers or privacy boards to ensure compliance with current privacy laws and regulations.

Step 5: Analyze and Compare Collected Data

The PI committee should compare aggregate satisfaction ratings on performance measures with previous trends within the organization or with satisfaction levels achieved by other organizations. Such comparisons may be conducted using patient satisfaction data collected within the enterprise or satisfaction ratings published by state departments of health, national accreditation agencies, or other national organizations specializing in healthcare quality assessment. For instance, AHRQ has released the CAHPS® Hospital Survey (HCAHPS) to the public domain, making it available for use by hospitals and others. HCAHPS and its benchmarking database can be accessed on the Internet at https://www.cahps.ahrq.gov/ or the Department of Health and Human Services' (HHS) Hospital Compare Web site at http://www.hospitalcompare.hhs.gov. (The vendors of patient satisfaction surveys listed in table 6.1 can also provide national data.) As noted in chapter 5, an organization's published performance data on national or regional benchmarking criteria today are often referred to as a "report card," providing the public with information on the quality of care provided in the organization.

Step 6: Identify Opportunities for Improvement

Finally, the committee should develop a list of areas that need improvement based on its comparisons with aggregate satisfaction ratings on quality measures. PI teams should be implemented to define appropriate performance expectations and design or redesign processes.

Real-Life Examples

The following two examples help illustrate the process of measuring customer satisfaction. The first example looks at a PI measure involving external customers. The second example addresses both internal and external customers.

External Customers of a Food Services Department

Virginia Mullen, RHIA, is the director of quality and service excellence for a large US health-care corporation. She was working with one of her corporation's smaller facilities, an acute care hospital with 80 beds. To evaluate the service excellence of the facility, Mullen and the administration decided to use a satisfaction survey. The survey was to be mailed to patients after they had been discharged from the hospital.

One part of the survey asked for patient feedback on inpatient food services. The quality of food services was rated on a five-point scale, with 5 indicating very satisfied and 1 indicating very dissatisfied. The survey contained the following items:

- Taste of the food

- Temperature of the food

- Appearance of the food

- Variety of menu items

- Overall satisfaction with the food

After administering the survey for several months, Mullen and the administration noted that only 10 to 30 percent of patient ratings of food services fell within the excellent category.

Mullen considers the percentage of responses in the excellent category to reflect the loyalty of a facility's customers. Customers who ranked food service as less than excellent may or may not return to the facility for care in the future. In a highly competitive environment, developing market loyalty is extremely important to the survival of a facility.

Historically, institutional food does not get rave reviews. Upon review of the literature for institutional nutrition services, the investigators found the research noted that assessment of food quality is highly subjective. Everyone has his or her own idea about what is high quality. The fact that the respondents are hospitalized further complicates the assessment because illnesses and medications often significantly affect taste sensation. Food services have traditionally received the lowest ratings across the healthcare industry. Yet, despite this historical precedent, administration and management of the food services department decided to see if they could improve ratings in this area.

Using PI methodology, the PI team developed an entirely new approach to menu selection for inpatients. The team focused on lunch and dinner, leaving breakfast as it was, providing the usual standard breakfast items. The directors had read about a few hospitals that use a method similar to hotel room service. They contacted a hospital in Washington

State that had implemented a similar program and invited the staff to give a presentation about the pros and cons of the program. Following the presentation, the team did additional research to locate other facilities that used the system, and identified the system's successes and challenges. It became apparent that every facility needed its own process for designing this service. The service features needed to be based on the specific organization's patient population, staffing, equipment, and financial resources. The pilot hospital assembled a multidisciplinary team to identify possible issues that could arise with such a change. The food services team needed the support of the administration, staff, ancillary staff, and especially nursing.

The program was implemented as planned. Patients on regular diets had a 3½-hour window during which they could order from a menu similar to a hotel room-service menu. Patients on therapeutic diets were visited by the dietitian, who helped them develop appropriate diets for their medical conditions.

Over the following months, Mullen and the administration saw the ratio of very satisfied ratings increase from the 10 to 30 percent range to more than 50 percent. The ratio of ratings in the satisfied and very satisfied responses rose to more than 80 percent. Annual projected costs in food services decreased $30,000 thanks to a decrease in the amount of wasted food. Patients could now eat what they wanted, when they wanted it, and they were more likely to eat all of it.

Long term, the system has worked extremely well. Food services staff members who were initially skeptical would not go back to the old way of doing things. Patient satisfaction scores have remained high. There is less food waste, and the nursing staff keeps all liquid diet products on the units so that patients have access to them whenever they want them. Nursing staff also knows when patients are moving from a liquid diet to a solid diet, and they can help their patients order appropriate food.

The food services department at the hospital has become a revenue-generating unit because the room-service menu has been expanded to serve visitors. Families are thrilled to be able to have meals with the patients, and they are willing to pay for the meals. This service has recently been expanded to the hospital staff. The hospital cafeteria is closed on weekends, and the staff can call for room service at any time. They love it, and the program has improved employee satisfaction as well.

A copy of a patient satisfaction survey is provided in figure 6.5.

Internal and External Customers of a Pathology Laboratory

Dr. Lagios has been chief pathologist at Western States University Hospital for two months. He moved to the university setting from a large, tertiary care, private hospital in a metropolitan community because he wanted to expand the scope of his responsibilities. As many managers do when they come into new positions, he began an inventory of the pathology laboratory's functioning and examined each of its processes.

In general, the lab appeared to be functioning well, particularly in the area of processing surgical specimens. But in the area of autopsy report dictation, he found a huge backlog of reports that had not been dictated and finalized. The backlog of 40 reports extended back more than two years. When he asked his secretary for an explanation of the backlog, she reacted with amazement and said she was totally unaware of the situation. No one had been monitoring the status of the autopsy reports on a continuing basis.

Figure 6.5. Example of a patient satisfaction survey

Patient Satisfaction Survey

Instructions:
 Use a pencil or black pen to fill in your answers to the questions on the survey.
 Mark your answers in the circles provided.
 Answer only the questions that apply to your stay in the hospital.

Please choose one of the responses provided for the following questions.

1. Was this the first time you came to this hospital for inpatient care?
 ○ Yes ○ No

2. Would you recommend this hospital to a friend or family member who needed inpatient care?
 ○ Yes ○ No

3. Where were you admitted into the hospital?
 ○ Registration Area ○ Emergency Department ○ Other

4. How long did you wait before you were taken to your room?
 ○ Less than 20 minutes ○ 21 to 30 minutes ○ 31 to 60 minutes ○ More than 1 hour

5. Did you have surgery while you were hospitalized?
 ○ Yes ○ No

6. Were you in an intensive care unit at any time during your stay?
 ○ Yes ○ No

Fill in the circle to the right of each statement that best describes how satisfied you were with the care and services you received while you were in the hospital.

Registration Process	Very Dissatisfied	Somewhat Dissatisfied	Neutral	Somewhat Satisfied	Very Satisfied
7. Courtesy and friendliness of the registration staff	○	○	○	○	○
8. How well the registration staff answered your questions	○	○	○	○	○
9. Amount of time needed to complete the registration process	○	○	○	○	○
10. Overall satisfaction with registration procedures	○	○	○	○	○

Nursing Staff

11. Caring and concern of the nurses who cared for you	○	○	○	○	○
12. Skill of the nurses who cared for you	○	○	○	○	○
13. Time it took for nurses to respond to your calls	○	○	○	○	○
14. Willingness of your nurses to listen to your concerns	○	○	○	○	○
15. Amount of time your nurses spent with you	○	○	○	○	○
16. Overall satisfaction with nursing staff	○	○	○	○	○

PLEASE COMPLETE THE SURVEY ON THE REVERSE SIDE OF THIS PAGE.

(Continued on next page)

Figure 6.5. *(Continued)*

Medical Staff	Very Dissatisfied	Somewhat Dissatisfied	Neutral	Somewhat Satisfied	Very Satisfied
17. Caring and concern of the doctors who cared for you	○	○	○	○	○
18. Availability of your doctors	○	○	○	○	○
19. Ways your doctors worked together and with your nurses	○	○	○	○	○
20. Information your doctors provided about your condition	○	○	○	○	○
21. Amount of time your doctors spent with you	○	○	○	○	○
22. Overall satisfaction with medical staff	○	○	○	○	○
Housekeeping Services					
23. Cleanliness of your room	○	○	○	○	○
24. Overall cleanliness of the hospital	○	○	○	○	○
25. Overall satisfaction with housekeeping services	○	○	○	○	○
Food Services					
26. Taste of the food	○	○	○	○	○
27. Temperature of the food	○	○	○	○	○
28. Appearance of the food	○	○	○	○	○
29. Variety of menu items	○	○	○	○	○
30. Overall satisfaction with food services	○	○	○	○	○
Other Hospital Services					
31. Overall satisfaction with x-ray services	○	○	○	○	○
32. Overall satisfaction with respiratory therapy services	○	○	○	○	○
33. Overall satisfaction with rehabilitation services	○	○	○	○	○
34. Overall satisfaction with emergency department services	○	○	○	○	○
35. **Overall satisfaction with the care and services you received**	○	○	○	○	○

36. What did we do really well? (Please be specific.) _____

_____

_____

37. What do we need to improve? (Please be specific.) _____

_____

_____

REMEMBER: ALL OF YOUR RESPONSES ARE CONFIDENTIAL.
THANK YOU FOR PARTICIPATING.

Dr. Lagios began his investigation by interviewing his fellow pathologists. Each of them told a similar story: An autopsy was usually performed the day after the death of a patient, and the remains were picked up by a mortician. Organ specimens were harvested during the procedure, and microscopic slides were processed in the days immediately following. During the autopsy procedure, the pathologist would dictate notes about the findings to the *diener* (the nonphysician assistant who managed the remains and specimens). The diener would write the notes on a photocopied form that outlined the order in which the autopsy was performed. But then the report never got dictated because the pathologist had so many surgical specimens to process that he or she never made time to finalize the autopsy report. When a physician needed the autopsy findings to fill out a death certificate, he or she had to call the assigned pathologist, who would verbally report the results.

There was definite room for improvement in this process. Dr. Lagios decided to convene a PI team to examine the situation and come up with a better process for dictating and finalizing autopsies. He asked two of his fellow pathologists who had been on staff longer than he, as well as the diener, to serve on the team. In addition, he requested the participation of the director of health information services, who managed pathology and autopsy report transcription processing, and two internal medicine physicians whose deceased patients had been autopsied most frequently in the past two years.

Using the interview technique of information gathering at the first meeting (see the discussion of interview design later in this chapter), the two internists talked the most. There was clearly a fair amount of suppressed frustration about the current situation. If the two internists on the team were unhappy, then other physicians were probably unhappy, too. The internists had morticians contacting them to get the cause of death to put on the death certificates, and tracking down the pathologists to get the autopsy findings considerably delayed the death certificate process.

Mrs. Castle, director of health information services, reported that it was becoming difficult to tell which autopsies had been done and which had not, because there were so many of them. She was very willing to try to find a solution, if the pathologists were willing to accept some changes in the procedures. She thought that because this was an information management problem, an information management solution might be available.

The group decided to reconvene to determine whether new procedures could be developed. Mrs. Castle volunteered to contact the local dictation equipment vendor representative to see whether he had any suggestions. The representative introduced her to the concept of simultaneous dictation—dictating the details of a procedure during the procedure itself. The representative proposed installing a planetary microphone, which is designed to record circumferentially around the entire room. With a planetary microphone installed above the autopsy table where the gross dissections are performed, the pathologists, unhampered by cords or handheld recording devices, could move around the table as necessary during the procedure. Foot pedals under the table would allow the pathologists to turn the recording device on and off as they proceeded through the autopsy. The representative also proposed a similar setup for the pathologists' offices. Microphones would be mounted to the desktops in positions that would capture dictation while the pathologists looked at the prepared slides on the microscopes. Foot pedals under the desks would allow the pathologists to turn the recording devices on and off during their reviews. This would keep the pathologists from having to take notes regarding findings on the slides and dictate using the traditional handheld microphones attached to the dictation machines.

At the next meeting of the PI team, Mrs. Castle reviewed her findings with the team members. All of the pathologists were delighted with the proposal from the dictation equipment vendor representative. They immediately saw that simultaneous dictation would streamline their report production operations. They also recognized that the benefits would extend to their dictation of the surgical specimen reports as well, which was accomplished completely at the desk microscopes. The cost of installing the equipment was not exorbitant, so the team decided to move forward with the proposed solution.

With the time freed up by using simultaneous dictation systems and the commitment of the pathologists, the backlog of autopsy dictations was cleared in a few weeks. The pathologists were all happy with the new processes, and the attending physicians now routinely get their autopsy preliminary diagnoses in time to prepare death certificates.

QI Toolbox Techniques

Surveys and interviews are two data collection techniques commonly used to measure customer satisfaction. As mentioned earlier in this chapter, direct observation of behavior can be used as well, but behavior is difficult to analyze, because it often changes when people realize that they are being observed. However, all three methods can be used to measure outcomes and processes. A discussion of some design considerations for surveys and interviews follows.

Survey Design

When designing a survey, the PI team must define the goal of the survey in clear and precise terms, keeping the purpose and audience of the survey in mind. The team must carefully consider the questions asked on the survey and must have a reason to include every item on the survey. It should avoid asking for information that is interesting but not necessary for measuring process capabilities.

Survey items should be arranged from the general to the specific. For example, demographic data should be followed by process-specific questions. It is helpful to identify the broad categories of necessary information and then determine their order. The first question should not attempt to elicit emotionally charged or sensitive information. For example, if physicians are surveyed about the quality of the transcription system, the first question should not ask whether they are happy with the transcription system. The initial questions should ask how much they use the system, what types of reports they generate, and so on. The next set of questions can be used to determine their level of satisfaction with the system.

After the team has determined the broad categories of information it needs, it should think about individual questions or items. The single most important factor in item construction is clarity (Jagger 1982). Item format and content should be consistent. Similar questions should be formatted in the same way using the simplest sentence structure possible. (See figure 6.6.)

The survey should be written at the reading level of the respondents. The average reader in the United States reads at the sixth-grade level, so vocabulary should be simple, rather than sophisticated medical or technical terminology that the average person would not understand. Furthermore, the items should be written in an objective manner so that they do not imply that any particular response is either desired or correct. (See figure 6.7.)

Surveys may incorporate a variety of question types. Open-ended questions allow respondents to construct a free-text answer in their own words. Responses to open-ended questions, however, are difficult to score, and response data are difficult to aggregate because there is no defined scale of responses. So responses may show no clear connection or pattern.

Open-ended questions should be used only at the end of the survey, and they should not be used to elicit information that could be more easily collected in a structured format. (See figure 6.8.) When the researcher wants specific information about a particular

Figure 6.6. Example of inconsistent format and consistent format

Inconsistent Format	Consistent Format
What is your ZIP code? _____	Check which ZIP code you live in: ___ 84065 ___ 84070 ___ 84092 ___ 84094 ___ Other (specify): _____
Sex (circle one): Male Female	What is your sex? ___ Male ___ Female

Figure 6.7. Example of poor wording and appropriate wording of survey items

Poor Wording	Simple Wording
Why were you admitted to the hospital? To deliver a child ___ To have a C-section ___ To have a surgical procedure___ For medical reasons ___ Other (specify): _____	Why were you in the hospital? ___ To have my baby ___ To have an operation ___ To obtain medical treatment ___ Other (specify): _____

Figure 6.8. Example of an open-ended question and a more structured question

Open-Ended Question	More Structured Question
How has your coronary artery disease affected your lifestyle?	Now that you have heart disease, are you exercising: ___ More than before ___ Same as before ___ Less than before ___ Not at all, before or now

area of investigation, the items must be worded precisely so that comparable data can be collected.

The use of structured questions on a survey limits the number of possible responses and thus standardizes the data collected. Care should be taken to include all possible responses to each question. Respondents must be able to select their answers from the choices provided. One method of ensuring this is to include a choice of "Other (specify)" so that respondents can write in an answer when the desired answer is not among the choices offered. Even then, it is important to provide as many of the common answers as possible to minimize the number of write-in responses. When items include categories of responses, the categories must be mutually exclusive; that is, categories should not overlap. (See figure 6.9.)

Another important issue in survey design involves the use of terms, phrases, and words that are known to both the PI team and the respondent. Careful word choice reduces ambiguity. This clarity of terminology is called an *operational definition* (Jagger 1982). (See figure 6.10.)

A survey may be personally administered or mailed to the respondents. Either method is effective, but the response rate decreases and turnaround time is greater when the survey is mailed.

Figure 6.9.   Example of poor question construction and good question construction

Poor Question Construction	Good Question Construction
What is your present age?	What is your present age?
0–17 ___	___ 20 or younger
17–35 ___	___ 21–30
35–45 ___	___ 31–40
45–60 ___	___ 41–50
60–75 ___	___ 51–60
	___ 61–70
	___ 71 or older

Figure 6.10.   Example of unclear and clear terminology

Unclear Terminology	Clear Terminology
Have you received treatment in the ambulatory surgery unit?	Have you had surgery at this hospital for which you came to the hospital in the morning and left after surgery in the afternoon or evening?
Yes ___	___ Yes
No ___	___ No
Don't know ___	

Interview Design

Whether an interview is conducted face-to-face or over the telephone, it can provide important insight into quality issues in healthcare. Interviews may be unstructured or structured. In an unstructured interview, the sequence of questions is not planned in advance. Instead, the interview is conducted in a friendly, conversational manner. This type of interview is helpful when the interviewer is trying to uncover preliminary problems that may need in-depth analysis and investigation.

By contrast, a predetermined list of questions is used in a structured interview. The team knows exactly what information is needed, and the interviewer must know and understand the purpose and goal of each question so that a meaningful response can be recognized.

During the interview process, the interviewer must establish rapport with the respondent. Without this trust, the respondent may not reveal his or her true opinions. Some techniques to keep in mind during the interview process include funneling, using unbiased questions, and clarifying responses. *Funneling* is the process of moving questions from a broad theme to a narrow theme in an unstructured interview. This technique helps the interviewer establish trust with the respondent and address the pertinent quality issues. For example, if a supervisor in health materials management wanted to discuss service to the emergency department with the nursing coordinator from that unit, he or she might use the following series of questions, which get more specific as the interview proceeds:

Question: Overall, how do you rate our service to the department?

Response: Overall, I think your department is doing a better-than-average job.

Question: A better-than-average job? Where have you experienced problems?

Response: There have been problems at times getting cath packs when we need them.

Question: Cath packs. Any particular shift?

Response: Definitely in the late afternoons of the day shift.

The interviewer must state each question in a clear and somewhat benign manner so that bias is not introduced. If a specific word or phrase were overemphasized, it might elicit a different response than if all the words were spoken in the same tone. The interviewer should restate each response for clarification. This ensures the correct interpretation of each response.

Sometimes the interviewer may choose to use closed-ended questions, with all of the possible responses specified. In such cases, the interviewer must examine each question carefully to ensure that the wording and delivery do not bias the response. Questions should begin with broader issues and work toward more specific areas of concern.

Case Study

As previously discussed, one common method of measuring customer satisfaction in healthcare involves conducting a survey. Figure 6.11 shows a survey that was used in a healthcare organization. Students should critique this survey against the criteria listed in

Figure 6.11.   Sample survey instrument for the case study

SSS Questionnaire

Date of Short-Stay Surgery _____
    Type of Procedure _____

Your general impression of the hospital:
___ Excellent   ___ Good   ___ Average   ___ Poor

When you spoke with the staff prior to surgery, were they courteous?   ___Yes   ___ No

Did they answer your questions about SSS satisfactorily?
___Yes   ___ No   Comments: _____
_____

Were your accommodations in the SSS room:
a.   Clean   Yes ___   No ___
b.   Comfortable   Yes ___   No ___

Treatment by other hospital personnel:

Recovery	exc	good	needs improvement	poor
Concern	☐	☐	☐	☐
Efficiency	☐	☐	☐	☐
Courtesy	☐	☐	☐	☐
Adequate Explanation	☐	☐	☐	☐

Surgery

	exc	good	needs improvement	poor
Concern	☐	☐	☐	☐
Efficiency	☐	☐	☐	☐
Courtesy	☐	☐	☐	☐
Adequate Explanation	☐	☐	☐	☐

X-ray

	exc	good	needs improvement	poor
Concern	☐	☐	☐	☐
Efficiency	☐	☐	☐	☐
Courtesy	☐	☐	☐	☐
Adequate Explanation	☐	☐	☐	☐

When you were discharged, did you receive adequate information and instructions?   __Yes   ___ No

If your surgery was delayed, was an explanation given?
___Yes   ___ No

What determined your selection of Community Hospital of the West as a hospital?
☐ Physician   ☐ Convenience   ☐ Insurance
☐ Friend   ☐ Previous experience
☐ Other:_____

How did you choose the physician who provided your care? _____

Given a choice of hospitals, would you return to Community Hospital of the West?
___Yes   ___ No

In your opinion, how could we improve or add to our services?
_____
_____
_____
_____
_____
_____
_____
_____
_____
_____
_____
_____
_____
_____

We appreciate your confidential opinion of our services. It provides us with the valuable feedback we need in order to continually improve our patient care.

the preceding discussion of survey design, giving careful consideration to factors such as format, wording, and appearance.

Project Application

In the project application for chapter 2, students identified a process needing improvement. They should now identify the expectations of internal and external customers regarding the process being examined. Then, the students should design a survey, an interview, or a combination of the two to collect data on the process. Students should either collect a minimum of 30 responses for a survey or conduct five interviews. Student surveys and interviews should be critiqued by the instructor before they are administered. A subject consent clause must appear in the introductions to the surveys.

Summary

In healthcare PI, decisions about process or product improvements must be based on meaningful customer satisfaction data. Customers may be either internal or external to the organization. Many aspects of quality must be considered for each process. Effective ways to collect customers' opinions include surveys and interviews. These tools must be constructed carefully to collect relevant and unbiased data.

References

Agency for Healthcare Research and Quality (AHRQ). 2008. CAHPS® Hospital Survey (HCAHPS). https://www.cahps.ahrq.gov/.

Atlantic Information Services. 1995. *A Guide to Patient Satisfaction Survey Instruments*, 2nd ed. Washington, DC: Atlantic Information Services.

Hospital Consumer Assessment of Healthcare Providers and Systems. 2011. HCAHPS Survey. http://www.hcahpsonline.org/Files/HCAHPS%20V6%200%20Appendix%20A%20-%20HCAHPS%20Mail%20Survey%20Materials%20(English)%202-16-2011.pdf.

Jagger, J. 1982. Data collection instruments: Side-stepping the pitfalls. *Nurse Educator* (5–6):25–28.

Resources

Bowling, A. 2009. *Research Methods in Health*, 3rd ed. Philadelphia: Open University Press.

Department of Health and Human Services. 2011. Hospital compare. http://www.hospitalcompare.hhs.gov.

Sekaran, U. 2009. *Research Methods for Business*, 5th ed. New York: John Wiley & Sons.

Shelton, P.J. 2000. *Measuring and Improving Patient Satisfaction*. Baltimore: Aspen Publishers.

Vavra, T.G. 1997. *Improving Your Measurement of Customer Satisfaction*. Milwaukee, WI: ASQ Quality Press.

Chapter 7
Refining the Continuum of Care

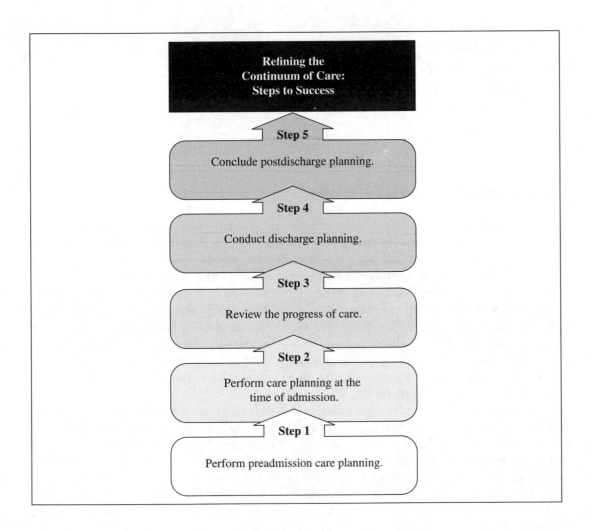

Refining the
Continuum of Care:
Steps to Success

Step 5
Conclude postdischarge planning.

Step 4
Conduct discharge planning.

Step 3
Review the progress of care.

Step 2
Perform care planning at the
time of admission.

Step 1
Perform preadmission care planning.

Learning Objectives

- To explain that processes were developed to optimize the continuum of care
- To discuss the method used to develop a continuum of care in a community health-care setting
- To identify and discuss the steps in the case management function
- To describe how criteria sets and core measures contribute to the management of care in the US healthcare system

Key Terms

Case management
Community needs assessment
Continuum of care
Critical Pathway
Gantt chart
Indicator

Background and Significance

Today, American consumers are demanding more extensive and complete healthcare services in the hope of improving the quality and longevity of their lives. Third-party payers, both private and governmental, are trying to maximize profits, minimize costs, and address healthcare fraud. Public and private purchasers, such as businesses buying health insurance for their employees, are looking for comprehensive coverage at affordable premium rates. Many physicians are struggling to pay for insurance premiums for their businesses because liability issues and legal awards have driven the cost of malpractice insurance to new heights. The lack of direct accountability for peer-to-peer medical practice was in large part responsible for the increasing liability suits and rising insurance costs. Medical groups were slow to develop means for handling malpractice within their own medical field and lawsuits against their members.

The mission of healthcare organizations is to make a positive contribution to the health of their communities by providing safe, cost-effective, and ethical treatment. The increasing nature of litigation in healthcare, coupled with the increased cost of malpractice insurance for providers, places an additional financial burden on healthcare organizations and physicians. In the United States, these conflicting objectives and values have led to a variety of attempts to control the healthcare market, none of which has been entirely successful. The goal of this chapter is not to review the history, successes, and failures of the US healthcare system but to provide a basic understanding of the system's history, successes, and failures that will allow you to understand the issues surrounding the concept of the continuum of care. **Continuum of care** can be defined as the totality of healthcare services provided to a patient and his or her family in all settings, from the least extensive to the most extensive.

The emphasis is on treating individual patients at the level of care required by their course of treatment. Figure 7.1 shows various types of treatment settings available along the continuum of care.

Healthcare in the United States

In discussions of healthcare in the United States, there are many common viewpoints, including public and private regulation, healthcare economics, and the human desire to benefit personally and collectively.

Throughout the past century, attempts have been made to balance the competing needs and expectations of consumers, providers, and payers. At different times, each group has dominated the marketplace, though none has been on top for long. The products of this competition have included the voluntary hospital system, the finest healthcare technological infrastructure in the world, private health insurance plans, the broadest range of the most effective pharmaceuticals available, Medicare, Medicaid, preferred provider arrangements, and health maintenance organizations, to name a few. The culmination has come in the most recent experimental solution: managed care. Students of healthcare quality and performance improvement (PI) should review the economic and policy issues inherent in US approaches to delivering healthcare.

The overall goal of the US healthcare system is to achieve equilibrium between health and spending, as illustrated in figure 7.2. As the figure shows, a finite level of optimal collective health can be realized in US society. Although many factors influence collective health, the system today seeks to identify the optimal level of spending that will achieve the optimal level of collective health. Expenditures are funded by a combination of public and private resources: public health, Medicare, Medicaid, insurance, private payers, public sanitation, and others. But there comes a point where more spending does not mean more collective health.

Figure 7.1.   The continuum of care

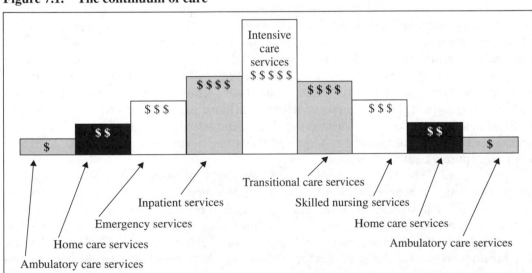

Figure 7.2. Optimal spending for optimal health

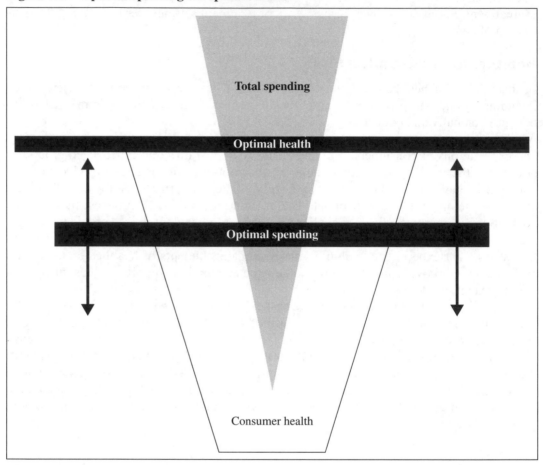

In figure 7.2, the shaded triangle that represents total spending extends above the black line that represents optimal health. This representation acknowledges the realization that all of the healthcare spending a society could possibly do would not necessarily achieve the goal of optimal collective health. At some point for every patient within the healthcare system, no additional health benefit would be achieved by further spending. Any additional expenditure would, in effect, be wasted. The money could have been used for another patient who might still have benefited. Because millions of Americans never approach the optimal health condition, that waste is considered intolerable. The continuum of care system seeks to provide benefits up to the point of optimal health for each individual, thereby realizing optimal health collectively.

For example, Mr. Abraham Smith is a 90-year-old Caucasian male who has, in recent years, developed a heart condition known as chronic ventricular fibrillation. The condition is manageable with medication, but patients often continue to experience occasional periods of the arrhythmia (irregular heart rhythm) even when taking their medication as prescribed. Mr. Smith experiences such arrhythmias. Each time the fibrillation begins, Mr. Smith feels weak and unwell, his face flushes, and he can feel his heart fluttering in his chest. He is afraid that he is going to die. Immediately, he calls to his wife to take him to the emergency department of his local hospital. By the time the couple drives to the hospital and Mr. Smith is checked by a physician, the fibrillation has subsided, and his heart has returned to a normal sinus rhythm. The emergency department physician on duty examines him, performs an EKG, and draws blood studies, all of which are negative. Each time, the symptoms could be those of a heart attack, but they are not.

Mr. Smith does not want to accept the fact that his heart condition cannot be managed any better than it currently is managed. His demand for services at the emergency department accomplishes nothing, but no one is prepared to tell him not to go when he experiences arrhythmias, especially in light of the litigious nature of US society. Yet emergency visits are among the most expensive types of ambulatory care. Every time Mr. Smith visits the emergency department, he wastes services that could have been used by someone for whom the emergency visit would have been more helpful. Mr. Smith's use of healthcare services is not optimal, either for him or for society.

Regulatory approaches seek to control expenditures on individuals such as Mr. Smith in the hope that more resources will be available for those who can still benefit. Medicare regulations mandated utilization review in the mid-1960s. The system required physician committees to review the practice patterns of their colleagues at institutions receiving Medicare dollars. The difference between those who could afford good healthcare coverage and those who could not was very wide. As a result, directives were issued to the effect that organizations receiving federal Medicaid and Medicare monies must provide the same care to all patients without differentiation as to their ability to pay.

In the 1970s, Medicaid programs in most states trained their own reviewers to visit hospitals and make sure that Medicaid patients met set criteria for hospitalization and were staying in the hospital only as long as absolutely necessary. In the mid-1980s, the prospective payment system was implemented for Medicare and Medicaid patients. Under this system, standardized payments are made to hospitals according to the diagnosis-related group (DRG) into which a patient falls. In the 1990s, the private and public sectors wrestled with the sometimes unfortunate decisions of managed care officials. All of these efforts have attempted to accomplish a balance between health benefits and health spending.

The issue remains important in the administration of healthcare organizations today. Services are to be accorded to, and expenditures made for, individuals who can still benefit. Organizations must be able to demonstrate that rational decisions were made about a patient's care and that those decisions were in the patient's and society's collective best interests. Healthcare organizations must be able to demonstrate as well that the services provided to the patient were safe and appropriate to the patient's physical and quality-of-life needs across the continuum of care. The continuum of care consists of all the possible settings in which patients may receive care. (See figure 7.1.) Today, care is delivered in patients' homes, physicians' offices, ambulatory care centers, hospitals, long-term care facilities, and residential care facilities. Each of these care settings provides a more or less complex set of services, all of which depend on the identified needs of the patient during the initial assessment when presenting for services. In addition, each patient's needs may change, depending on the time that the needs are identified: prior to hospital admission, during the admitting process, during the hospital stay, during the discharge process, and during any immediate subsequent care episode. The expectation of the public and private regulatory agencies is that patients' needs will be identified, prioritized, and provided for in the setting most appropriate to their requirements for care.

Understanding that the patient-centered approach to care (table 7.1) has evolved from a very unilateral, authoritarian system of care (figure 7.3) is an important starting point. In the past, medicine was practiced as an art, with most information for treatments based on the individual practitioner's skill and knowledge. Most patients expected their physicians

Table 7.1. Patient-centered approach to care

	Admissions office	MD	RN	LCSW	Treatment team	Discharge planner/ UR	Educator
Prescreen	X	X				X	
Admission	X	X	X			X	
Assessment		X	X	X			
Care/ Treatment		X	X	X	X	X	X
Patient teaching			X	X			X
Discharge		X	X	X	X	X	X
Follow-up		X					

Figure 7.3. Authoritarian approach to care

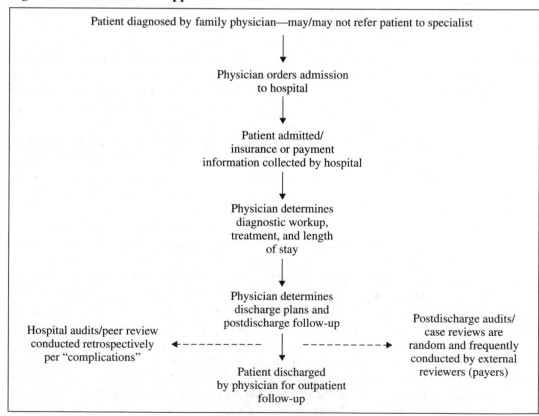

to tell them what to do regarding their own health. A physician was seen either as a separate, individual provider who treated only one aspect of a patient's illness or as the family practitioner who treated everything. For example, a surgeon practiced only surgery, and if the patient had other health issues, he or she was referred to another physician for care of those issues. Physicians ordered the tests they felt were necessary for treatment, and patients did not question physicians' diagnoses or whether a test was required. There was little review of whether tests and care were necessary and little supervision or assessment of how one physician initiated and treated a patient compared with how another physician might have treated the same patient for the same illness. Best-practice standards were not a common approach to care. Sometimes patient care and hospitalization were provided on the basis of the patient's ability to pay. Some physicians and clinics provided free care for indigent patients, but this was at their own discretion.

Each individual physician maintained medical files on each patient, and physicians had to make formal requests to get patient information from another treating physician. Transfer of information was not always reliable and was often a cumbersome and lengthy process that required a written request to be mailed and the requested information then returned by mail. The concept of a seamless patient health record entered the picture as the pace of healthcare and the complexities in providing total care necessitated better communication among treating physicians and entities.

As treatments and technologies developed, the costs of research and knowledge-based care began to rise. As the cost of treatment rose, insurance companies began to experience higher payouts for treatments and interventions that were sometimes duplicated and not always best for the patient. For example, at one point, it was routine practice for OB/GYN physicians to remove both the ovaries and the uterus during a hysterectomy to prevent future problems. It was later discovered that women seemed to fare better hormonally when healthy ovaries were allowed to remain after surgery. Research demonstrated the importance of maintaining ovaries in young women who were not menopausal as a protection against early onset of menopause. Insurance companies then stepped in to state that they would no longer reimburse physicians for the additional surgery unless there was clear indication of a need to remove the ovaries.

The increased awareness of duplication of services increased the drive to determine the medical necessity for treatments and care. Purchasers and payers of healthcare services began to demand a more comprehensive approach to care—one that decreased costs and improved the quality of care provided. Along with this demand came standards intended to ensure that the services provided were timely, cost-efficient, and appropriate to the patient's medical condition. As patients were stuck with medical bills that insurance companies refused to pay and providers were unwilling to write off because they were not deemed medically necessary, new processes were developed to address these concerns. Insurance companies and healthcare organizations developed a role for case managers who worked with physicians and hospital employees to ensure that the care ordered was appropriate to the diagnosis and that it was a payable covered item under the patient's insurance policy. Thus, the continuum of care model was developed to meet the needs of patients, providers, and payers. A review system was put into place to address medical necessity issues and fraudulent billing practices that began to occur as a result of the treatment restrictions placed on providers. Still, millions of dollars are lost in Medicaid and Medicare fraud each year because billing practices and systems are not carefully audited.

One product of these changes was the establishment of health maintenance organizations (HMOs). These organizations provide their members with many levels of care at reduced costs through an extensive network of healthcare providers contracted by the HMO. Members of HMO plans are rewarded with lower premiums for utilizing only those services provided by the HMO's group of physicians, hospitals, and pharmacies. These organizations strive to keep all patient care within their own continuum of services. Since the HMO functions as both insurer and provider, it can offer many different services at substantial savings because of the ability to contract for them to meet the needs of its substantial number of members.

One of the performance tools utilized to help HMOs address their specific members' needs is a **community needs assessment.** A team composed of community members, HMO members, and community leaders compiles this assessment. A needs assessment allows researchers to become acquainted with a community, identify the community's characteristics as a healthcare client, and assess that set of clients by collecting and analyzing information about community needs. The assessment also identifies the target members of the interventions and their interest in change. Data from these assessments provide HMO decision makers with significant information regarding the community's health-related needs and possible solutions to those needs. Such data also expand the existing body of knowledge relating to behavior changes that promote healthier lifestyles and have the potential to promote wellness in at-risk populations. The needs assessments may also address important subsystem issues such as the physical environment, education, transportation, healthcare and social services, and mechanisms available in the community for coping with and solving problems. For example, if an HMO contracted with a community to provide care, and a majority of clients were of childbearing age, the HMO may complete a needs assessment for that population and, based on the information identified from the assessment, add new or expanded components of obstetric and pediatric care to its contracts.

Refining the Continuum of Care: Steps to Success

The principal process by which organizations optimize the continuum of care for their patients is **case management.** Case managers review the condition of patients to identify each patient's care needs and to integrate patient data with the patient's course of treatment. The case manager in many organizations matches the patient's course with a predetermined optimal course (also known as an integrated care map, **critical pathway**, or practice guideline) for the patient's condition. This map or pathway is a multidisciplinary outline of anticipated care within an appropriate time frame to aid a patient in moving progressively through a clinical experience that ends in a positive outcome. The case manager identifies, in conjunction with the treatment team, the actions to be taken when the patient's care is not proceeding optimally. The same concept, under the name *managed care*, is used by many payers to clearly define when a patient may have a procedure or to stipulate a particular course of treatment that the payer believes will be equally effective but less costly.

Step 1: Perform Preadmission Care Planning

Preadmission care planning is initiated when the patient's physician contacts a healthcare organization to schedule an episode of care service. The case manager reviews the patient's projected needs with the physician. Admission criteria are established on the basis of a suggested diagnosis. The manager also may contact the patient directly to obtain further information.

In addition, the manager may contact the patient's payer to confirm that all necessary preadmission authorizations have been obtained, that admission criteria have been met, and that the payer will pay for the patient's services. This process is called *preauthorization*. As part of preauthorization, the payer's representative will have compared the planned services with the payer's criteria of care for the patient's diagnosis. Some payers will pay 80 to 100 percent for care provided in their preferred provider list of agencies. If a patient opts to go to an "out-of-contract" facility or provider, he or she may have to pay a higher reimbursement rate for services. Some insurance plans allow the patient to choose the treating facility and physician, but these plans usually have a lower reimbursement rate.

Step 2: Perform Care Planning at the Time of Admission

When the patient is admitted to the hospital, the case manager will review all of the information gathered by the clinicians assigned to the case to confirm that the patient meets the admission criteria for an admitting diagnosis. The manager will confirm that the patient requires services that can be performed at the facility. If it is determined that the facility cannot perform the services needed, the case manager will arrange for the patient to be transferred to another facility.

If the facility utilizes care-mapping methodology, at this time the case manager will assign the case to the appropriate critical pathway (see figure 7.4) and verify that all of the services stipulated in the critical pathway have been initiated.

Step 3: Review the Progress of Care

The case manager periodically reviews the patient's progress throughout the entire episode of care. When a critical pathway is being used, the manager will reintegrate care data each time the case is reviewed and compare the patient's progress with the pathway. When variations from expected progress occur, the case manager coordinates interventions among the clinicians and therapists assigned to the case to move the patient along the path.

From the beginning of the episode of care, the case manager continuously monitors the patient's acuity level and requirements for services. At the same time, he or she plans—in conjunction with the patient, the patient's family, and the clinical team—for the services the patient will need after discharge. The manager will arrange for the patient to be transferred to another facility or nursing unit to meet the patient's care needs. Ultimately, the goal is to maintain the patient in the least costly level of care possible based on his or her assessed needs.

Step 4: Conduct Discharge Planning

As the patient's requirements for care decrease and the patient moves toward discharge, the case manager undertakes final discharge planning. In this step, the patient's continued

Figure 7.4.   Sample Gantt chart format in an excerpt of a critical pathway

Western University Regional Medical Center **Department of Nursing** **Case Management Plan**	

Diagnosis: Idiopathic pediatric scoliosis, with surgery, without complications   **Unit:** 9 East   **DRG:** 215

Average Length of Stay: 7 days   **Usual OR Day (admission day = 1):** 2

Clinical Milestones:

	Prior to Admission	Day 1	Day 2	Day 3	Day 4	Day 5	Day 6	Day 7	Day 8	Day 9	Day 10	Day 11	Day 12
Self-donation of blood	X												
Chest x-ray, chem panel	X												
Labs, EKG, blood type & crossmatch	X												
PM admission		X											
H&P		X											
Care planning		X											
Surgery			X										
Surgical ICU			X										
Catheter removed				X									
Patient sits up in bed					X								
Transfer to surgical floor					X								
Physical therapy					X	X	X						
Patient walks down corridor					X								
Patient education for self-care							X						
Patient receives meds and instructions for follow-up care								X					
Outpatient physical therapy scheduled						X							
Patient discharged to home								X					

Health Outcomes:

Diagnosis	Outcome (The patient . . .)	Day–Visit	Intermediate Goal (The patient . . .)	Day–Visit	Process (The nurse . . .)	Day–Visit	Process (The physician . . .)
Fluid-electrolyte imbalance: third space shifting secondary to large volume loss and replacement	Has stable vital signs consistent with base-line at admission	5–6 4–14	Is afebrile	4	Takes vital signs every 2 hours	PTA	Arranges for self-donation of blood before surgery
		4–6	Maintains urine output over 1 cc/kg/hr while catheterized	4	Measures and records urine output every hour	1	Assesses patient's cardiac status on admission
	Has a baseline nor-mal voiding pattern	6–8	Voids 8 hours after Foley is discontinued			1	Orders lab workup
		4–14	Maintains specific gravity under .1020	4	Monitors specific gravity		
	Has no edema	8–9	Returns to baseline skin turgor	4–8	Balances IV and oral intake to achieve maintenance fluid requirements		

care after discharge is planned. Many times, family members and significant others are an active part of this process because they will often assist with care after discharge. Postdischarge medications are prescribed and therapies are scheduled. In accordance with the National Patient Safety Goals, copies of the detailed list of current medications are forwarded to the providers in the next step of the continuum. Arrangements to transfer the patient to a subacute facility are made when necessary. Effective discharge planning often begins at the time of admission to ensure that the patient will be prepared to leave the facility as scheduled.

Step 5: Conclude Postdischarge Planning

Once the patient has been discharged, the case manager conveys information about the patient's course of treatment to the clinicians who will continue to care for the patient. At this point, the case management function is returned to the patient's physician and office staff. Some healthcare organizations, however, follow up with patients after discharge to ensure that the transition has gone smoothly and that the patient is receiving all of the services required. Procedures to address the flow of information from one practitioner to another (also known as discharge planning) became a part of the continuum of care when the federal government instituted EMTALA (Emergency Medical Transfer and Active Labor Act) regulations. Efforts were made to ensure that information could be easily shared between practitioners and providers so that continuing care postdischarge could be coordinated effectively. Discharge planning became an integral part of the clinical team's decision making regarding length of stay, services rendered, and provision of benefits. PI monitoring of the utilization of healthcare services began in many facilities when efforts to control costs and ensure quality were initiated. Table 7.2 demonstrates the change in access to care before and after implementation of the healthcare utilization management (UM) function.

Real-Life Example

Information collected in the form of valid and reliable data is the starting point for the management of the continuum of care. Established criteria for care and clinical paths are crucial to the quality of patient care. Such guidelines, coupled with the clinical expertise of the case manager, can make the process of case management more effective.

At one hospital, care guidelines used internal criteria as well as external criteria for the process of utilization review and case management. It also used the feedback information provided by third-party payers. Unfortunately, the organization lacked the ability to share that information.

The quality leadership had noted through data collection that the process of admission, treatment, and discharge planning was not well coordinated among the associated caregivers and the business operations of the organization. Key issues included the following:

- Patients were admitted to the hospital for diagnosis and treatment in cases where the patients could have received appropriate care in a less intensive care setting.

Table 7.2. Examples of hospital standard measures

Measure of process	Type Out/Proc	Measured Y/N	Indication/Formula	Benchmark	How often measured	Owner	Source of data	Results given to
Discrepancies—Pre-op/Post-op/Path	O	Y	# cases with discrepancy / # of pathology cases	0%	Quarterly	OR	OR data sheet	QC, Med Exec & the Board
Complications of post-procedure care	P	Y	# pts w/complications / # patients operated on	0%	Quarterly	OR	OR data sheet	QC, Med Exec & the Board
Preparing and dispensing: Dispensing errors	O	Y	# dispensing errors / # inpatient days	0%	Quarterly	Pharmacy	Pharmacy tracking system	P&T
Monitoring the effects on patients: Adverse drug reactions	O	Y	# ADRs / # of admissions	0%	Quarterly	Pharmacy	Incident report	Med Exec
Administration: Blood hung within 20 minutes of dispensing	P	Y	# units hung within 20 minutes / # units dispensed	100%	Quarterly	Lab	Blood slips	QC & Med Exec
Monitoring effects on patients: Potential transfusion reactions	O	Y	# of true reactions / # transfusion episodes	0%	Quarterly	Lab	Transfusion reaction investigations	QC & Med Exec
Utilization management: Patients admitted to observation who should have been inpatients	P	Y	# pts not admitted as IPs who met inpatient criteria / # pts admitted	0%	Quarterly	UR	Utilization management form	QC & Med Exec
Adverse events during anesthesia	O	Y	# adverse events / # pts given anesthesia	0%	Quarterly	OR	OR data sheet	QC & Med Exec
VBAC rate	O	Y	# VBAC / # repeat C-sections	36%	Quarterly	Labor & Delivery	Obstetric report	QC & Med Exec
Joint replacements with complications	O	Y	# joint replacements with complications / # joint replacements	0%	Quarterly	OR	Patient record & surgical stats	QC & Med Exec
Notice of intent	O	Y	# for current quarter	1%	Quarterly	Risk Mgmt.	Receipt of atty letter or notice	QC & Med Exec
Patient/Family complaints—care	O	Y	# complaints / # patient days	1%	Quarterly	Risk Mgmt.	Complaint system	QC & Med Exec
Medical device reporting (manufacturer)	O	Y	# complaints / # patient days	<0.1%	Quarterly	Risk Mgmt.	Complaint system	QC & Med Exec
Patient satisfaction: Inpatient	O	Y	Percentage reported only	93%	Quarterly	QRS	Gallup results	QC, Med Exec & the Board
Completion of competency testing of employees	O	Y	# employees completing competency testing / # of employees	100%	Annually	Human Resources	Results of tests	QC, Med Exec & the Board
Hospital-acquired infection rate	O	Y	# hospital-acquired infections / # patients	<1%	Quarterly	Infection Control	Culture reports & Pt records	QR, IC Committee
Surgical wound infection rate	O	Y	# post-op infections / # surgeries	0.8%	Monthly/ Quarterly	Infection Control	Culture reports & Pt records	QR, IC Committee
Medical record delinquency: Overall	O	Y	# charts 21 days delinquent / # discharges for month	<50%	Quarterly	HIM	Record report	QC, Med Exec & the Board
Suspensions	O	Y	# suspensions / # physicians	0%	Quarterly	HIM	Record report	QC, Med Exec & the Board

- Hospital stays were continued after symptoms and treatment had reached a point where the patient could have received appropriate care in a less intensive care setting.

- Families were not involved in the decisions regarding discharge placement options or care plans. Home health agencies, skilled nursing care facilities, and hospices were not being contacted early enough in the patient's stay to facilitate postdischarge transition to other levels of care.

- Insurance carriers and Medicare were denying payment because services had not been preauthorized and had been rendered after discharge criteria had been met and documented.

- Health records contained inadequate documentation of medical conditions, interventions, and outcomes.

At first, hospital utilization and quality department personnel organized themselves to better communicate the needs, problems, and obstacles of an effective case management system. It quickly became apparent, however, that they alone could not make the kinds of differences necessary to improve the ailing system.

A PI team was formed. The team included a representative from the admissions and registration department, business office and financial counselors, the admissions nurse, the operating room scheduler, the operating room manager, a representative from outpatient services, representatives from the nursing units, discharge planners, the utilization review/case managers, and the director of the utilization/quality department.

The team implemented Shewhart and Deming's (1986) PI model. The team discovered, however, that it had not included all of the individuals and departments that were closely associated with the process. The team realized that it also needed representatives and participants from physicians' offices. It invited key office personnel to participate on the team.

The newly composed team spent several weeks working on team building. Leading this group of people to form a cohesive team was a difficult task. Accusations and feelings of failure ensued. But eventually, an important breakthrough occurred. After repeated reinforcement of the concept that improving this process would benefit all departments, the team was able to break down departmental barriers, focus on its common mission and goals, and get to work.

Team members found more purpose and pleasure in their work and felt more powerful and less frustrated. The team collected, analyzed, and reported the information to those persons who could directly make a difference. The medical staff was educated regarding the problems and proposed solutions that could help develop an effective case management model. Other office personnel and service departments were included to complete the circle of participants.

The team's achievements included the following:

- Critical information was shared about postdischarge planning (such as treatment plans and care goals) and financial information (including benefits, limits, out-of-pocket expenses, and deductibles).

- Primary care providers were included in the decision-making process and were given information that benefited not only patients and their families but also the physicians' practices and the hospital.

- Coordination of services was improved, and access to specialists and special services was provided in a timely manner, including options for alternative care placement and the wise use of financial resources. Often, with completed care plans, the payers were willing to discontinue the patient's insurance contract and pay for services that would complete the healing process and avoid readmission or duplicate extended care and testing.

- The number and dollar amounts of payment denials decreased. The organization's fiscal situation improved, thus allowing staff to purchase equipment and expand services.

- The quality of health records documentation improved, as did access to records and reports. Some forms and the flow of some medical information were changed.

- Having a proven method of case management served as an asset in subsequent contracting with new providers and payers.

- Departments, personnel within the organization, and provider offices became more unified. The team approach served as a catalyst for change within the organization. Individuals realized that they could make a difference and that they had the ideas and power to make change happen. The PI activity strengthened the employees' commitment to the mission and vision of the organization.

QI Toolbox Techniques

Indicators, or criteria, and Gantt charts are often used in assessments of continuum of care issues.

Indicators

An **indicator,** or criterion, is a performance measure that enables healthcare organizations to monitor a process to determine whether it is meeting requirements. The criteria may be established and implemented internally, externally, or generically.

Internal criteria are usually developed by an interdisciplinary team made up of physicians, nurses, and other clinical staff from the healthcare organization. This type of criterion is developed to monitor specific processes within the organization.

External criteria are created by an organization outside the healthcare facility. Insurance companies, peer review organizations, the Centers for Medicare and Medicaid Services (CMS), and other regulatory agencies develop healthcare criteria.

Generic criteria have been developed by many of the same agencies for use across the continuum of care and in various regions of the country. The term *generic* implies that the criteria are applicable across many organizations and with many different kinds of patients.

One of the most common applications of generic criteria measures is in the area of admission certification. Admission criteria are used to establish that each patient requires care at the level at which he or she has been admitted. Usually, admission criteria in acute care settings have two categories: intensity of service and severity of illness. For a patient to meet the admission criteria, he or she must meet a clinical measure in both categories. *Intensity of service* refers to the type of services or care the patient requires. *Severity of illness* refers to how sick the patient is or what level of care the patient requires, such as intensive care or general medical care. (See the list of admission criteria in the following case study.)

Each indicator, written in the form of a ratio, is used as a tool for monitoring care and service. An indicator for the number of admissions that meet set admission criteria might be the following ratio:

$$\frac{\text{Number of admissions meeting criteria}}{\text{Total number of admissions}}$$

A target or goal set by a healthcare facility might be, "Admission criteria met 99 percent of the time." Meeting such high expectations is very important to healthcare organizations today because care rendered to patients who do not meet admission criteria is generally not reimbursed.

Monitoring these indicators allows the organization's leadership to identify the cases in which a patient did not receive the best care. The indicators also identify excessive numbers of cases in which this was true, thus providing an opportunity for improvement in organizational processes. A set of hospital standard measures (or indicators) utilized by one community hospital is provided in table 7.2. These indicators were used to provide standardized reporting. (See the discussion on standardized reporting in chapter 16.) The formula for each criterion is given, along with the benchmark the organization wants to meet, how often the indicator is measured, which organizational unit is responsible for the measure, where data are pulled from to compute the measure, and where the results are reported.

Recently, the Joint Commission and CMS joined forces in an effort to standardize the core measures that each organization utilizes to make the data collection and assessment process cleaner and more easily interpreted statistically. The hope is to streamline the data that are collected and prevent duplication of data that have no standard measures from one agency to the next.

Gantt Charts

A **Gantt chart** is a project management tool used to schedule important activities. Gantt charts divide a horizontal scale into days, weeks, or months and a vertical scale into project activities or tasks.

Gantt charts are used in clinical process improvement to depict clinical guidelines or critical pathways in the treatment of common medical conditions. The tool provides a graphic method for showing the simultaneous and interdependent treatments for a clinical condition that are most likely to result in the best possible outcome. Figure 7.4 is an example of a Gantt chart. The chart depicts the clinical guidelines used for cases of idiopathic pediatric scoliosis at a large medical center.

Case Study

Table 7.3 is a set of admission criteria for medical and surgical admissions. Figure 7.5 shows an example of one patient's history and physical report. Students should compare the patient's history with the admission criteria and determine whether the patient meets the criteria for admission to the hospital. The patient must meet at least one criterion in severity of illness and one criterion in intensity of service.

Project Application

Students should refer to chapter 6 and the customers and their requirements that were identified for their student project application. Students then should identify the performance measure that could capture data about those customer satisfaction issues. For example, if students were looking at bookstore services, some of the criteria might be book pricing, availability of books, and buy-back percentage.

Table 7.3.   Admission criteria

Severity of Illness	Intensity of Service
Sudden onset of unconsciousness or disorientation	Intravenous medications and/or fluid replacement
Pulse rate: <50/min or >140/min and not typical for patient	Inpatient-approved surgery or procedure within 24 hours of admission
Blood pressure: systolic <90 or >200 mm Hg or diastolic <60 or >120 mm Hg *and* not typical for patient	Vital signs every 2 hours or more often
Acute loss of sight or hearing	Chemotherapeutic agents requiring continuous observation
Acute loss of ability to move body part	Treatment in an ICU, if indicated
Persistent fever	Intramuscular injection every 8 hours
Active bleeding	Respiratory care at least every 8 hours
Severe electrolyte/blood gas abnormality	Glucose monitoring at least 4 times daily
EKG evidence of acute ischemia	
Wound dehiscence or evisceration	
Widely fluctuating blood glucose levels	
Hemoglobin levels 1.4 times upper limit of normal	

Figure 7.5.   Example of a history and physical report

Reason for Admission: Severe, short-distance, lifestyle-limiting right lower extremity claudication

History of Present Illness: This is a 32-year-old woman who developed new-onset right lower extremity claudication following right transfemoral cardiac catheterization for routine follow-up 10 years after cardiac transplantation. The catheterization was approximately 10 days ago. Since that time, she describes symptoms of pain in her calf after walking approximately 20 yards or less. If she walks too far, she develops paresthesias and complete numbness in the right foot. The pain is relieved by rest. She does not have rest pain at night. She has never had any symptoms similar to this or any symptoms in the contralateral leg.

She underwent cardiac transplantation 10 years ago. Since that time, she has had annual routine evaluation by transfemoral cardiac catheterization. Dr. Smith, who reviewed the films from the catheterization, reports that there is evidence of mild narrowing in the common femoral artery, possibly due to prior catheterizations. There is also some concern regarding the possibility of arterial dissection more proximally, although this may be an artifact on the angiogram.

Allergies: No known drug allergies

Past Medical History: (1) History of hypertrophic cardiomyopathy, now status post cardiac transplantation. (2) Intermittent episodes of rejection. (3) History of herpes zoster.

Past Surgical History: Cardiac transplantation

Medications: Pepcid® 20 mg po bid, Vasotec 5 mg po bid, magnesium oxide 400 mg po bid, aspirin 81 mg po bid, CellCept® 1 gm po bid, Neoral® 100 mg qam and 75 mg qpm

Social History: The patient is a schoolteacher.

Habits: She drinks alcohol occasionally and does not smoke cigarettes.

Review of Systems: The patient has no active cardiopulmonary symptoms of which she is aware and no history of hepatorenal dysfunction. She has had no other episodes of bleeding or thrombotic disorders.

Physical Examination:

HEENT:	Unremarkable
CHEST:	Clear throughout to auscultation
CARDIOVASCULAR:	Regular rhythm without murmur, gallop, or rub
ABDOMEN:	Soft, nontender with no obvious masses or organomegaly
GENITALIA/RECTAL:	Deferred
EXTREMITIES:	No clubbing, cyanosis, or edema. There is no dependent rub or pallor on elevation. The patient has normal sensation and motor function in the lower extremities. Pulses are 3/3 except in the right lower extremity, where no palpable pulses are present.
LABORATORY DATA:	Potassium 3.8; hematocrit 45; sodium 142
TEST RESULTS:	Angiography demonstrated occlusion of the external iliac artery from near the bifurcation to the distal common femoral artery, which reconstitutes just above its own bifurcation. A guide wire passed easily through this, suggesting soft thrombus. There is excellent collateralization and no evidence of distal abnormalities.
	Duplex ultrasonography performed earlier demonstrated no evidence of deep or superficial thrombophlebitis. Noninvasive vascular studies also suggested aortoiliac/femoral occlusive disease with good collateralization distally.

Impression:
1. Occluded right external iliac and common femoral artery following transfemoral cardiac catheterization
2. Status post cardiac transplantation for hypertrophic cardiomyopathy
3 History of herpes zoster

Plan: The patient will be admitted to the hospital to undergo operative intervention to repair the femoral artery injury. Several possibilities exist, including possible dissection of the artery and injury to the artery during the catheterization or development of a collagen plug post angiography. I have discussed these possibilities with the patient, and I plan to perform an exploration of the right femoral area and, if necessary, a right lower quadrant, retroperitoneal incision to expose the proximal bifurcation and a bypass if necessary. Discussed the possibility of vein patch angioplasty as well. We also discussed the risks of the operation including MI, CVA, death, infection, bleeding, nerve injury, embolization and tissue loss, bowel injury, etc. She understands all these things as well as the indications for operative intervention. We plan to operate tonight as soon as an operating room is available.

Summary

Appropriate utilization of healthcare services has been a major issue in the United States with costs for healthcare services the highest they have ever been. Utilization management strategies led to the managed care approach, which was common in the last decade of the 20th century. Various approaches, including admission criteria, critical pathways, and disease-specific care standards, have been developed to assist reviewers in determining the nature and extent of required care. Part of the added cost of healthcare can be directly attributed to this level of utilization management that has arisen. While it may have helped prevent inappropriate charges and care, the cost to maintain this system is passed on to the patient in the form of higher deductibles for insurance coverage. Management and analysis of these issues remains a major component of PI activities in every healthcare organization in the nation.

Reference

Shewhart, W.A., and W.E. Deming. 1986. *Statistical Method from the Viewpoint of Quality Control*. New York: Dover Publications.

Resources

Abdelhak, M., E. Jacobs, S. Grostick, and M.A. Hanken. 2007. *Health Information: Management of a Strategic Resource*, 3rd ed. Philadelphia: W. B. Saunders.

Groopman, J. 2000. *Second Opinions*. New York: Viking Penguin Publishing, Member of Penguin Putman.

Joint Commission. 2011. *Hospital Accreditation Manual*. Oakbrook Terrace, IL: Joint Commission Resources.

US Food and Drug Administration. 2011. Critical Path Initiative. http://www.fda.gov/ScienceResearch/SpecialTopics/CriticalPathInitiative/default.htm.

Chapter 8
Improving the Provision of Care, Treatment, and Services

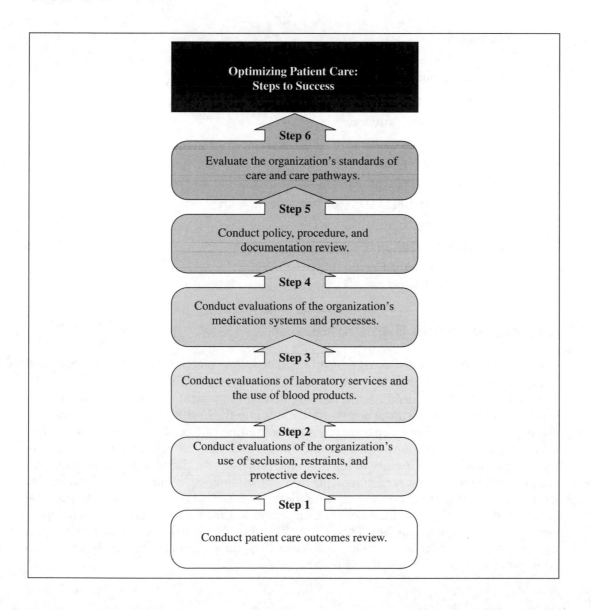

Optimizing Patient Care:
Steps to Success

Step 6
Evaluate the organization's standards of care and care pathways.

Step 5
Conduct policy, procedure, and documentation review.

Step 4
Conduct evaluations of the organization's medication systems and processes.

Step 3
Conduct evaluations of laboratory services and the use of blood products.

Step 2
Conduct evaluations of the organization's use of seclusion, restraints, and protective devices.

Step 1
Conduct patient care outcomes review.

Learning Objectives

- To identify four core processes or elements in the care, treatment, and service of patients and to recognize the common means by which healthcare organizations monitor and improve the quality of these elements of care

- To describe how the National Patient Safety Goals interface with the performance improvement cycle during the patient care process

- To describe the roles that clinical practice guidelines and evidence-based medicine play in standardizing patient care

- To explore how partnering with agencies and consumer groups has improved the quality of patient care

Key Terms

Clinical guidelines

Clinical Laboratory Improvement Amendments (CLIA)

Clinical practice standards

Core processes

Evidence-based medicine

Facility quality-indicator profile

Minimum Data Set (MDS) for Long-Term Care

Patient-centered care

Standards of care

Transfusion reaction

Background and Significance

The preceding chapters discussed the performance improvement (PI) model, its goals, and some of the factors involved in working with PI processes. This chapter focuses on a systematized approach to PI that can ultimately benefit the patient. The care of patients is a complex process that begins at any point of entry into the healthcare system and may last from one brief emergency department visit to a lifetime of frequent outpatient visits and hospitalizations for a patient with a chronic illness. Every interaction within the healthcare system provides an opportunity to improve care processes for patients and their families.

The individual medical requirements of a single patient can initiate the PI cycle. The critical factor in optimizing the care of patients is the organization's ability to improve patients' understanding of their health, their ability to care for themselves, their independence, and their quality of life. The goal of PI in healthcare is to design and implement systems that provide consistency and quality in all of the patient care processes performed to improve each individual patient's health.

With respect to the provision of care, treatment, and services, PI efforts provide a process for evaluating every service, provider, setting, and outcome that patients, residents, and clients expect in a healthcare organization. The **core processes** involved in care, treatment, and services to patients are *assessing* patient needs; *planning* care, treatment, and services; *providing* the care, treatment, and services that the patient needs; and *coordinating* care, treatment, and services. Activities utilized in providing these four core processes include assessing and providing appropriate access to levels of care; providing interventions based on the plan of care developed in conjunction with the patient and significant others; teaching patients what they need to know about their care, treatment, and services; and coordinating care, treatment, and services when the patient is referred, transferred, or discharged. The greatest responsibility for care lies within these processes.

The Patient Care Process Cycle

In practice, the core patient care processes actually become part of a cycle that begins with the patient's initial assessment and concludes with his or her discharge or referral to another care provision venue. (See figure 8.1.) Most patients probably will have to go

Figure 8.1. Patient care process cycle

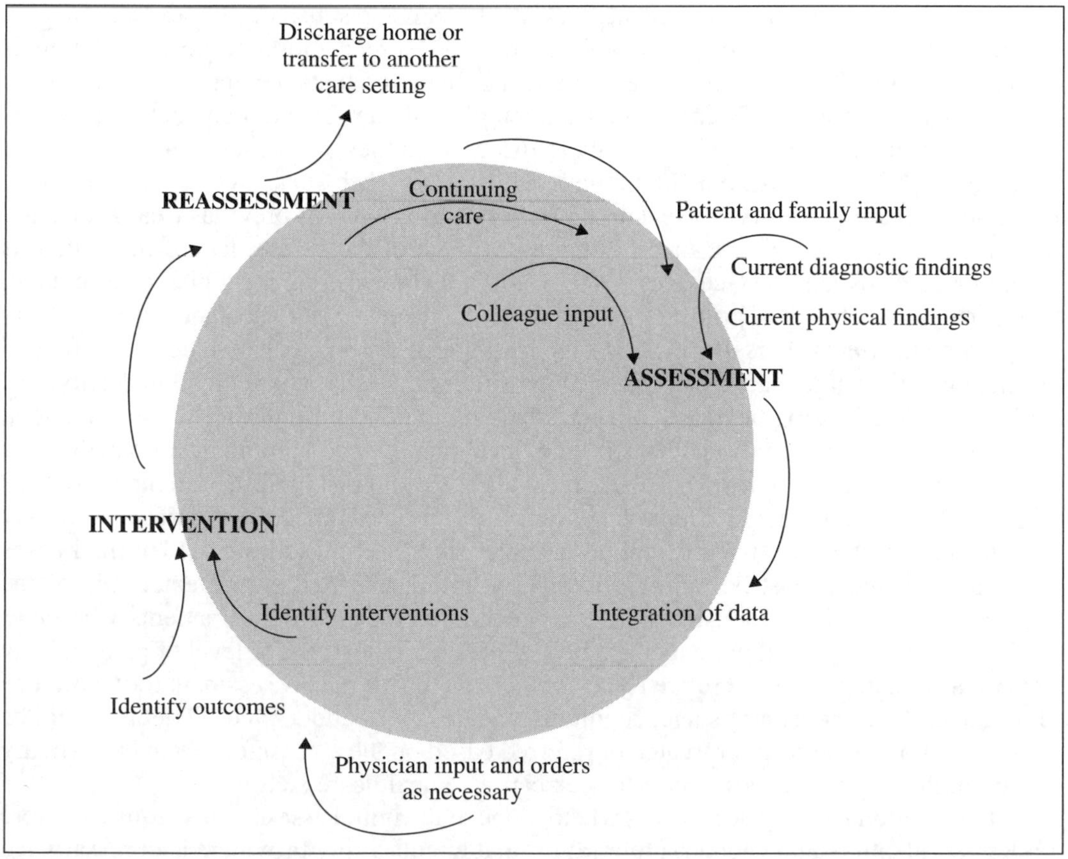

through this cycle several times during the duration of an illness, and the cycle may occur in one facility or across the continuum of facilities involved in the patient's care.

Core Process 1: Assessing the Patient's Needs

The cornerstone of good patient care is the initial assessment, which determines the patient's appropriateness for admission to the facility and the level of care to be rendered. Specific admission criteria based on defined services help caregivers determine which patients will benefit most from services the facility offers during the assessment and reassessment period. Community standards and thus accrediting and licensing entities require collection of the following information in the initial patient assessment for admission:

- Physical, psychological, and social assessment
- Nutrition and hydration status
- Functional status, that is, how well an individual performs activities of daily living
- Social, spiritual, and cultural variables that influence the patient's and family members' perceptions of their lives

In addition to physical conditions, patients are assessed for issues related to legal or correctional status, victim abuse and neglect, alcoholism and substance use disorders, presence of pain, and emotional or behavioral disorders. The organization may refer individuals who are emotionally ill or who suffer from alcoholism or substance abuse for care, treatment, and services as consistent with its written plan of care. If the organization provides services for alcoholism and substance abuse disorders, a thorough assessment will need to be conducted. That assessment should include history of each substance use, age at onset, duration, intensity, patterns of use, consequences of use, types of previous treatments, and responses to those treatments. In the initial assessment of these disorders, if the patient is receiving psychosocial services, he or she would also be assessed for a history of mental, emotional, and behavioral problems and their co-occurrence with substance use disorders and treatment. Items typically included in this type of assessment include religious and spiritual beliefs, values and preferences, living situation, leisure and recreational activities, military service history, peer group, social factors, ethnic and cultural factors, financial status, vocational or educational background, legal history, and communication skills.

A history of physical or sexual abuse must also be evaluated in this assessment. Victims of possible abuse and neglect must be assessed on the basis of defined criteria and may be referred for care to private or public agencies that treat these issues. Identified cases of abuse or neglect must be reported internally within the facility and externally to the proper agency. A comprehensive pain assessment is completed on all patients who enter the healthcare system. All patients must be assessed on admission for level of pain and any pain management tools used regularly to alleviate pain. The pain assessment tool would be coordinated with the patient's age, condition, and ability to understand. Patients would be reassessed for pain and either treated or referred based on the assessment. Pain is a primary symptom that motivates individuals to seek care in a healthcare setting.

Organizational policy determines whether one of the initial assessments requires a more in-depth evaluation and whether a referral for that to consulting providers is necessary. All facilities have policies that outline the required information to be collected for an adequate assessment and initial treatment plan. Policies also outline who is authorized to collect this information. Family members may be a source of data collection for an initial assessment if the patient is not capable of providing coherent information.

Diagnostic testing and procedures are performed as ordered in the initial assessment period in compliance with specified time frames as defined by organizational policy.

Regulatory and licensing agencies usually also define the education, training, and experience required of team members to perform an adequate assessment. Only licensed and competent caregivers are allowed to assess patients. For instance, most hospital medical staff rules and regulations require a medical history and physical examination be completed by a physician on a patient within 24 hours of inpatient admission or within 30 days prior to the admission. If the physical exam is within 30 days, an updated physical to note any changes in the patient's condition needs to be done within 24 hours of admission. A registered nurse completes a nursing assessment within 24 hours of a patient's inpatient admission and determines the patient's need for nursing care on the basis of this assessment. A functional screening is also completed for each patient within 24 hours of admission.

The care team, patient, and family, if available, establish priorities for treatment. If this is done early in the course of treatment, it is classified as an initial treatment plan. This plan is usually a blueprint for a more complex plan that will follow and addresses the most emergent need of the client. An initial problem list is also developed to reflect the most critical problems to be managed. Some treatment issues may be delayed or postponed on the basis of urgency or immediacy of care needs. For example, a patient admitted to an emergency department with active upper gastrointestinal bleeding and diabetes may undergo treatment for the acute bleeding first and evaluation of the diabetes later. The diabetes may be listed as a problem on the treatment plan and documented as deferred to a later time. Goals and interventions are developed by the team to address the patient's need for services and to evaluate clinical improvement. Staff are assigned to accomplish interventions for each goal, and a time frame for completion or frequency of intervention is identified.

Core Process 2: Planning Care, Treatment, and Services

If an appropriate need for admission has been determined, the establishment of an interactive, written care plan that is specific, individualized, and based on a thorough assessment of the patient's physical, emotional, social, cognitive, and cultural needs is the next step in the care process. In the case example of the diabetic patient treated in the ER for gastrointestinal bleeding, the ER treatment team will begin an initial treatment plan addressing the patient's most critical needs. For example, this patient's treatment plan may have a goal of stabilizing his body fluid level and preventing further blood loss since this could be a life-threatening issue for him. The objectives for this goal would include stopping his blood loss through gastric lavage with ice water, intravenous fluids to balance fluid loss, and hourly lab values to ensure blood loss is stabilized. The interventions would be listed as hourly hemoglobin and hematocrit draws, D5NS at a rate of 200 cc per hour, NPO status, and gastric lavage until bleeding ceases. Most of these immediate interventions are defined best-care standards that have been researched to provide the most expedient and lifesaving measures.

The collaborative written plan of care for patients is begun at the time of admission by the interdisciplinary admitting team, the patient, and perhaps the family and is revised as the patient's condition changes. Healthcare facility policy will determine when the written plan of care is due and will be based on the patient's goals and the time frames, settings, and services required to meet those goals. With the use of disease-specific care plans or care paths, many of the objectives and goals will be determined on the basis of researched and established guidelines in the care pathway.

Core Process 3: Providing Care, Treatment, and Services

In many of today's healthcare settings, the care pathway has become the model for the documented outline of patients' progression of treatment. A multidisciplinary team using data developed through team assessment processes initiates the care pathway. (See figure 8.2.)

The goals of the care pathway are broad in scope and set the overall direction for care. The pathway defines the specific treatment and its timing and frequency. Many healthcare facilities use a system of care based on established national clinical standards for treatment interventions, which have been extensively researched. The care pathways also have become the basis for the core measures monitoring program currently required for Joint Commission accreditation and Centers for Medicare and Medicaid Services (CMS) participation. In addition, organizations can now prepare for and seek special accreditations as centers of excellence in the evaluation and treatment of specific commonly occurring conditions such as stroke or myocardial infarction, or specialized procedures such as myocardial revascularization.

Much of a patient's care is provided by several professionals operating as a collaborative team. Risser and his colleagues (2000) advocate the use of team approaches in every care process. They identify the team approaches as contributing significantly to improving patient care and to decreasing the number of patient care errors. According to Risser and colleagues (241–242), the teamwork approach:

> teaches team members to actively coordinate and support each other in the course of clinical task execution using the structure of work teams. Teams and teamwork behaviors do not replace clinical skills but rather serve to ensure that clinical activities are properly integrated and executed to deliver effective . . . care. Teamwork is a management tool to expedite care delivery to patients, a mechanism to give caregivers increased control over their constantly changing environments, and a safety net to help protect both patients and caregivers from inevitable human failings and their consequences. The goal of each core team is to deliver high-quality clinical care to the set of patients assigned to it. To achieve this goal, team members coordinate directly and repeatedly with each other to ensure proper and timely clinical task execution and to detect and help overloaded teammates. Each team member works to maintain a clear understanding (a common situation awareness) of the care status and care plan for each patient assigned to the team and the workload status of each team member. Teams hold brief meetings to make team decisions, assign/reassign responsibilities and tasks, establish/reestablish situation awareness, and learn lessons. The team oversees and directly manages the use of all care resources needed by the patient assigned to the team.

Once the care pathway has been developed, implementation begins. The patient's status is continuously monitored for signs of stabilization, improvement, or destabilization. Revisions of the care pathway and treatment interventions are developed in response to changes in the patient's clinical status. Most care teams meet daily to evaluate patient data,

Figure 8.2. Integrated care pathway

Example of an integrated care pathway for the management of adults with MRSA

Guidance for use

This ICP represents usual practice, and variations are expected as clinical staff use their own professional judgement.

ICP developed 1.2.2000 **Review date 1.2.2001**

The main source of information for this ICP was the Hospital Infection Society (1998) Working Party Report. Revised guidelines for the control of methicillin-resistant *Staphylococcus aureus* infection. *J Hosp Infect* 1998; 39: 253–290

Local protocols may differ as the guidelines must be adapted to fit in with local circumstances

Decision to treat
Following a positive result of MRSA from the pathology department, an informed decision is to be made to treat or not treat the patient. Please complete all the boxes and sign at the bottom of the page.

Outcomes:
Use this page only when managing a colonised infection.

Management plan for treatment of adult patient colonised with MRSA
Use this page only when managing a colonised infection.

Outcomes:
1. Infection is contained to patient identified with MRSA
   Outcome 1 achieved   yes □   no □
2. Treatment is successful
   Outcome 2 achieved   yes □   no □

Management plan for systemic treatment of patient infected with MRSA
Use this page only when managing a systemic infection.

Outcomes:
1. Treatment is successful
   Outcome 1 achieved   yes □   no □
2. Renal, hepatic, liver function tests and clinical checks are monitored
   Outcome 2 achieved   yes □   no □

Recording of variance
Variance from the planned care must be recorded, signed and dated, together with the reason why this happened and the alternative plan of care.

Signature   Date   /   /

Decision to treat

Patient name: Hospital number:

Please remember:
*Staff hands are the main route of cross-infection in wards.
*Early communication is essential in minimising spread of MRSA.

If there are **any** variances to ICP, please sign and date the reason(s) and alternative action taken.

Site	Colonised (Organism is present but not causing signs or symptoms of infection)	Infected (Organism is present and has resulted in signs and symptoms of infection)
Nose		
Throat		
Perineum/groin		
Skin lesion		
Burn		
Catheter urine		
Indwelling intravascular catheter		
Central line		
Intravenous infusion		
Tracheostomy		
Sputum		

Low risk
Medical ward, general and acute elderly care, non-neonatal paediatrics

Moderate risk
General surgery, urology, neonatal, gynaecology/obstetrics, dermatology

High risk
Intensive care unit, special care baby unit, transplantation, cardiothoracic, orthopaedic, trauma, vascular, regional, national/international referral centres

• Isolate if possible
• Basic infection control measures
• Full screen of index case
NB: screening of other patients is not necessary

As above plus:
• Isolate in single room
• Screen other patients in the unit
• Treat patient topically (and systemically if necessary)
• Policy of admission screening is advised

As above plus:
• Isolate in single room
• Screen other patients to the event of two or more cases

Isolation precautions
Hand washing following contact
Gloves when dealing with infected site(s)
Apron for close contact

Decision to treat
Colonisation yes □ no □
Infected site yes □ no □

Treatment of adult patient colonised with MRSA

Patient name: Hospital number:

Please remember:
• Re-emergence of resistant strains is common; these patients should always be screened as carriers
• If surgery is required, systemic prophylaxis may be necessary
• Treatment may be decided upon due to risk and re-availability of other patients
• A carrier may become a heavy dispenser of *Staphylococcus* if he/she develops an upper respiratory tract infection
• The throat is more likely to be infected if the patient has dentures

If there are **any** variances to ICP, please sign and date the reason(s) and alternative action taken.

Management: five-day topical treatment plan

		1	2	3	4	5
Nasal	**Nasal preparation** Bactroban Apply to nose three times a day					
Axillae and groin	**Skin preparation** Hexachlorophane powder (Ster-Zac) Apply daily					
Broken skin	Bactroban Apply to any small broken skin sites daily					
Daily bathing	Triclosan 2% Apply to wet skin					
Shampoo	Triclosan 2% Apply on days 1 and 3					

Is this the 1st □ or 2nd □ treatment?

Doctor's signature:

Screening schedule

	Date taken	Results due	Positive/ negative
48 hours after treatment ends (day 7)			
48 hours after 1st screen (day 9)			
48 hours after 2nd screen (day 11)			

Patient is clear only when 3rd set of swabs are negative.
If any of these screens positive, start 2nd treatment cycle.
If positive after 2nd treatment cycle, contact infection control team for further advice.

Transfer/discharge of patients
Inform relevant people
Wear gloves and apron, and wash hands
Send curtains for cleaning
Decontaminate non-disposable equipment with detergent and/or water hypochlorite solution
Allow all surfaces to dry before using equipment/room again
Place last on list for OPD or surgery

Systemic treatment of adult patient infected with MRSA

Patient name: Hospital number:

Please remember:
• Early but including effective MRSA therapy is a significant mortality risk factor
• Intensive care patients have a higher risk of developing MRSA infection than medical patients
• A combined medical and surgical approach may be necessary

Drug 1	Dose	Route	Duration	Frequency	Signature and date

Monitoring

Drug 2	Dose	Route	Duration	Frequency	Signature and date

Monitoring

Caution

Side-effect	Present (time)	Drug stopped (specify)	
Inflammation			
Pain			
Oedema			
Nausea/vomiting			
Diarrhoea			
Rash			
Headache			
Pruritus			

Treatment of side-effect(s)

If there are **any** variances to ICP, please sign and date the reason(s) and alternative action taken.

Isolation precautions
Hand washing following contact
Gloves when dealing with infected site(s)
Apron for close contact

Systemic treatment of adult patient infected with MRSA (continued)

Vancomycin or teicoplanin, possibly combined with rifampicin, may be used for severe infections
For continuing treatment or less severe infection, a combination of rifampicin and fusidic acid may be used (if organism susceptible)
Quinupristin/dalfopristin should be reserved for unresponsive severe infections or for when IV therapy is appropriate

Drug	Dose	Route	Frequency	Guidance on dosage until levels available
Vancomycin	1,000 mg	IV, given over at least 100 mins	12-hourly	CrCl (ml/min): >50: 12-hourly 30–50: 24-hourly <30: load, then measure levels*

Monitoring
Plasma levels
Pre-dose 'trough' 5–10 mg/l checked at 48 hours
If >10 mg/l increase dose interval/perhaps omit a dose
Monitor every two days when previous level satisfactory

Renal function tests may be helpful

Clinical checks on hearing (eg, tinnitus)

*Discuss with microbiologist

Drug	Dose	Route	Frequency	Guidance on dosage until levels available
Teicoplanin	400 mg (reduced from day 4 in renal impairment)	IV	12-hourly for three doses, then daily	Reduced renal function: CrCl (ml/min): 40–60: reduce by 50% <40: reduce by 66%**

Monitoring
Plasma levels helpful in complex cases
Pre-dose ('trough') >10 mg/l
Post-dose ('peak') 20–50 mg/l

**Discuss with microbiologist if patient on renal support

Drug	Dose	Route	Frequency	Caution
Rifampicin	600–1,200 mg	Oral or IV	Daily (divided doses)	Rifampicin must always be combined with another agent active against MRSA in order to prevent emergence of resistance

Monitoring   Liver function tests

Drug	Dose	Route	Frequency	Caution
Fusidic acid	500 mg	Oral	8-hourly	

Monitoring   Liver function tests

interventions, and improvement. The flow of patient care is cyclical and integrated in the following way (see figure 8.1):

- Assessment to treatment planning

  —Treatment planning to care or service

  —Care or service to reassessment

- Coordination of care when improvement is demonstrated or reassessment when the patient is referred, transferred, or discharged

As the patient's care proceeds, some key care procedures are implemented. These procedures involve such services as laboratory, radiology, pharmacy, dietary, nursing, and physical and respiratory therapy. Each of the departments in a facility that provides these ancillary services has licensing requirements for monitoring and data collection for quality verification. Each of these services must also ensure that the service it provides is specific to the patient's written plan of care and accommodates the patient's cultural, religious, or ethnic needs.

Patients and families should be involved in this process and should be actively encouraged to take part in the ongoing cycle of planning care. The patient's strengths and limitations should be considered when developing the treatment plan and completing the goals. Care pathways need to reflect the cultural values that affect a client and family in the care setting as well. For instance, in some Asian countries, certain types of cold and hot foods must be served to a newly delivered mother to ensure her health and well-being. Making dietary accommodations to meet an Asian client's needs can ease the transition and improve the client's perception of holistic, individualized care. Family members and other significant persons should be encouraged to become involved and should be educated about the patient's treatment process and care needs, recognizing that adult patients need to approve of such involvement in compliance with federal and state privacy laws.

Core Process 4: Coordinating Care, Treatment, and Services

The expected eventual outcome of this flow of care is an improvement in the patient's condition that allows discharge to the patient's home or to a different care setting. The coordination of patient services and care is often discussed among care team members. There is a defined process in the healthcare facility to receive or share patient information when the patient is referred to another internal or external provider of care, treatment, or services. A clear picture of the patient's requirements must be developed for:

- The primary care provider
- Community resources that will be involved following discharge, such as home health agencies or social workers
- Family or friends who will assist the patient at home following discharge
- Rehabilitation or long-term care settings to which the patient is transferred from a hospital

Coordinating care services includes resolving conflicts in scheduled appointments, preventing duplication of services, and ensuring care is administered within a time frame that meets the patient's needs. Specific information must be given to the patient regarding exercise and activity levels, medication regimens, weight monitoring, sexual activity, and acceptable dietary habits, as well as what to do if his or her condition deteriorates following discharge. Information regarding diagnoses and procedures performed must also be transmitted to primary care physicians or other follow-up providers.

Optimizing Patient Care: Steps to Success

The treatment and care of a patient in a healthcare system can be measured in many ways. Different measures can be used to identify problems, demonstrate compliance with regulations, or reflect improvement in patient care processes. However, some problems are more easily measured than others. For example, it is easier to measure the number of patients who receive a preoperative dose of antibiotics to prevent postoperative wound infection than it is to measure that particular intervention's effect on the occurrence of infection in a specific individual. Different people respond differently to medication interventions. Such differences create variation in the overall response to medication. The focus of improvement processes, therefore, must be tied to patient-specific data about the care processes provided at any given facility.

Several common improvement processes are discussed in the following steps.

Step 1: Conduct Patient Care Outcomes Review

Patient care outcomes are reviewed to improve the safety and quality of care as well as to identify issues related to medical necessity for treatment and appropriateness of care. One means of outcomes review is the ORYX initiative, introduced by the Joint Commission in 1997. This initiative has evolved to include core measure sets based on the services the healthcare organization provides and is now also required of Medicare participants by CMS. The intent of requiring organizations to collect performance data on their outcomes of care allows the Joint Commission, CMS, and the healthcare organizations themselves to review and compare data trends and patterns in treatment among like organizations to help improve patient care processes. Available core and noncore measure sets include:

- SCIP Core Measure Set

- Heart Failure Core Measure Set

- Acute Myocardial Infarction Core Measure Set

- Pneumonia Core Measure Set

- Pregnancy Core Measure Set

- ORYX Risk Adjustment Guide

- Hospital Outpatient Department Quality Measures

- Children's Asthma Care

- Hospital-Based Inpatient Psychiatric Services

Accrediting and licensing entities expect that healthcare organizations will choose appropriate measures for the services they offer and that the data collected will be reported through the PI systems in the organization. The Joint Commission uses the core measure data as part of its scoring mechanism for accrediting facilities. Core measure information can be obtained in detail from the Joint Commission Web site (http://www.jointcommission.org/) or from the CMS (2011) Web site (http://www.cms.gov/QualityMeasures).

Step 2: Conduct Evaluations of the Organization's Use of Seclusion, Restraints, and Protective Devices

The facility must have written behavior management policies approved by the facility's clinical leaders and an external expert that define which behavior management procedures can and cannot be used. Procedures that may physically harm a patient or place the individual at psychological risk are not allowed, such as:

- Denial of a patient's basic needs, food, and water

- Denial of shelter

- Denial of essential, safe clothing

- Use of corporal punishment

- Use of fear-eliciting techniques

- Use of mechanical restraint and seclusion

- Any procedure that allows a patient to implement behavior management and treatment techniques on other patients

Because a restraining device may be part of the patient's written plan of care, all facility, state, and federal guidelines must be complied with and defined in the plan of care. Protective restraint devices include wrist restraints, jacket restraints, chairs with restraining tables, restraints to stabilize a patient's body during surgery, and side rails on hospital beds. Such protective restraint devices prevent something from happening. One example is the use of head stabilization devices for dental procedures.

The use of restraints involves an increased risk of client deaths with pursuant legal risks and, therefore, requirements for monitoring during their use. On admission, an initial assessment of the patient's need for restraint should occur, including a discussion with the patient and his or her family about a least-restrictive progression of interventions prior to the possible use of restraint; this assessment and discussion should be documented. Independent licensed practitioners should be credentialed for the privilege of assessing and applying restraint and seclusion. Continued training and staff competency for seclusion and restraint procedures and protective devices must be documented. It is also very important to document leadership philosophy, education, and commitment to the facility-wide elimination of the use of seclusion and restraint. The primary focus of training for facilities includes staff competency in a number of de-escalation techniques and safety procedures as well as facility philosophy about restraint and seclusion. The Joint Commission wants to reduce the frequency of seclusion and restraint across all facilities through use of the PI process to identify opportunities to reduce the risks associated with these procedures. It is particularly concerned about the use of restraint and seclusion and protective devices in long-term care and rehabilitation settings because the procedures may infringe on patients' rights and have been identified through the sentinel event alert process as high risk.

Written policies must outline the use of restraint for *nonbehavioral* purposes, such as for an emergency room patient. These policies are approved by the medical staff and nursing leadership of the facility. Common items in these policies include:

- Protection of the patient's rights, dignity, and well-being

- Use of restraint based on the patient's assessed needs

- Use of the least-restrictive method of restraint

- Safe application and removal of restraints

- Monitoring and reassessment of patients who are restrained

- Methods for meeting the physical needs of patients who are limited by restraint

- Risks posed by restraints to vulnerable patient populations such as ER and pediatric patients or patients who are cognitively or physically challenged

- Discussion of the use of restraint with the patient and family

- Written orders for restraint limited to licensed independent practitioners

- Renewal of orders in accordance with law and regulation

- Frequency and content of entries in the patient's health record for each episode of restraint

Use of restraint for nonbehavioral purposes is usually initiated by an individual order from a licensed independent practitioner (LIP) or by written approved protocol. A registered nurse (RN) may initiate the order based on an assessment of the patient, but the LIP must be notified immediately and must provide a verbal or written order within 12 hours of initiation of the use of restraint. Within 24 hours of the initiation of the order for use of nonbehavioral restraint, the LIP must examine the patient. Each 24 hours of continued use of nonbehavioral restraint requires an order from the LIP based on his or her examination of the patient.

Written protocols for the use of restraint for nonbehavioral health purposes include the following items: guidelines for assessing the patient, criteria for the use of restraint, criteria for monitoring the patient and reassessing the need for restraint, and criteria for when the restraint can be discontinued. Only authorized staff educated in restraint standards and hospital protocols can maintain and discontinue restraint for nonbehavioral purposes. Any patient restrained for nonbehavioral health purposes must be monitored at a minimum of every two hours and more frequently based on the individual assessment of the patient's needs. All facilities are required to collect and analyze data on the use of nonbehavioral restraint, and these data are analyzed statistically and reported based on the facility's policies. Opportunities for improvement of care in this area are based on statistical analysis of the data. Facilities are required to act when planned improvements in the use of nonbehavioral restraint are not achieved or not sustained.

Restraint and seclusion for behavioral health purposes have different guidelines and policies for care. The hospital's approach to the use of restraint and seclusion for behavioral health purposes includes the following:

- Its commitment to work to eliminate the use of restraint and seclusion

- The need to prevent emergencies that could potentially lead to the use of restraint and seclusion

- The use of nonphysical intervention as the preferred intervention

- Limitation of the use of restraint and seclusion to emergencies involving imminent risk of a patient causing self-harm or harm to others, including staff

- The responsibility to discontinue restraint or seclusion as soon as possible

- The need to raise awareness among the staff about what restraint or seclusion may feel like to the patient

- Preservation of the patient's safety and dignity when restraint or seclusion is used

Written policies and procedures guide the use of restraint and seclusion for behavioral purposes. These policies address staffing levels and staff competence. Each patient must be assessed during the initial examination for any concerns related to physical or sexual abuse, or any physical disabilities or limitations that may cause harm or place the patient at increased risk. Techniques that would help the patient control his or her behavior should be noted in the assessment. Family members may be educated about the facility's approach to restraint and seclusion and, unless their participation is contraindicated by the patient's condition, may be asked to help in minimizing the need for restraint and seclusion. Staffing levels for restraint and seclusion are based on staff qualifications, the physical design of the environment, patient diagnoses, patient co-occurring conditions, patient acuity level, and age and developmental functioning. Other items addressed in these policies are as follows:

- The patient's initial assessment

- The role of nonphysical techniques in behavior management

- Limiting restraint or seclusion to emergencies

- Notifying the patient's family when restraint or seclusion is initiated

- Ordering of restraint or seclusion by an LIP; no PRN (as needed) orders

- In-person evaluation of a patient in restraint or seclusion by an LIP or a qualified, trained individual authorized by the hospital to perform this function: four hours for ages 18 and older, two hours for ages 9 through 17, and one hour for younger than age 9

- Initiation of restraint or seclusion by staff other than an LIP

- Time-limited orders to four hours for ages 18 and older, two hours for ages 9 through 17, and one hour for younger than age 9

- The patient's reassessment for continued need for restraint or seclusion by an LIP at least once in 8 hours for ages 18 and older and every four hours for 17 and younger

- Monitoring of a patient in restraint and seclusion (15-minute intervals) and in-person observation by an assigned staff member who is competent and trained in the use of restraint and seclusion

- Discontinuing restraint or seclusion occurs as soon as the patient meets criteria for its discontinuation

- Debriefing a patient after each use of restraint or seclusion occurs within 24 hours of the episode and identifies what led to the restraint or seclusion and what could have been done differently; ascertainment that physical well-being, psychological comfort, and the right to privacy were maintained; counseling of the patient for any physical or psychological trauma that may have resulted; and modification of the plan for care

- Reporting injuries and deaths to the hospital's leadership and appropriate external agencies in accordance with law and regulation

- Documentation

- PI activities include the notification of clinical leaders of extended use or multiple episodes of restraint or seclusion for behavioral health purposes, defined as restraint or seclusion longer than 12 hours, or experiences of two or more separate episodes of restraint or seclusion of any duration within 12 hours. Data collection is done on each episode of restraint and seclusion that addresses the shift in which the episode occurred; the setting, unit, or location; staff who initiated; length of episode; date and time of episode; day of week; type of restraint; injuries sustained by staff or patient; patient identifier, age, and gender; and use of psychoactive medications as an alternative to restraint or seclusion or to enable its discontinuation.

Restraint and seclusion standards are highly defined by the Joint Commission, CMS, and state licensing agencies. There is clear distinction in the regulations about the use of restraint and seclusion for nonbehavioral health patients versus behavioral health patients. There are multiple PI monitors required for any use of restraint or seclusion in all facilities. Restraint or seclusion is limited to emergencies in which there is an imminent risk of a patient inflicting physical harm to himself or herself, staff, or others and in which nonphysical interventions would not be effective. Most of the monitors are directed toward patient safety, timeliness, care, dignity, and least-restrictive use. In the ER patient's case, he is a nonbehavioral patient, and the use is for medical purposes to prevent him from accidentally removing his tube during sedation. This intervention would include temporary immobilization for a medical procedure (gastric lavage) and would, therefore, be required to meet all the nonbehavioral restraint and seclusion standards.

Staff training for management of restraint and seclusion is intensive, and staff must demonstrate competency in several areas as well as be trained in CPR and available at all times. The list of training needs is as follows:

- Recognition of when to contact emergency medical assistance to evaluate or treat the patient's physical status

- Recognition of signs of restraints applied incorrectly

- The taking of vital signs and the interpretation of their relevance to the patient's physical safety

- Recognition of the patient's nutrition and hydration needs

- How to check the patient's circulation and range of motion in his or her extremities

- How to address the patient's hygiene and elimination

- How to address the patient's physical and psychological status and comfort

- How to help the patient meet criteria for discontinuing restraint and seclusion

- Recognition of the patient's readiness for discontinuing restraint and seclusion

Step 3: Conduct Evaluations of Laboratory Services and the Use of Blood Products

The organization's compliance with established standards related to the use of laboratory equipment and the handling of laboratory specimens must be monitored. Laboratory services are regulated by established protocols from the **Clinical Laboratory Improvement Amendments (CLIA)** and the Centers for Disease Control and Prevention (CDC). Equipment calibration and other parameters of laboratory values must be monitored daily.

The handling of blood and blood products for transfusions is also regulated and monitored. Measuring, assessing, and improving the ordering, typing, matching, dispensing, and administering of blood and blood products are a standard part of continuous monitoring for most clinic and hospital settings. The review process seeks to validate the need for transfusion, the use of the appropriate type of blood product, and effective procedures for blood product administration.

The National Patient Safety Goal (NPSG) 01.01.01 (Joint Commission 2011a) states that two patient identifiers are used when administering medications, blood, or blood components. (For more information, see "Ongoing Developments" in this chapter.) Two identifiers must also be used when collecting blood samples and other specimens for clinical testing. In addition, one of the goals is that containers used for blood and other specimens are labeled in the presence of the patient. Following are common current implementation expectations:

1. Before a blood product transfusion is initiated, the patient is matched to the blood product, and the blood product is matched to the order using either a two-person verification process or an automated identification technology such as bar coding.

2. When using a two-person verification process, one individual conducting the identification verification must be the qualified transfusionist who will administer the blood product to the patient.

3. When using a two-person verification process, the second individual conducting the identification verification must be qualified to perform this task.

The cause of every **transfusion reaction** must be investigated. Most deaths resulting from hemolytic transfusion reactions were primarily attributable to incomplete patient identification processes for blood verification. Some were a result of improper handling and processing of samples for many patients at the same time in the same location. Some risk-reduction strategies identified through the analysis of these events are in-service training on transfusion-related processes, revision of staffing models for these work areas, improved patient identification processes for blood verification, environmental redesign to accommodate fewer specimens in one location, and procedures to restrict simultaneous cross-matching of many patients.

Step 4: Conduct Evaluations of the Organization's Medication Systems and Processes

Over the course of the last few years, several advocacy groups have noted that medication use is one of the most complex healthcare processes and also one fraught with the greatest possibilities for error. This situation has made a healthcare organization's medication systems and processes one of the aspects most examined by accreditation and licensing agencies. Because of its complexity and impact on the patient care process cycle, we acknowledge it as one of the most important areas for examination with respect to PI. Details of that examination can be found in chapter 11 of this text.

Step 5: Conduct Policy, Procedure, and Documentation Review

The development of policies on standard practices in a facility should be multidisciplinary in nature and design. Most facilities operate within a standard set of policies developed by a multidisciplinary team of clinical and administrative professionals who meet regularly. Policies are updated and revised as national standards of care and NPSGs change. The governing board and leadership of an organization are ultimately responsible for the services provided in the facility and generally recommend changes and set time frames for the review of every policy and procedure to be followed. Some facilities operate with a separate policy and procedure committee.

A key quality performance concern is the adequate and reliable documentation of care. Poor documentation leads to the largest number of risk management and legal situations in the industry. Accreditation and licensing agencies have standards on the documentation of patient care and expect that a sample of clinical documentation will be regularly reviewed as part of an organization's PI activities. The expectation is that all records have been authenticated and contain the necessary reports and that they appropriately document the condition and treatment of the patient. An example of this type of standard would be the timeline requirement for signing off on a verbal order from a physician to a nurse in the client record. Each licensing agency will have a directive regarding this standard. Verbal order sign-offs for seclusion and restraint orders must be completed by a physician within 24 hours of the order. Facility policies will direct the time frame for other verbal order sign-offs based on the facility and type of care provided.

Step 6: Evaluate the Organization's Standards of Care and Care Pathways

For a healthcare organization to define optimal care, it must first establish **standards of care** and care policies. Some healthcare organizations have moved from a policy and procedure format to a **clinical practice standards** model. This model defines practice based on diagnosis. The flow of treatment interventions and the patient's progress are evaluated on the basis of nationally accepted standards of care for the diagnosis. As each standard is developed and approved, a baseline for performance in the healthcare setting develops. Variations from the standards of care; sentinel events; and high-risk, problem-prone activities must be examined. Action plans are then developed to improve care in areas identified through the monitoring process. A decline in performance or a lack of improvement may require further evaluation and redesign of care processes. One way to facilitate this is through comparing organization performance with that of other organizations on core measures discussed earlier.

Ongoing Developments

It is important to recognize that the PI processes discussed in the preceding section are part of a continuum of development in the evaluation of patient care. This continuum of development began, effectively, with the initiation of accreditation and standardization programs decades ago and will continue in the future. In addition, major national developments that must be monitored by healthcare administrators will eventually affect all healthcare organizations. Discussion of some of these developments follows.

Focus on Patient Safety: NPSGs

It is significant to note that in spite of the tremendous amount of data collection that has occurred in healthcare, there continues to be a tremendous number of errors in care administration that occur on a daily basis in organizations across the country. The development of the Patient Safety and Quality Improvement Act of 2005 and the NPSGs (Joint Commission 2011b) have demonstrated a national focus on improving safety for patients. All healthcare organizations are effectively mandated to examine care processes that have a potential for error that can cause injury to patients. The concern for safety may be numbers driven, but it has become process oriented as well. The *Salt Lake Tribune*, on August 19, 2008, related the death of a man from a transfusion reaction. "Tragedies like that are never supposed to happen. But these so-called 'never events,' the most serious medical errors, occurred at least an average of once every six days in Utah hospitals and surgical centers, with 57 reported last year. And what happened to the patients? Twenty-seven died and twenty-eight were severely injured, losing physical or mental function, according to health department data requested by the *Salt Lake Tribune*" (May 2008).

NPSGs for hospitals, established by the Joint Commission at the time of publication of this text, are presented in figure 8.3. Sets for other settings, for example, long-term care or behavioral health organizations, are similar. The long-term care set adds preventing residents from falling and preventing the development of bed sores.

In previous iterations of the NPSGs, one of the goals was to prevent wrong-person, wrong-site, and wrong-procedure surgeries. This has been pulled out of the NPSGs and made a universal protocol by the Joint Commission, similar to the universal protocol used

Figure 8.3. Joint Commission 2011 Hospital NPSGs

In the first decade of the 21st century, a new emphasis on patient safety has arisen in response to analysis by independent organizations like the Leapfrog Group, the Institute of Medicine, the Joint Commission, and others. Research has revealed that hundreds of thousands of individuals are injured or killed in healthcare organizations every year from mistakes or miscommunications involving the care they are receiving, particularly that involving medication administration and provision of surgical procedures.

In response to the significant body of data elucidating this problem, the Joint Commission began the National Patient Safety Goals initiative, which all organizations participating in accreditation must promote and train their staff members to adhere to. In 2009 standards preparation, the Commission began to further focus attention on the nature of these unsafe occurrences with its Robust Process Improvement initiative.

Listed below are the 2011 Hospital National Patient Safety Goals as formatted for the general public, which are the latest revision and promulgation of the safety goals made by the Joint Commission prior to publication of this text. The safety goals are reviewed and revised each accreditation year, some moved off to become permanent standards in the various chapters of the applicable accreditation manual. Please note that since the 2009 Accreditation Manual for Hospitals, the National Patient Safety Goals have been accorded their own chapter because of their significant impact on patient safety and care outcomes that must be examined in the process of institutional review for Joint Commission accreditation.

- Identify patient correctly
  - Use at least two ways to identify patients. For example, use the patient's name and date of birth. This is done to make sure that each patient gets the medicine and treatment meant for him or her.
  - Make sure that the correct patient gets the correct blood type when he or she gets a blood transfusion.
- Improve staff communication
  - Read back spoken or phone orders to the person who gave the order.
  - Create a list of abbreviations and symbols that are not to be used. Quickly get important test results to the right staff person.
  - Create steps for staff to follow when sending patients to the next caregiver. The steps should help staff tell about the patient's care. Make sure there is time to ask and answer questions.
- Use medicines safely
  - Create a list of medicines with names that look alike or sound alike. Update the list every year.
  - Label all medicines that are not already labeled, for example, medicines in syringes, cups, or basins.
  - Take extra care with patients who take medicines to thin their blood.
- Prevent infection
  - Use the hand-cleaning guidelines from the World Health Organization (WHO) or Centers for Disease Control and Prevention (CDC).
  - Report death or injury to patients from infections that happen in hospitals.
  - Use proven guidelines to prevent infections that are difficult to treat.
  - Use proven guidelines to prevent infection of the blood.
  - Use safe practices to treat the part of the body where surgery was done.
- Check patient medicines
  - Find out what medicines each patient is taking. Make sure that it is OK for the patient to take any new medications with his or her current medicines.

(Continued on next page)

Figure 8.3.   *(Continued)*

> —Give a list of the patient's medicines to the next caregiver or to the patient's regular doctor before the patient goes home.
>
> —Give a list of the patient's medicines to the patient and his or her family before the patient goes home. Explain the list.
>
> —Some patients may get medicine in small amounts or for a short time. Make sure that it is OK for those patients to take those medicines with their current medicines.
>
> • Prevent patients from falling (long-term care)
>
> —Find out which patients are most likely to fall. For example, is the patient taking any medicines that might make him or her weak, dizzy, or sleepy? Take action to prevent falls for these patients.
>
> • Prevent bed sores (long-term care)
>
> —Find out which residents are most likely to have bed sores. Take action to prevent bed sores in these patients. From time to time, recheck residents for bed sores.
>
> • Identify patient safety risks
>
> —Identify suicidal patients.

Source: Joint Commission 2011c, 2011d.

Figure 8.4.   Universal protocol for surgery

> • Wrong-person, wrong-site, and wrong-procedure surgery can and must be prevented.
>
> • A robust approach using multiple complementary strategies is necessary to achieve the goal of always conducting the correct procedure on the correct person, at the correct site.
>
> • Active involvement and use of effective methods to improve communication among all members of the procedure team are important for success.
>
> • To the extent possible, the patient and, as needed, the family are involved in the process.
>
> • Consistent implementation of a standardized protocol is most effective in achieving safety.

Source: Joint Commission 2011e, 11.

to prevent the spread of hospital-acquired infection. The elements of this universal protocol are outlined in figure 8.4.

National Standardization of Care Processes

The evaluation of patient care across all settings is extremely difficult. The expectation is that healthcare will be individualized because what works well for one patient may not work well for another. Some healthcare researchers, particularly those working in the federal government, have spent millions of dollars and years of research to develop **clinical guidelines** that attempt to standardize the care of a single condition across the entire country. Many clinical practitioners, however, find the guidelines difficult to implement or even contraindicated in some cases because of comorbid conditions or social ramifications in a patient's clinical presentation. (The use of **critical pathways** was discussed in detail in chapter 7.)

Other healthcare researchers have developed the concept of **evidence-based medicine.** Evidence-based medicine attempts to identify the care processes or interventions that achieve the best outcomes in different types of medical practice. Researchers perform large population-based studies. Such studies are difficult to do without a well-developed information infrastructure to provide data for analysis. The United States does not yet have a well-developed information infrastructure.

CMS has begun to address some of these issues in its "Pay for Performance" (P4P) initiative (2006). P4P is an emerging movement in healthcare reimbursement. Providers under this arrangement are rewarded for meeting preestablished targets for delivery of healthcare services that improve quality and efficiency. This is a fundamental change from fee-for-service payment. "CMS' strategic objective is to shift to a quality-oriented, patient-centered payment system. Because payment for care should be based on a patient's needs rather than on the type of facility that provides the care, we are developing a single assessment instrument for hospitals, nursing homes and home health agencies" (CMS 2006, 31). CMS collaborated with many public and private organizations, the National Quality Forum, the National Committee for Quality Assurance (NCQA), the American Medical Association (AMA), and the Joint Commission, to name a few, in an effort to improve quality of care while containing and decreasing the costs of care. For examples of some of these initiatives, see figure 8.5.

In California, the initiative to improve care by restricting payment for adverse events occurring during patient care has been codified by the state legislature in a list of adverse events reportable to the state health facilities licensing division of the California Department of Public Health (SB 1301, Alquist, Chapter 647, Statutes of 2006). The California list expands the list developed by CMS to 28 "never events" (that is, events that should never occur in healthcare in the state). Patient cases during which any of these events occur will not achieve routine standardized reimbursement from state programs under the P4P initiative of CMS. The list of all 28 reportable adverse events can be found in figure 8.6. Note that the CMS elements are included in bold, italic type.

The process of data collection and reporting is complicated and critical. Numbers are just numbers unless they can be compared equitably—apples to apples, so to speak. It is significant to note that "the Joint Commission and the Centers for Medicare and Medicaid Services announced the signing of an agreement to work together in completely aligning current and future common Hospital Quality Measures in their condition-specific performance measure sets. The specification manual can be found on the Joint Commission Web site [http://www.jointcommission.org]" (Joint Commission 2011f).

Figure 8.5. P4P initiatives

Hospital Quality Initiative

The Hospital Quality Initiative is part of the Department of Health and Human Services' (HHS) broader National Quality Initiative that focuses on a set of quality measures by linking reporting of those measures to the payments the hospitals receive for each discharge. Hospitals that submit the required data receive the full payment update to their Medicare severity diagnosis-related groups (MS-DRGs) payments.

http://www.cms.hhs.gov/HospitalQualityInits/

Hospital Inpatient Value-based Purchasing Program

The hospital value-based purchasing program, which would apply beginning in FY 2013 to payments for discharges occurring on or after October 1, 2012, would make value-based incentive payments to acute care hospitals based either on how well the hospitals perform on certain quality measures or on how much the hospitals' performance improves on certain quality measures from their performance during a baseline period. The higher a hospital's performance or improvement during the performance period for a fiscal year, the higher the hospital's value-based incentive payment for the fiscal year would be.

http://www.cms.gov/HospitalQualityInits/

(Continued on next page)

Figure 8.5. *(Continued)*

Physician Practice

Physician Quality Reporting. To participate in the 2011 Physician Quality Reporting, individual eligible professionals may choose to report information on individual Physician Quality Reporting quality measures or measures groups: (1) to CMS on their Medicare Part B claims, (2) to a qualified Physician Quality Reporting registry, or (3) to CMS via a qualified electronic health record (EHR) product. Individual eligible professionals who meet the criteria for satisfactory submission of Physician Quality Reporting quality measures data via one of the reporting mechanisms above for services furnished during a 2011 reporting period will qualify to earn a Physician Quality Reporting incentive payment equal to 1.0% of their total estimated Medicare Part B Physician Fee Schedule (PFS) allowed charges for covered professional services furnished during that same reporting period.

http://www.cms.gov/pqri/

Home Health Care

Home Health Agencies (HHAs) collect and report Outcome and Assessment Information Set (OASIS) data. CMS evaluates home healthcare quality by continuing to rely on the submission of OASIS assessments. Continuing to use the current OASIS instrument ensures that providers will avoid any additional burden of reporting through a separate mechanism and any related costs associated with the development and testing of a new reporting mechanism. There are currently 41 Home Health Quality Measures, and tying a portion of reimbursement to delivery of care is currently in demo and based on Home Health Compare measures.

http://www.cms.hhs.gov/HomeHealthQualityInits/01_Overview.asp#TopOfPage

---

Nursing Home Initiatives

The nursing home quality measures come from resident assessment data that nursing homes routinely collect on the residents at specified intervals during their stay and are posted on Nursing Home Compare (http://www.medicare.gov/NHCompare/Include/DataSection/Questions/SearchCriteria. asp?version=default&browser=IE|6|WinXP&language=English&defaultstatus=0&pagelist= Home&CookiesEnabled Status=True). These measures assess the residents' physical and clinical conditions and abilities, as well as preferences and life care wishes. The assessment data have been converted to develop quality measures that give consumers another source of information that shows how well nursing homes are caring for their residents' physical and clinical needs. A pay for performance demonstration in nursing homes is under consideration but has not been detailed at the time of this publication.

http://www.cms.hhs.gov/NursingHomeQualityInits/

ESRD Quality Initiatives

The End Stage Renal Disease (ESRD) Quality Initiative promotes ongoing CMS strategies to improve the quality of care provided to ESRD patients. This initiative supports quality improvement efforts among providers and makes available quality information that will enable patients to participate in making healthcare decisions. Quality measures for dialysis facilities are available to consumers on the Dialysis Facility Compare Web site (http://www.medicare.gov/Dialysis/Include/DataSection/Questions/ SearchCriteria.asp?version=default&browser=IE%7C7%7CWinXP&language=English&defaultstatus= 0&pagelist=Home).

http://www.cms.hhs.gov/ESRDQualityImproveInit/01_Overview.asp

Figure 8.6.   California reportable adverse events

Surgical events

1. Surgery on the wrong body part
2. Surgery on the wrong person
3. Wrong surgical procedures
4. *Retention of foreign object in a patient after surgery or other procedure**
5. Death during or up to 24 hours after induction of anesthesia post-surgery on an otherwise healthy patient

Product or device events

6. Patient death or serious disability associated with use of a contaminated device, drug, or biologic provided by the facility
7. Patient death or serious disability associated with use or function of a device in patient care in which the device is used or functions other than as intended
8. *Patient death or serious disability associated with intravascular air embolism that occurs while being cared for in a facility**

Patient protection events

9. Infant discharged to the wrong person
10. Patient death or serious disability associated with patient disappearance for 4 hours or longer
11. Patient suicide or attempted suicide resulting in serious disability

Care management events

12. Patient death or serious disability associated with a medication error
13. *Patient death or disability associated with incompatible blood**
14. Maternal death or serious disability associated with labor or delivery in a low-risk pregnancy
15. Patient death or serious disability directly related to hypoglycemia
16. Death or serious disability associated with failure to identify and treat hyperbilirubinemia in neonates during the first 28 days of life
17. *A Stage 3 or 4 ulcer, acquired after admission to a health facility, excluding progress from Stage 2 to Stage 3 if Stage 2 was recognized upon admission**
18. Patient death or serious disability due to spinal manipulative therapy

Environmental events

19. Patient death or serious disability associated with electric shock
20. Any incident in which a line designated for oxygen or other gas to be delivered to a patient contains the wrong gas or is contaminated by a toxic substance
21. Patient death or serious disability associated with a burn
22. *Patient death or serious disability associated with a fall**
23. Patient death or serious disability associated with the use of restraints or bedrails

Criminal events

24. Any instance of care ordered by or provided by someone impersonating a physician, nurse, pharmacist, or other licensed healthcare provider
25. Abduction of a patient of any age
26. Sexual assault on a patient within or on the grounds of a health facility
27. Death or significant injury of a patient or staff member resulting from a physical assault that occurs within or on the grounds of a facility

Other (not National Quality Forum [NQF]-endorsed)

28. An adverse event or series of adverse events that cause the death or serious disability of a patient, personnel, or a visitor

*Event included on CMS's list of nonreimbursable events.

Source: Managed Risk Medical Insurance Board (California) 2008.

Patient-Centered Care Initiatives

Scattered throughout the new legislation passed at the federal level in 2010 and discussed in previous chapters is renewed emphasis on the concept of **patient-centered care.** Most of the central and most important processes inherent in patient-centered care were discussed earlier in the chapter, in the section entitled "The Patient Care Process Cycle," with an emphasis on respect for patient values, preferences, and expressed needs and an emphasis on the providers' cultural competence, information and education regarding the patient's conditions under treatment and the modalities of treatment being utilized, access to care at levels appropriate to the patient's current progress, involvement of family to the level that the patient desires, pain management, and continuity and coordination of care as the patient progresses from one level of care to another and from one type of provider to another. The concepts have actually been emphasized for a good many years, but healthcare organizations across the country have not universally put them into action or made planned improvements where necessary to accomplish them. The new legislation seeks to give the development of patient-centered care principles a boost.

Underpinning much of the new emphasis on patient-centered care is the stimulus that the federal government seeks to inject into the situation with advancements in the use of health information technologies. "A patient-centered healthcare system gives patients the ability to communicate effectively and immediately with their providers. It provides patients access to information that is important and useful for them, when they need it. Finally, patient centered health[care] allows providers to look holistically at an individual and treat them through the coordination of their care across the spectrum of providers that may be involved" (Dimick 2011). All three of these aspects require access to information about the patient in a real-time mode of operations. Examples of recent research that underscores the need for this type of development reveals projects like:

- Reti et al. (2010), "Improving Personal Health Records for Patient-Centered Care," in which the authors assessed personal health record applications in a variety of US healthcare settings, including hospitals, ambulatory care organizations, payers, and commercial entities.

- Effken and Abbott (2009), "Health IT-Enabled Care for Underserved Populations," in which the authors discuss the use of information technologies to improve the care provided to those living in highly rural areas and advocate the development of new collaborative models for coordinating care in these areas, the capture of relevant nursing data across the continuum of care to facilitate care in these areas, preparation of technology-competent nurses to serve in these areas, and the stimulation of nursing informatics research focused on the provision of care in these areas and populations.

- And Roblin et al. (2009), "Disparities in Use of Personal Health Records in a Managed Care Organization," in which the authors explore the various levels of utilization of a personal health record by patients in the Kaiser-Permanente delivery system.

Development of organization-specific advances in the continuing deployment of patient-centered care processes will be at the forefront of accreditation and regulatory monitoring activities for the foreseeable future even if radical redirection occurs with changes in the political scene at the national level.

Measuring the Effectiveness of Managed Care Organizations

The NCQA (2011) began accrediting managed care organizations in 1991 in response to the need for standardized objective information about the quality of the services provided by managed care organizations. The NCQA introduced the Health Plan Employer Data and Information Set (HEDIS™) in the early 1990s as a means of gathering information about care, outcomes, and member satisfaction with managed care organizations and other health plans. HEDIS gathers a significant amount of information about the ambulatory care experiences of millions of health plan members from across the country. Specifically, HEDIS gathers data in the following areas:

- Measures of quality, such as immunization, cholesterol screening, mammography, and prenatal care

- Measures of access, with at least one visit to a provider within three years used as an indicator of assessment of healthcare need

- Measures of membership, with particular attention to coverage cancellation as an indicator of dissatisfaction

- Measures of utilization, including factors such as high-occurrence, high-cost, and diagnosis-related groups; frequency of procedures; general hospital acute care; outpatient and emergency visits; cesarean section rates; complicated neonatal care; and outpatient drug utilization

- Measures of financial performance, such as cost per member, cost per member plus dependents, and indicators of financial stability

The NCQA reports these findings to employers, who use the information to make decisions about contracts with health plans. In this way, the NCQA influences the kind of care offered by managed care plans and provides consumers with information about the healthcare offerings of different plans.

Consumer Advocacy Groups

Other important efforts are also made by consumers and consumer advocacy groups. The December 1, 2005 news release from the National Academies (http://www.nationalacademies.org) stated, "If pay for performance initiatives and public reporting systems are to be effective in improving the quality of healthcare in the United States, a comprehensive, universally accepted system is needed to measure and report on the performance of healthcare providers and organizations." This news release further reported that "one of the biggest obstacles to overcoming shortfalls in the quality of healthcare is the absence of a coherent, national system for assessing and reporting performance of providers and organizations." As the number of agencies and organizations that provide patient advocacy and monitor performance grows, the more complex the issues become. One outcome of this complexity has been the development of patient advocacy services. The focus of the patient advocacy role has been to offer education, consultation, conflict resolution, and support to patients and families. This role for advocacy developed out of necessity due to numerous complaints received by agencies about the quality of healthcare.

Advocacy groups have provided much of the impetus for change in the industry today. Some of the larger groups include the American Association of Retired Persons (AARP), the Council on Aging, the Women's Policy Group, and state advocacy groups like Georgia Watch. Some of these groups provide patient advocacy in the form of financial and legislative support, while others view themselves as public educators or researchers. Federal regulations, such as the Americans with Disabilities Act (ADA), and state and local laws regulate compliance. For instance, the federally mandated Occupational Safety and Health Administration's (OSHA) primary goal is to keep the employee safe in the work environment. The current requirements for needle safety precautions and bloodborne pathogen policies developed from this agency. Noncompliance with the safety regulations from federal, state, and local agencies can result in great cost to a facility.

An increase in seclusion- and restraint-related deaths began to be documented during the early 1980s. The death of a developmentally delayed young man who suffocated during a restraint process caused a riptide of reaction in mental health communities across the country. The parents of this young man took their concerns to the American Association of People with Disabilities organization, which lobbied for change in the psychiatric industry at the federal level regarding the care of patients who are in seclusion and restraint. The standards for care regarding seclusion and restraint that are now used by agencies such as CMS and the Joint Commission are a direct result of this political effort. Seclusion and restraint standards related to documentation, staff training, patient and family education and involvement, and patient rights have all become required for facilities. In addition, there has been a big move to reduce or eliminate the use of restraint in many settings, similar to the zero-tolerance policy many schools utilize regarding weapons. All these changes are directly related to one family's loss and an organization with enough political leverage and data to make change a legislated reality.

The Joint Commission Consumer Protection Initiatives

Another private organization that has provided a drive to change patient care is the Joint Commission. This agency created a data collection process on incidents it believes to be sentinel in nature. A sentinel event is an unexpected occurrence involving death or serious physical or psychological injury, or the risk thereof. The data are identified by number and definition, and in 2003, the Joint Commission began a voluntary reporting process with all agencies it accredits. Any sentinel event requires a credible root-cause analysis (see chapter 9) to be completed within 45 days of the incident. It is from these credible root-cause analyses that the Joint Commission has begun to identify ways to correct errors. The result has been the identification of 35 processes that carry a high risk of death or injury. These processes are researched by experts, and a regular Joint Commission notification titled "Sentinel Event Alert" defines these processes and identifies measures that can be used to prevent errors and improve outcomes (Joint Commission 2011g). The potential for the occurrence of errors in healthcare is tremendous, and the associated costs of errors to facilities and individuals have concomitantly driven up the price of care. These sentinel event alert processes, when incorporated into healthcare systems, are some of the most economical and research-driven models for care improvement.

Long-Term Care and Home Healthcare Monitoring

Another approach to monitoring care and identifying opportunities for improvement within healthcare organizations has arisen in the long-term care setting. In June 1998, the federal government mandated the use of the **Minimum Data Set (MDS) for Long-Term Care** to plan the care of long-term care residents. The MDS 3.0 version became effective in 2010. This data set structures the assessment of long-term care residents in the following areas:

- Delirium
- Cognitive loss/dementia
- Communication
- Vision function
- Activities of daily living (ADL) function and rehabilitation potential
- Urinary incontinence and indwelling catheter status
- Psychosocial well-being
- Mood and behavior symptoms
- Activity-pursuit patterns
- Falls
- Disease diagnoses
- Oral/nutritional status
- Oral/dental status
- Dehydration/fluid maintenance
- Pressure ulcer
- Medication use
- Treatments and procedures
- Pain
- Return-to-community referral

The federal government requires that long-term care facilities receiving Medicare or Medicaid funding transmit the patient-specific data to the state departments of health for processing and use in the long-term care certification and survey review process. The certification and survey review process is carried out by the state departments of health on behalf of the federal government to certify that facilities receiving Medicare or Medicaid funds are complying with federal regulations. The departments of health pay special attention to data on the occurrence of decubitus ulcers in low-risk patients (those who can ambulate, can turn over in bed, are not cognitively impaired, and so on), dehydration, and fecal impaction.

On the basis of the data gathered via the MDS, the facility is provided a **facility quality-indicator profile** that shows what proportion of the facility's residents have deficits in each area of assessment during the reporting period and, specifically, which residents have which deficits. The profile also provides data comparing the facility's current status with its preestablished comparison group. Data from the facility quality-indicator profile are also forwarded to CMS. An example of a facility quality-indicator profile is provided in figure 8.7.

Figure 8.7.   Example of a facility quality-indicator profile for a long-term care facility

Facility Characteristics
Run Date: 2/1/09   12:36:15 p.m.   **Report Period:** 8/1/08 to 1/31/09
Facility: Western Gardens   **Date Submitted:** 1/31/09
Comparison Group Used: **Facility Login ID:** AT 4763
All State Facilities,
October–December 2008

Resident Population	Number of Residents	Facility Percentage*	Comparison Group Percentage*
Gender			
Male	19	28.8	33.7
Female	47	71.2	66.2
Age			
<25 years	1	1.5	0.5
25–54 years	4	6.1	7.5
55–64 years	2	3.0	6.5
65–74 years	13	19.7	14.8
75–84 years	23	34.8	32.7
85+ years	23	34.8	38.0
Payment source (all that apply)			
Medicaid per diem	48	72.7	45.1
Medicare per diem	11	16.7	22.1
Medicare ancillary part A	18	27.3	19.2
Medicare ancillary part B	6	9.1	5.8
Self-pay/family-pay per diem	4	6.1	16.3
Medicaid resident liability			
or Medicare copayment	1	1.5	6.1
Private insurance per diem	3	4.5	8.1
All other per diem	1	1.5	2.6
Diagnostic characteristics			
Psychiatric diagnosis	8	12.1	9.7
Mental retardation	2	3.0	2.5
Hospice	0	0.0	0.7
Type of assessment			
Admission	12	18.2	34.0
Annual	7	10.6	11.0
Significant change in status	0	0.0	4.6
Significant correction of prior			
full assessment	1	1.5	0.5
Quarterly	42	63.6	49.7
Significant correction of			
prior quarterly	4	6.1	0.2
All other	0	0.0	0.0
Stability of conditions			
Conditions/disease make resident unstable	5	7.6	35.6
Acute episode or chronic flare-up	2	3.0	4.6
End-stage disease, ≤6 months to live	2	3.0	1.3
Discharge potential			
None	44	66.7	56.6
Within 30 days	2	3.0	15.3
Within 31–90 days	5	7.6	3.9
Uncertain	14	21.2	21.6

Figure 8.7. *(Continued)*

<table>
<tr><td colspan="6">

Facility Quality Indicator Profile
Run Date: 2/1/09   12:36:15 p.m.   **Report Period:** 8/1/08 to 1/31/09
Facility: Western Gardens   **Date Submitted:** 1/31/09
Comparison Group Used: **Facility Login ID:** AT 4763
  All State Facilities,
  October–December 2008

</td></tr>
</table>

Domain/Quality Indicator	Number in Numerator	Number in Denominator	Facility Percentage*	Comparison Group Percentage*	Percentile
Accidents					
1. Incidence of new fractures	0	53	0.0	1.1	0
2. Prevalence of falls	1	54	1.9	14.4	0
Behavioral/emotional patterns					
3. Prevalence of behavioral symptoms affecting others	13	54	24.1	28.2	41
High risk	10	40	25.0	32.7	34
Low risk	3	14	21.4	16.9	70
4. Prevalence of symptoms of depression	8	54	14.8	21.1	42
5. Prevalence of symptoms of depression without antidepressant therapy	1	54	1.9	8.7	18
Clinical management					
6. Use of nine or more medications	21	54	38.9	37.7	56
Cognitive patterns					
7. Incidence of cognitive impairment	1	14	7.1	12.5	41
Elimination/incontinence					
8. Prevalence of bladder or bowel incontinence	27	51	52.9	52.0	51
High risk	13	13	100.0	88.6	100
Low risk	14	38	36.8	39.9	38
9. Prevalence of occasional or frequent bladder or bowel incontinence without a toileting plan	9	18	50.0	55.7	40
10. Prevalence of indwelling catheter	3	54	5.6	4.9	60
11. Prevalence of fecal impaction	0	54	0.0	0.7	0
Infection control					
12. Prevalence of urinary tract infection	0	54	0.0	0.7	0
Nutrition/eating					
13. Prevalence of weight loss	1	54	1.9	2.5	54
14. Prevalence of tube feeding	1	54	1.9	2.5	54
15. Prevalence of dehydration	0	54	0.0	0.9	0
Physical functioning					
16. Prevalence of bedfast residents	1	54	1.9	6.1	29
17. Incidence of decline in late-loss activities of daily living	3	43	7.0	14.7	23
18. Incidence of decline in range of motion	7	47	14.9	9.8	79

(Continued on next page)

Figure 8.7. *(Continued)*

Domain/Quality Indicator	Number in Numerator	Number in Denominator	Facility Percentage*	Comparison Group Percentage*	Percentile
Psychotropic drug use					
19. Prevalence of antipsychotic drug use in the absence of psychosis or related conditions	8	50	16.0	18.7	46
High risk	4	9	44.4	35.4	75
Low risk	4	41	9.8	13.9	38
20. Prevalence of antianxiety/hypnotic use	9	50	18.0	18.6	61
21. Prevalence of hypnotic use more than two times in past week	1	54	1.9	3.4	50
Quality of life					
22. Prevalence of daily physical restraints	11	54	20.4	9.4	91
23. Prevalence of little or no activity	33	54	61.1	36.1	86
Skin care					
24. Prevalence of stage 1–4 pressure ulcers	4	54	7.4	7.9	65
High risk	4	23	17.4	13.5	81
Low risk	0	31	0.0	2.8	0

*Percentages may not total 100 owing to missing data.

Note: Original form designed by the Center for Health Systems Research and Analysis at the University of Wisconsin–Madison.

CMS (2005) has developed and maintains data for the Outcome and Assessment Information Set (OASIS), which is used in home health agencies. The OASIS lists a core of items for the comprehensive assessment of an adult home care patient. The data also help measure patient outcomes for outcome-based quality improvement. Home health agencies are required to electronically submit these data to the state standard system, and they become part of the *Conditions of Participation* for CMS.

Real-Life Example

A typical example of an improvement effort might begin with an assessment of an overweight adolescent who is being treated for psychosis with the antipsychotic drug Zyprexa. One side effect of Zyprexa is a decrease in satiety factors in the brain, which creates a sense of hunger even when adequate food is provided. Upon assessment of the patient, based on national standards for height and weight of adolescents (body mass index [BMI]), the individual might be identified as being in a high-risk category for obesity. An evaluation of the causative factors might reveal a genetic component, a disease component, medication side effects, poor personal habits, or a knowledge deficit regarding healthy nutrition. A multilayered action plan would be initiated after an investigation of all aspects of the contributing factors. This plan might include a nutritional consult, a dietary regimen, a medication evaluation, or a psychiatric consult. At some point in the process, an activity therapist might be consulted to direct physical exercise as an intervention to increase and support muscle strengthening as the patient loses weight. This example demonstrates how the PI process may be individualized for a patient.

A system-wide PI measure could be instituted in a care setting in regard to the problem of obesity in adolescents. If treating physicians noted significant weight increases over a brief period of time in many adolescent patients started on medications with the side effect of promoting weight gain, they might standardize their case management. Baseline evaluations of weight and height could be mandated for all patients started on this type of medication. Significant weight gains could be tracked, and interventions could be instituted for the most effective outcomes. The outcomes may result in a change in treatment that would lead physicians to order dietary consults and weight monitoring for all patients taking this medication. Other preventive measures could be instituted early in treatment to avoid excessive weight gain and alleviate the patient's risk of cardiac disease related to obesity. The potential outcome from this PI process could lead to healthier patients who require fewer medical services in the future.

QI Toolbox Technique

A common toolbox technique applicable to the improvement of patient care is the patient care outcome review criteria set. Criteria sets are used to identify opportunities for improvement with respect to the appropriateness, processes, and outcomes of medical care and surgical procedures in healthcare facilities.

The Joint Commission (2011h) Core Measures are an example of criteria sets that healthcare organizations use for ongoing patient care monitoring. The list of Joint Commission Core Measures includes Acute Myocardial Infarction, Heart Failure, Community-Acquired Pneumonia, and Pregnancy and Related Conditions. In table 8.1, a portion of the Joint

Table 8.1.   Joint Commission Core Measure criteria set—Heart Failure

Performance Measure Name	Numerator	Denominator
Discharge instructions	Heart failure patients with documentation that they or their caregivers were given written discharge instructions or other educational material addressing all of the following: activity level, diet, discharge medications, follow-up appointment, weight monitoring, what to do if symptoms worsen	Heart failure patients discharged home
LVS assessment	Heart failure patients with documentation in the hospital record that left ventricular systolic (LVS) function was assessed before arrival, during hospitalization, or is planned for after discharge	Heart failure patients
ACEI or ARB for LVSD	Heart failure patients who are prescribed an angiotensin-converting enzyme inhibitor (ACEI) or angiotensin receptor blocker (ARB) at hospital discharge	Heart failure patients with LVSD
Adult smoking-cessation advice/counseling	Heart failure patients who receive smoking-cessation advice or counseling during the hospital stay	Heart failure patients with a history of smoking cigarettes anytime during the year prior to hospital arrival

© Joint Commission 2011. Used with permission.

Source: Joint Commission 2011h.

Commission Core Measure criteria set for heart failure is listed. Cases are identified using the ICD-9-CM diagnosis codes, and then each data measure is captured in a retrospective review of the patient health record. These data are then monitored, rated, and ultimately compared with nationwide benchmarks to point to areas of potential improvement in patient care outcomes.

Case Study

Students should consider a personal healthcare experience in any setting. They should identify the key processes in relation to the areas discussed in this chapter (for example, pharmacy, medication administration, nutritional assessment, or special procedure).

Case Study Questions

1. How might the student monitor the processes he or she has experienced? What types of data would be useful? Describe variations and possible causes of variations in the care processes.

2. What worked and what did not work in the processes? Consider interviewing healthcare professionals to discuss these issues.

Project Application

Students should consider using a standardized criteria set in evaluating customer satisfaction for the student project.

Summary

The application of PI processes to patient care is varied and multifaceted. Opportunities for improvement can be identified at many levels, and organizations are limited only by constraints on their creativity and resources. Typical activities focusing on improvement of care include assessment of pharmacy and therapeutics usage; blood products usage; policy, procedure, and documentation; surgical case review; and special treatment procedures. Important work is being done at the national level in the areas of clinical practice guidelines, clinical pathways, evidence-based medicine, indicator monitoring, and data set analysis.

References

Centers for Medicare and Medicaid Services. 2005. Outcome and Assessment Information Set (OASIS). http://www.cms.hhs.gov/OASIS/.

Centers for Medicare and Medicaid Services. 2006. Centers for Medicare and Medicaid Service Strategic Action Plan for 2006–2009: Achieving a transformed and modernized healthcare system for the 21st century. http://www.cms.gov/MissionVisionGoals/Downloads/CMSStrategicActionPlan06-09_061023a.pdf.

Centers for Medicare and Medicaid Services. 2011. Quality measures overview. http://www.cms.gov/QualityMeasures.

Dimick, C. 2011. First steps to patient-centered care. *Journal of AHIMA* 82(2):20–24.

Effken, J.A., and P. Abbott. 2009. Health IT-enabled care for underserved populations. *Journal of AMIA* 16(4):439–445.

Joint Commission. 2011a. *2011 Hospital National Patient Safety Goals*. Oakbrook Terrace, IL: Joint Commission. http://www.jointcommission.org/assets/1/6/HAP_NPSG_6-10-11.pdf.

Joint Commission. 2011b. *Performance Measures Initiatives*. Oakbrook Terrace, IL: Joint Commission. http://www.jointcommission.org/Performance_Measurement.aspx.

Joint Commission. 2011c. *National Patient Safety Goals*. Oakbrook Terrace, IL: Joint Commission. http://www.jointcommission.org/assets/1/6/2011_HAP_NPSG_EASYTOREAD_docs_112-29.pdf.

Joint Commission. 2011d. *Long Term Care National Patient Safety Goals*. Oakbrook Terrace, IL: Joint Commission. http://www.jointcommission.org/assets/1/6/2011_LTC_NPSG_EASY.pdf.

Joint Commission. 2011e. National Patient Safety Goals. *Hospital Accreditation Standards*. Oakbrook Terrace, IL: Joint Commission Resources.

Joint Commission. 2011f. *Specifications Manual for National Hospital Inpatient Quality Measures*. Oakbrook Terrace, IL: Joint Commission. http://www.jointcommission.org/specifications_manual_for_national_hospital_inpatient_quality_measures/.

Joint Commission. 2011g. *Sentinel Event Alert*. Oakbrook Terrace, IL: Joint Commission. http://www.jointcommission.org/sentinelevents/sentineleventalert/.

Joint Commission. 2011h. Oakbrook Terrace, IL: Joint Commission. http://jointcommission.org/core_measures.

Managed Risk Medical Insurance Board (California). 2008. Adverse ("never") events. http://www.mrmib.ca.gov/MRMIB/Agenda_Minutes_080708/Agenda_Item_5.b_Never_Events.pdf.

May, H. 2008 (August 19). Bad errors alarm Utah hospitals. *Salt Lake Tribune*.

National Academies. 2011. http://www.nationalacademies.org.

National Committee for Quality Assurance (NCQA). 2011. Health Plan Employer Data and Information Set (HEDIS). http://www.ncqa.org.

Patient Safety and Quality Improvement Act of 2005. Public Law 109-41.

Reti, S., H.J. Feldman, S.E. Ross, and C. Satran. 2010. Improving personal health records for patient-centered care. *Journal of AMIA* 17(2):192–195.

Risser, D.T., R. Simon, M.M. Rice, and M.L. Salisbury. 2000. A structured teamwork system to reduce clinical errors. In *Error Reduction in Healthcare*. Edited by Spath, P.L., 235–278. San Francisco: Jossey-Bass.

Roblin, D., T.K. Houston, J.J. Allison, R.J. Embi, and E.R. Becker. 2009. Disparities in use of personal health records in a managed care organization. *Journal of the American Informatics Association* 16(5):683–689.

SB 1301, Alquist, Chapter 647, Statutes of 2006.

University of Wisconsin–Madison, Center for Health Systems Research and Analysis. n.d. Example of a long-term care facility quality-indicator profile.

Resources

Agency for Healthcare Research and Quality (AHRQ). 2003. What is cultural and linguistic competence? http://www.ahrq.gov/populations/cultcompdef.htm.

Agency for Healthcare Research and Quality (AHRQ). 2011. National Quality Measures Clearinghouse. http://www.qualitymeasures.ahrq.gov/.

Allison, J.J., T.C. Wall, C.M. Spettell, J. Calhoun, C.A. Fargason, Jr., R.W. Koylinski, R. Farmer, and C. Kiefe. 2000. The art and science of chart review. *Joint Commission Journal of Quality Improvement* 6(3):173–181.

American Society of Health-Systems Pharmacists (ASHP). 1999–2000. *Best Practices for Health-System Pharmacy: Position and Practice Standards of the ASHP*. Bethesda, MD: ASHP.

Committee on Redesigning Health Insurance Performance Measures, Payment, and Performance Improvement Programs. 2007. *Rewarding Provider Performance: Aligning Incentives in Medicare (Pathways to Quality Health Care Series)*. Washington, DC: The National Academies Press.

Directors of Health Promotion and Education. 2011. Addressing infectious disease threats. http://www.dhpe.org/infectintro.asp.

Institute for Family-Centered Care. 2010. FAQ. http://www.familycenteredcare.org/faq.html.

Joint Commission on Accreditation of Healthcare Organizations. 2004. *Joint Commission Perspectives: The Joint Commission and CMS Align to Make Common Performance Measures Identical*. November(24):11.

Wolf, D., L. Lehman, R. Quinlin, T. Zullo, and L. Hoffman. 2008. Effect of patient-centered care on patient satisfaction and quality of care. *Journal of Nursing Care Quality* 23(4):316–321.

Chapter 9
Preventing and Controlling Infectious Disease

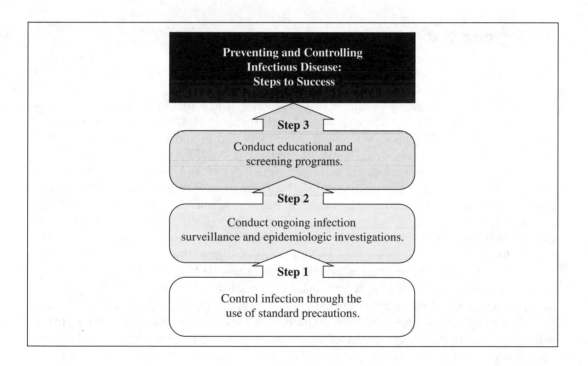

Preventing and Controlling
Infectious Disease:
Steps to Success

Step 3
Conduct educational and
screening programs.

Step 2
Conduct ongoing infection
surveillance and epidemiologic investigations.

Step 1
Control infection through the
use of standard precautions.

Learning Objectives

- To describe why the control of infection is so important in healthcare organizations

- To differentiate healthcare-associated infections from community-acquired infections

- To explain the various approaches that healthcare organizations use to incorporate risk reduction strategies regarding the occurrence of infection

- To identify the governmental organizations that develop regulations in this area, and explain the regulatory approaches often taken by healthcare facilities

- To explore the National Patient Safety Goals related to infectious disease and their impact on healthcare providers

Key Terms

Bloodborne pathogen

Community-acquired infection

Flow charts

Healthcare-associated infection (HAI)

Icons

Multiple drug-resistant organisms (MDROs)

Standard precautions

Background and Significance

Infectious diseases are generally unpleasant to experience, may be easy to catch, and may be deadly if not treated appropriately. Epidemics of infectious disease such as bubonic plague, tuberculosis, and cholera have resulted in major loss of life throughout the centuries. New diseases still erupt onto the world landscape: avian bird flu, severe acute respiratory syndrome (SARS), hanta virus, and pneumonia due to antibiotic-resistant strains of bacteria known as **multiple drug-resistant organisms** (MDROs).

"Societal costs of infectious diseases are staggering. In the United States, treatment of non-AIDS sexually transmitted diseases (STDs) alone costs $5 billion annually. The yearly price tags of other infectious diseases are $30 billion for intestinal infections, $17 billion for influenza, $1 billion for salmonella, and $720 million for hepatitis B. Altogether, the cost of treatment and lost productivity associated with illness from infectious agents tops $120 billion each year" (Directors of Health Promotion and Education 2005, 2). In 2002, the estimated number of healthcare-associated infections (HAIs) in US hospitals, adjusted to include federal facilities, was approximately 1.7 million (Klevens et al. 2007).

The discovery of pathologic organisms, such as bacteria, viruses, and parasites, as the causative agents of infection provided the human species with its most valuable tool in controlling and preventing disease. Currently, the most effective means of stopping the spread of disease is through education, preventive measures, and sanitation procedures. In 1865, Joseph Lister discovered that using carbolic acid during surgery could reduce infections after surgery. Understanding germ replication and disease vectors has allowed humans the critical opportunity to control and cure many diseases.

As a result of this understanding, procedures and vaccines were developed to limit the spread of infectious disease within a population, and antibiotics were created to help limit the growth and spread of pathologic organisms within the human body. Because of vaccinations, a much smaller portion of the world population today is affected by infectious disease than has been affected in historical times. The Bill and Melinda Gates Foundation has provided millions of dollars for vaccinations across the world, mostly in third-world countries where the death rate from many preventable diseases is still high. The tragedy of Hurricane Katrina in 2005 points to the devastation that can occur when large groups of people in crisis live in close contact under unsanitary conditions. Caring for victims who were trapped by sewage-filled waters carried a great risk to both survivors and rescuers.

In the United States, government agencies and professional associations such as the Centers for Disease Control and Prevention (CDC) and the Association for Professionals in Infection Control and Epidemiology (APIC) maintain national standards for disease prevention and treatment based on careful research. APIC and the American Public Health Association (APHA) are involved in training communicable disease specialists. In addition, most state licensing agencies and healthcare accrediting agencies publish standards of care for the management of infection and disease prevention within organizations. The Occupational Safety and Health Administration (OSHA) also has regulations that protect the worker in the workplace from exposure to infectious materials. These regulations can be found in the OSHA manual under standard 1910.1030 (Bloodborne Pathogens). Organizations that do not comply with OSHA's basic safety standards can be fined.

Infections and infectious disease processes play a prominent role in the management of quality and performance in every healthcare facility, whether it is an acute care hospital, a residential care facility, or a community day-care program for senior citizens. Consumers who hear about HAIs in facilities may be concerned about receiving services from those agencies. Patients who acquire an infection while hospitalized may spread the word about their experience to their families, friends, neighbors, and co-workers. Clearly, the infectious disease experience in healthcare facilities is of paramount importance in terms of its effect on patients' lives, costs of care, and a healthcare facility's reputation and accreditation status. If a patient is admitted for a minor procedure and dies from infection-related complications, the consequences to the facility carry beyond a bad patient outcome.

The Joint Commission has included unexpected deaths or unanticipated major loss of function from nosocomial (healthcare acquired) infections as sentinel events, which require review with use of a tool such as a credible root-cause analysis. This is such an important issue that the Joint Commission (2011a) established a National Patient Safety Goal (NPSG) to address the concern. Goal #7 is to reduce the risk of HAIs. Certainly, a death from an unexpected infection that occurred during hospitalization would fit this definition. The use of this approach is patient focused and evaluates systems and processes as well as disease clusters, providing a more balanced assessment of the cause of infection or death.

Because of the potential for rapid spread of infection in a healthcare setting, it is critical to have a team in place that can prevent or control the acquisition and transmission of infectious agents. This team must have the ability to move rapidly and assume its own authority to regulate care and employ resources if there is an influx of contagious patients. The governing board is required to determine and verify qualifications for an infection control (IC) team leader (frequently a doctor or epidemiologist) and ensure that the appropriate resources are granted to the leader and team so that the goals for the IC plan in the facility can be met. The governing board reviews the IC data on a quarterly basis and annually reviews the IC plan and goals for the year.

The IC team must report data to several agencies. All states have a health department with a division that is required to track and record communicable diseases. When a patient is diagnosed with one of the diseases from the health department's communicable disease list, the IC team must notify the public health department. (See figure 9.1 for a sample list.)

Figure 9.1.   Sample list of reportable diseases to public health departments

Definition

Reportable diseases are diseases considered to be of great public health importance. Local, state, and national agencies (for example, the Centers for Disease Control and Prevention) require that such diseases be reported when they are diagnosed by doctors or laboratories. This permits surveillance (that is, the collection of statistics on the frequency with which the disease occurs), which in turn allows these agencies to identify trends in disease occurrence as well as disease outbreaks.

Information

All states have a "reportable diseases" list. Although it is up to each state to decide which diseases are reportable, most of these lists are similar, with only a few variations depending on geographical location. The diseases are divided into several groups:

- Mandatory written reporting. Examples are gonorrhea and salmonellosis.
- Mandatory reporting by telephone. Examples are rubeola (measles) and pertussis (whooping cough).
- Report of total number of cases. Examples are chickenpox and influenza.
- Cancer. This is reported to the state cancer registry (not all states have cancer registries).

A typical state list may appear as follows:

Acquired immunodeficiency syndrome (AIDS)
Amebiasis
Anthrax*
Botulism*
Brucellosis
Campylobacteriosis
Cancer***
Chancroid
Chickenpox**
Chlamydial infections
Cholera*
Coccidioidomycosis
Colorado tick fever
Diphtheria*
Echinococcosis
Encephalitis (postinfectious, arthropodborne, and unspecified)
Foodborne illness, including food poisoning
Giardiasis
Gonococcal ophthalmia neonatorum
Gonorrhea
Granuloma inguinale
Hemophilus influenza, invasive disease (all serotypes)
Hepatitis A
Hepatitis B, cases and carriers
Hepatitis, other viral: Type C
Influenza**
Legionellosis
Leprosy

Figure 9.1.   *(Continued)*

Leptospirosis
Lymphogranuloma venereum
Malaria
Meningitis, aseptic and bacterial
Meningococcemia
Mumps**
Pelvic inflammatory disease
Pertussis*
Plague*
Poliomyelitis*
Q-fever
Rabies (human and animal)*
Relapsing fever (tickborne and louseborne)
Rheumatic fever
Rocky Mountain spotted fever
Rubella
Rubella, congenital syndrome
Rubeola*
Salmonellosis
Shigellosis
Staphylococcal diseases**
Syphilis
Tetanus*
Toxic shock syndrome
Trichinosis
Tuberculosis
Tularemia
Typhoid*, cases and carriers
Typhus*
Yellow fever*

*Telephone reporting required

**Report total cases only

***Cancer should be reported to (state) cancer registry

The state health department will attempt to find the source of many of these illnesses, such as food poisoning or amebiasis. In the case of sexually transmitted diseases, the state will attempt to locate sexual contacts to ensure they are disease-free or are appropriately treated if they are already infected.

The information obtained by reporting allows the state to make informed decisions and laws concerning activities and the environment, such as food handling, water purification, insect control, animal control, sexually transmitted disease (STD) tracking, and immunization programs.

The healthcare provider is bound by law to report these events. People with any of the diseases listed in the state's reporting schedule should make every effort to cooperate with the state health workers. Cooperation may help locate the source of an infection or prevent the spread of an epidemic.

Source: Dugdale et al. 2011.

The CDC is another agency that offers guidelines and disease management assistance to all healthcare facilities. Most IC plans have the CDC's protocol for hand washing as the key element of training and prevention.

In summary, the management of infectious disease is an organization-wide performance issue that involves every area of the facility and affects every employee, medical staff member, patient or client, and visitor. In most facilities, a multidisciplinary approach to infection management involves the patient's physician, a pharmacist, an epidemiologist, a clinical laboratory staff member, the patient's nurse or case manager, and the patient and family. The goal is to initiate appropriate treatment, which usually involves administering an appropriate antibiotic medication prescribed in an effective dosage. A certified professional, such as an epidemiologist trained to evaluate the appropriateness of infection management measures, may be assigned to review unusual cases of infection. For a more in-depth discussion of the complexities of tracking and managing HAIs in healthcare facilities, see CDC (2010).

Managing Infectious Disease: Steps to Success

Institutional settings are prime locations for transmission of communicable infections since they bring susceptible individuals together in one place. IC, surveillance, and management become critical to patient safety and wellness and can be performed in a variety of ways. In some facilities, an IC committee composed of physicians, nurses, and clinical laboratory staff performs weekly reviews of the facility-wide incidence of infectious disease. In others, one individual (or a specialized department of skilled staff, depending on the size of the organization), with training and expertise, is specifically assigned to infection surveillance and control and is authorized by the governing board of the organization to institute any measures needed to prevent the spread of infection. In large facilities, a physician usually heads this committee. In smaller organizations, a consulting physician or epidemiologist may provide clinical oversight. The number, competency, and skill mix of the IC staff are determined by the goals and objectives of the IC activities. The IC committee meets monthly to evaluate risks for the infectious diseases in the facility and to establish priorities and strategies for management of the risks. The committee reviews the data collected regarding IC and reports the information to the quality council. The IC performance data are reported on a quarterly basis to the leadership council as well as the governing body. Staff members involved in IC generally are licensed, such as registered nurses, physicians, epidemiologists, and pharmacists, or are certified laboratory technicians.

Data reporting for IC usually includes data related to HAIs, community-acquired infections, antibiotic usage, culture reports, immunization data, employee illness, bloodborne pathogen exposures, and staff and patient IC education. The goal of the reporting procedure is to identify any trends in infection and to develop effective strategies to reduce the risk of infections to patients, employees, volunteers, and families and visitors.

Infection management should be based on a written plan that is developed by the facility's clinical staff and that has clearly defined goals for the prevention and control of infectious diseases in the facility. The plan should be specific to that facility's identified and prioritized risks for acquiring and transmitting infections based on geographic location, community, and population served, as well as the care, treatment, and services it provides. The goals include limiting unprotected exposure to pathogens; limiting the transmission of infections associated with procedures; and limiting the transmission of infections associated with the use of medical equipment, devices, and supplies. Another important goal is improving compliance with hand hygiene guidelines. It should include methods of surveillance and tracking of infections in all hospital components and functions such as medical surgical units, dietary services, newborn nurseries, and clinical laboratories. The plan should address major communicable diseases that affect the facility's client population, such as tuberculosis, MDROs, community-acquired pneumonia (CAP), hepatitis B and C, and human immunodeficiency virus (HIV). In addition, the plan should outline the types of routine surveillance and procedures the organization will undertake to limit the transmission of infectious agents among licensed independent practitioners, patients, staff, and visitors and families. This plan should be established on "evidence-based" national guidelines or expert consensus.

Step 1: Control Infection through the Use of Standard Precautions

The mandate of applying standard precautions in healthcare services has been the cornerstone of IC since the 1980s. **Standard precautions** can be defined as the use of infection prevention and control measures to protect against possible exposure to infectious agents. The concept behind these general precautions is that every individual encountered in the healthcare setting should be treated as if he or she may have an active **bloodborne pathogen** disease. Bloodborne pathogens such as HIV and hepatitis B and C are transported through contact with infected body fluids such as blood, semen, and vomitus. The precautions are described as standard because any individual may potentially be infected or could potentially infect others. Each facility should define the employee level of risk for infection associated with their job classification and define the proper precautions needed to prevent exposure.

Transmission-based precautions, one aspect of standard precautions, are measures to protect against exposure to a suspected or identified pathogen based on the way the pathogen is transmitted. Vectors for transmission of infections include direct contact, droplet, airborne, insect-borne, or any combination of these. These precautions apply specifically to diseases such as tuberculosis, Vancomycin-resistant pneumonia, and SARS. Information regarding these precautions may be accessed at http://www.cdc.gov.

The Joint Commission's NPSG to reduce the risk of HAIs includes the following requirements:

- Comply with current hand hygiene guidelines of the World Health Organization (WHO) or the CDC

- Implement guidelines to prevent infections that are difficult to treat

- Implement guidelines to prevent central-line-associated bloodstream infections

- Implement safe practices for preventing surgical site infections (Joint Commission 2011a)

Standard precautions require that caregivers be educated about proper hand-washing techniques, including appropriate types of hand cleansers and proper hand-washing procedure. Proper hand washing has been identified by the CDC as one of the single most important methods for preventing the spread of infection. Employees should wash their hands between patients and wear gloves when they examine patients and administer thera-pies. Caregivers also must wear gloves, gowns, masks, and eye protection whenever they perform procedures that disrupt the patient's skin or mucous membranes. Standard pre-cautions assume that all patients carry infectious disease agents. Therefore, barriers are erected between patients and between patients and caregivers when blood or body fluids are involved in any way.

Step 2: Conduct Ongoing Infection Surveillance and Epidemiologic Investigations

A: Healthcare-Associated versus Community-Acquired Infections

Within the healthcare facility, any occurrence of infection should be evaluated to determine whether the infection was nosocomial (healthcare associated) or community acquired. A **healthcare-associated infection** is an infection occurring in a patient in a hospital or healthcare setting in whom the infection was not present or incubating at the time of admission, or the remainder of an infection acquired during a previous admission. A **community-acquired infection** is an infection that was present in the patient before he or she was admitted to a healthcare facility.

Specific guidelines have been developed to determine whether an infection is health-care acquired or community acquired. For example, if a child was admitted to a hospital with a fever and within 24 hours measles developed, this disease would be considered community acquired. The incubation period for measles is at least 14 days; therefore, it can be determined that the patient's exposure to the disease occurred prior to admission. If, however, a patient was admitted for treatment of an intervertebral disk injury and then a urinary tract infection with fever developed several days after undergoing surgery, the infection was probably acquired while the patient was hospitalized. This infection would be classified as an HAI, especially if a urinalysis done prior to surgery did not demonstrate indicators for infection at that time.

Both of these instances of infectious disease would be tracked and reported to the Per-formance Improvement and Patient Safety Council and to the required state agency, but for different reasons. The measles would be tracked to document that the facility's staff took appropriate action to prevent exposure to other patients. The urinary tract infection would be tracked to document initiation of appropriate treatment interventions and to identify any presurgical measures that might be taken to prevent such infections in the future.

The National Nosocomial Infections Surveillance (NNIS) system is a data collection organization that provides comparative data regarding rates for HAIs and their associated risk factors and pathogens. The CDC's Division of Healthcare Quality Promotion manages the NNIS system. The CDC Web site provides a descriptive list of HAIs.

It is important to track HAI rates for each area of the facility that works with patients. Rates of HAI vary greatly depending on the nursing unit and the types of patients for whom care is provided. For example, a look at central vascular catheter-related bloodstream infec-tions (CR-BSIs) in the intensive care setting shows rates varying from 2.1 per 1,000 central catheter days in the respiratory intensive care unit (ICU) to 30.2 per 1,000 central catheter days in the burn ICU (Jarvis, et. al., 1991). Other types of procedures commonly associated with HAI that should be tracked include the use of indwelling urinary catheters, surgical wounds, and mechanical ventilation devices.

Decubitus ulcers and surgical site infections are often associated with hospital care. Other possible sources of HAIs include exposure to clinical or nonclinical staff who may carry infectious diseases, substandard surgical or postsurgical care, noncompliance with standard precautions, and improper equipment sterilization techniques.

B: Surveillance of Employee Health and Illness

A different aspect of infection surveillance involves employee health and illness tracking. Employees are a critical vector for bringing community-acquired infections into health-care settings. Policies related to the tracking of employee absences exist for the specific purpose of preventing infection via healthcare workers. Reports of absences are tabulated and examined for any possible connection to cases of HAI. Employees who are absent from work for infection-related reasons are asked to verify their fitness for duty by bringing in a clearance from a treating physician or clinic. The Joint Commission has added new standards addressing employee or patient exposure to infectious diseases. These new standards make provisions for screening, assessment, testing, immunization, prophylaxis or treatment, or counseling for patients or staff members who have been exposed to an infectious disease in the hospital. An additional set of standards for employees requires an annual influenza vaccination program that offers education about the vaccine; nonvaccine control and prevention measures; and the diagnosis, transmission, and impact of influenza. There is a requirement for on-site vaccinations at sites accessible to staff and licensed independent practitioners (LIPs). Part of the PI aspect of this program is that the facility must evaluate staff vaccination rates and reasons given by staff for declining vaccinations (for example, the cost of the vaccine or fear of infection developing from the vaccine) (Joint Commission 2011b, IC-12, IC 02.04.01).

C: Surveillance of the Facility Vaccine Program

The key areas for surveillance are developing and implementing protocols for flu vaccine and pneumococcus vaccine administration and documentation, and implementing a protocol to identify new cases of influenza and ways to manage an outbreak. The Department of Health and Human Services (HHS) has developed a pandemic flu plan for use if the country has a flu epidemic. Each state health department must develop its own plan, and each facility's IC plan must include how it will manage an influx of flu patients who might need isolation and intensive care.

Most healthcare facilities require employee job descriptions to carry a definition of bloodborne pathogen risk associated with the job tasks. Employees in high-risk categories are required to have hepatitis B vaccinations. This vaccination is a three-part series that will accord the employee some degree of protection from exposure to hepatitis B. Documentation of employees' bloodborne exposures and tracking of the follow-up procedures are other aspects of employee health data collection, as is annual tuberculosis testing for all employees.

D: Surveillance of the Healthcare Environment

Monitoring the care environment is another aspect of infection surveillance. Facilities that have laboratories on-site must meet standards for safety and IC through a rigorous inspection process since these areas perform very high-risk procedures and deal with infectious body fluids and tissue samples regularly. Most laboratories have to be nationally certified to provide credible services to healthcare facilities. In many facilities, specimens from patient care areas are cultured monthly to identify any pathological bacteria growing in the care environment. The cultures are reported and tracked. When the presence of a significant infectious agent is identified, another specimen is cultured after the area has been cleaned to determine whether the area was sufficiently disinfected.

Many healthcare facilities have a team of providers who regularly inspect all areas in the facility for health and safety issues. The IC team usually provides someone to assist with identifying potential areas of concern related to IC, such as patient care rooms, laundry rooms, bathrooms, central supply areas, laboratory areas, the pharmacy, and food service areas. Results from these inspections are reported through the Infection Control Committee along with any necessary corrective actions.

E: Surveillance of Food Preparation Areas

The cleanliness of food preparation and service areas is also tracked, and records are kept to document that all local and state regulations regarding safe food-handling procedures are being followed. The training and safety performance of food service staff is also documented. Most food service and preparation areas in facilities must be inspected and certified annually by the state department of health. Records of cleaning are documented daily.

Food temperatures and refrigerator temperatures are tracked daily, as are records of the cleaning of food preparation and service areas. Refrigerators containing medications are kept separate from refrigerators containing food, and temperature logs must be kept for medication refrigerators as well.

Kitchen areas also are required to record water temperatures of dishwashing machines. Food that is received must be dated and stored in rodent-proof containers, and a rotating stock is tracked to prevent food spoilage.

The IC committee approves all substances used for cleaning in the facility. In many facilities, the IC coordinator conducts monthly environmental rounds to look for areas of noncompliance with standards. The governing body that grants authority for IC measures in an agency or facility may also review the results of the monthly rounds along with any actions for improvement suggested by the committee.

Step 3: Conduct Educational and Screening Programs

An effective IC program routinely evaluates all the means of transmission of infection throughout the facility and develops educational programs that promote disease prevention. These programs include tuberculosis testing, hand-washing campaigns, influenza vaccination programs, hepatitis B vaccinations for high-risk employees, sterile technique in-services, and needlestick prevention programs. Education on standard precautions is mandatory for all employees in healthcare facilities and frequently occurs before the employee is allowed access to the work environment, to ensure both the employee's and potential patients' safety.

Tracking exposures to bloodborne pathogens such as HIV is required by all states and is outlined in OSHA (29 CFR 1910.1030) regulations, which require the monitoring of employees after exposure for at least one year, with HIV testing at 1 month, 6 months, and 12 months postexposure. HIV testing and screening for employees known to have been exposed to HIV require the informed consent of individual employees. OSHA also mandates that specific education on the risks and outcomes of testing be provided to employees by a certified HIV instructor or physician.

When state law requires the facility to report positive test results to the state department of health, the employee involved must be notified ahead of time. Many state departments of health provide programs to test, treat, and educate employees, clients, and patients regarding the HIV/AIDS disease process. With the advent of new Health Insurance Portability and Accountability Act of 1996 (HIPAA) regulations, client and patient rights of protection and notification related to infectious diseases have increased. Most states require facilities to outline a tuberculosis prevention plan that involves the careful screening of employees, clients, and patients to identify those who have active tuberculosis, as well as those who may have been exposed but do not have an active disease process. Annual mandatory testing of workers is required by state licensing agencies as an occupational safety measure for employees, but testing of patients and clients varies considerably from state to state. Often the testing of patients and clients is required in long-term rehabilitative settings. The tuberculosis plan for most facilities outlines the testing process; training and education of staff, clients, and patients; and required treatment interventions. Monthly reporting of the number of employees tested and the number of employees who convert to positive is required in many states. A positive tuberculin (TB) test result must be reported to the department of health in all states. A positive TB test requires an x-ray to further delineate whether there is active tuberculosis or simply exposure to the bacteria. Individuals who test positive may be required to wear a mask until a chest x-ray can be completed and results are known. If there is no active disease present in the lungs (the first site of possible infection in the body), the test-positive individual will be referred to his or her private doctor or the public health department for follow-up and may be placed on antibiotics specific to TB. The usual course of treatment varies from four to nine months, depending on age and exposure. This individual is not capable of exposing others to TB since the disease is not in active form. Once an individual has received antibiotic treatment for TB, he or she should never be retested. Subsequent testing of the individual can lead to potentially harmful local reactions to the skin where he or she is tested. An annual x-ray to ensure that there is no active disease is the usual standard for evaluation.

An individual with a positive chest x-ray will be immediately referred to a hospital for further sputum testing and treatment. This individual will require intense treatment in a negative pressure room that is isolated from others to prevent airborne transmission of the disease.

Some states that have populations at high risk for tuberculosis are now requiring a two-step testing process. This involves a skin test for tuberculosis followed by a second test seven days later to confirm a negative result. Positive results are followed up with a chest x-ray. The state department of health can help any facility determine whether it serves clients who are at high risk for tuberculosis. Such facilities should institute two-step testing. Facilities that treat patients with active tuberculosis also should provide negative-pressure rooms specially designed for the treatment of tuberculosis to prevent the airborne transmission of the disease.

Real-Life Example

At one time, Marilyn Nelson, RN, RHIA, worked as the nurse manager of the outpatient clinics at the Western States University Hospital. She was responsible for managing PI activities in the clinics, facilitating PI teams, and supporting PI activities with the various resources available to her. At that time, the medical center had recently embarked on a benchmarking program. Benchmarking, discussed in chapter 2, is the systematic comparison of one organization's outcomes or processes with the outcomes or processes of similar organizations.

Marilyn and some of her colleagues began the benchmarking process by comparing the outcomes of the clinic's patients with published information on the outcomes of other organizations and with clinical trends apparent in the literature. In the course of examining pharmacy and therapeutics data, Marilyn and her clinical colleagues recognized that their organization appeared to be treating a significantly higher number of urinary tract infections (UTIs) than other, similar organizations. To identify the reason for the apparent discrepancy, the team first examined the published literature on the frequency of UTIs in ambulatory care practice. Next, they contacted clinicians at other ambulatory care centers in the country to gather information on their experiences. The team's investigations confirmed that, while the sex-specific distribution of the incidence of UTI was similar to other institutions (mostly occurring in females), the overall incidence was significantly higher at Western States University Hospital than at any of the other medical centers contacted. The situation appeared to provide an excellent PI opportunity—the kind of improvement that clinicians would see as important and valuable to patients as well as one that had important cost implications for the organization.

Marilyn convened a PI team, which included the director of the outpatient pharmacy, the director of the outpatient clinic laboratories, and leaders of the nursing teams from each of the ambulatory clinics in which patients with UTIs were commonly treated: internal medicine, family practice, obstetrics/gynecology, urology, general surgery, and pediatrics.

The team's initial discussion of the situation revealed the complexity of the processes in place to evaluate urinary tract function. Because the clinics are affiliated with a major university medical center, a number of caregivers might be involved in any one patient's care. First, there were the attending physicians from a variety of specialties and areas of expertise. Next, there were the nurses and medical assistants in each clinic. Because the medical center was a teaching facility, there also were any number of house staff rotating through the clinics on a monthly basis. Finally, there were the technicians who performed urinalysis procedures in the clinical laboratory. Where, when, and by whom a patient's urinalysis was performed could take any one of a number of paths in the organization.

Marilyn and her colleagues decided to develop flow charts for the various care paths. (See figures 9.2 through 9.6.) They collected data on the outcomes of each of the paths to see whether they could identify the organization's true experience with UTIs.

QI Toolbox Technique

The use of **flow charts** allows a PI team to examine the process under investigation from all directions. The technique makes it possible for the team to gather the most important details so that everyone on the team can understand the process and its contributing subprocesses in the same way. When a flow chart is well designed, few misconceptions can survive.

Flow charts are used to represent standard functions within processes. Following is a discussion of representative and commonly used **icons**:

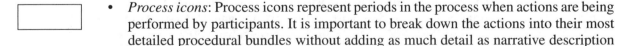

- *Process icons*: Process icons represent periods in the process when actions are being performed by participants. It is important to break down the actions into their most detailed procedural bundles without adding as much detail as narrative description would include. For example, in Marilyn Nelson's first flow chart, the first process icon reads "Nurse triage of patient needs." The concept of triage is represented by the icon, but the description does not specify all the steps that the nurse would have to go through to triage a patient.

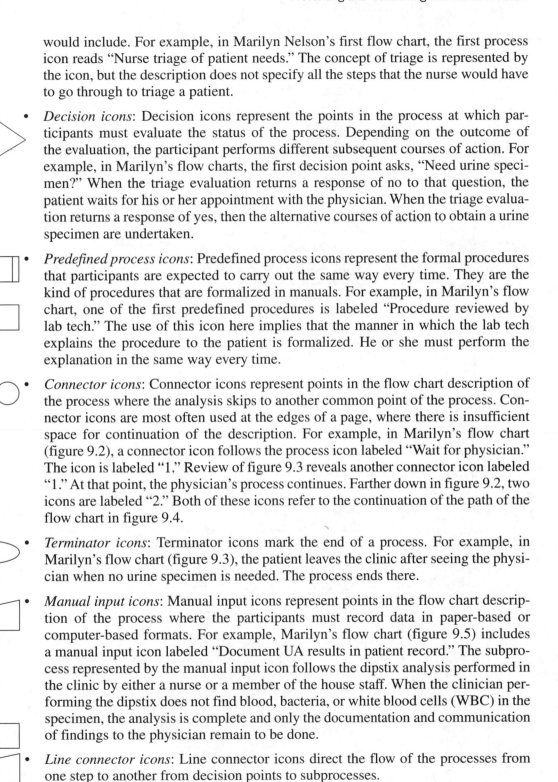

- *Decision icons*: Decision icons represent the points in the process at which participants must evaluate the status of the process. Depending on the outcome of the evaluation, the participant performs different subsequent courses of action. For example, in Marilyn's flow charts, the first decision point asks, "Need urine specimen?" When the triage evaluation returns a response of no to that question, the patient waits for his or her appointment with the physician. When the triage evaluation returns a response of yes, then the alternative courses of action to obtain a urine specimen are undertaken.

- *Predefined process icons*: Predefined process icons represent the formal procedures that participants are expected to carry out the same way every time. They are the kind of procedures that are formalized in manuals. For example, in Marilyn's flow chart, one of the first predefined procedures is labeled "Procedure reviewed by lab tech." The use of this icon here implies that the manner in which the lab tech explains the procedure to the patient is formalized. He or she must perform the explanation in the same way every time.

- *Connector icons*: Connector icons represent points in the flow chart description of the process where the analysis skips to another common point of the process. Connector icons are most often used at the edges of a page, where there is insufficient space for continuation of the description. For example, in Marilyn's flow chart (figure 9.2), a connector icon follows the process icon labeled "Wait for physician." The icon is labeled "1." Review of figure 9.3 reveals another connector icon labeled "1." At that point, the physician's process continues. Farther down in figure 9.2, two icons are labeled "2." Both of these icons refer to the continuation of the path of the flow chart in figure 9.4.

- *Terminator icons*: Terminator icons mark the end of a process. For example, in Marilyn's flow chart (figure 9.3), the patient leaves the clinic after seeing the physician when no urine specimen is needed. The process ends there.

- *Manual input icons*: Manual input icons represent points in the flow chart description of the process where the participants must record data in paper-based or computer-based formats. For example, Marilyn's flow chart (figure 9.5) includes a manual input icon labeled "Document UA results in patient record." The subprocess represented by the manual input icon follows the dipstix analysis performed in the clinic by either a nurse or a member of the house staff. When the clinician performing the dipstix does not find blood, bacteria, or white blood cells (WBC) in the specimen, the analysis is complete and only the documentation and communication of findings to the physician remain to be done.

- *Line connector icons*: Line connector icons direct the flow of the processes from one step to another from decision points to subprocesses.

Figure 9.2.   Example of a flow chart—page 1

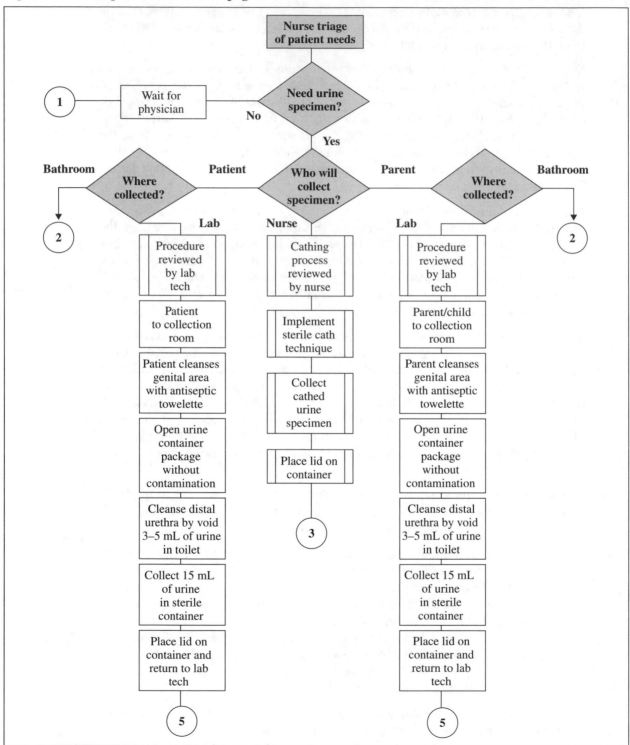

Figure 9.3.   Example of a flow chart—page 2

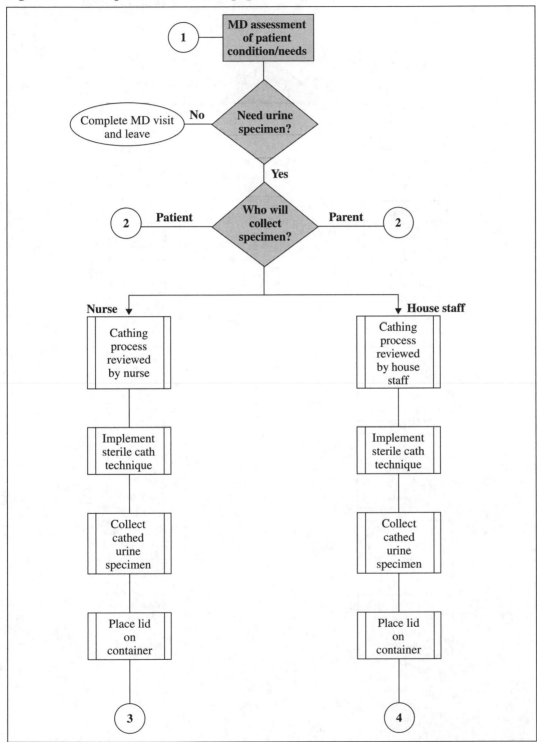

Figure 9.4.   Example of a flow chart—page 3

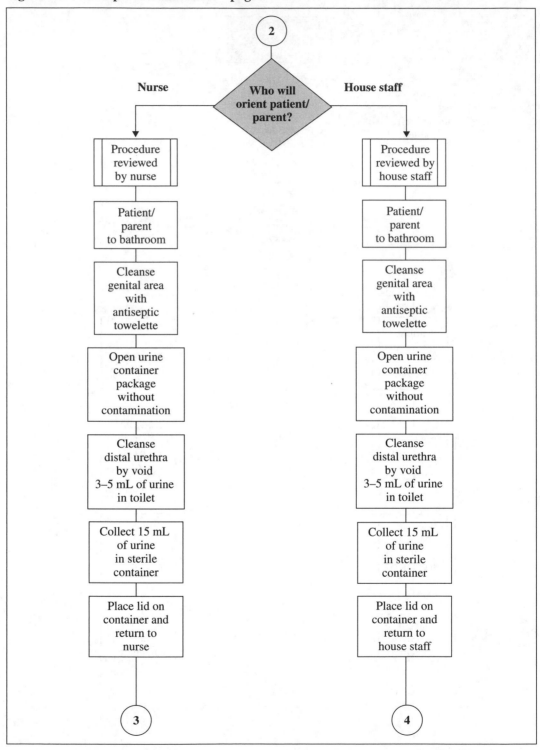

Figure 9.5.   Example of a flow chart—page 4

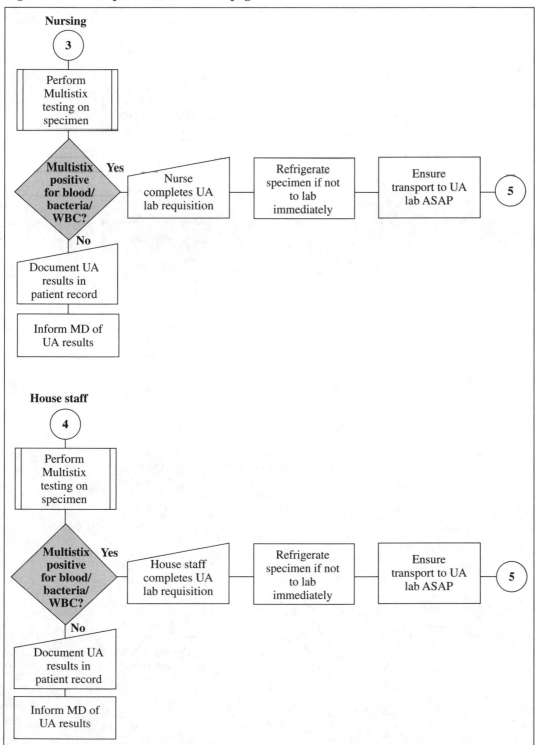

Figure 9.6.   Example of a flow chart—page 5

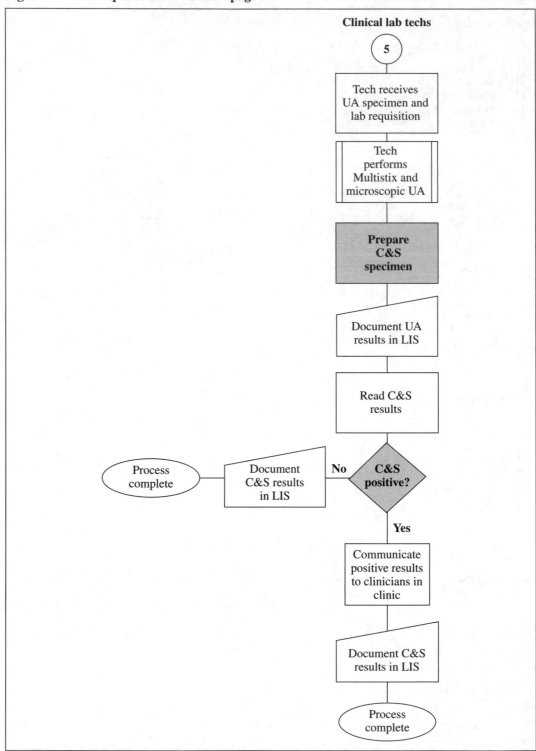

Case Study

The case study for this chapter is a continuation of Marilyn Nelson's investigation of the UTI issue in the ambulatory clinics of the Western States University Hospital.

After flowcharting the process for collecting urine specimens (depicted in figures 9.2 through 9.6), Marilyn and her colleagues recognized how complex the issue was within their organization. They decided to collect data from all process paths evident in the flow chart. Because so many people were involved in the processes and because significant delays could be involved, they also began to wonder what part contaminated specimens played in the situation.

Although it was an expensive project, the team designed an investigative study to collect data. Urine specimens were routinely tested by nursing personnel or house staff in the clinic to determine each specimen's pH and specific gravity and to classify each specimen according to its color, clarity, and presence of gross hematuria. Each specimen was then tested with Multistix to determine whether microscopic bacteria, red blood cells, or WBCs were present. When a specimen failed any of the Multistix screens, it was referred to Clinical Laboratory Services for microscopic analysis, culture, and sensitivity analysis by a laboratory technician.

First, the team collected data regarding time elapsed between collection of the specimen, point-of-care testing with Multistix, and receipt of the specimen in Clinical Laboratory Services. In addition, the team investigated the sequence of events that occurred in the interim. A summary of the data collected is provided in table 9.1.

Second, on a temporary and random basis, the team obtained urine specimens from each clinic immediately following collection and had a complete analysis performed STAT in the clinic labs. This analysis identified pH, specific gravity, color, clarity, cell counts, and bacterial counts almost immediately after the specimen was delivered by the patient or collecting clinician. All specimens that showed microscopic bacteria either on Multistix or on microscopic analysis were cultured. A summary of the data collected is provided in table 9.2.

Third, the team compared the incidence of UTI identified in the randomly collected specimens with the incidence identified in specimens going through the usual process. A summary of the data collected is provided in table 9.3.

Questions for Case Study

1. Upon examination of the data sets, Marilyn Nelson and her colleagues identified several areas where the analysis revealed situations that were probably contributing to the clinic's high UTI rate. Look at the UTI rate for children whose parents had collected the specimen versus the rate for children who had been catheterized by nursing personnel to collect the specimen. What do you see? What might be the reason for the higher rate in children whose parents had collected the specimen?

2. Are there any other areas in the data that reveal important aspects that may be contributing to the high UTI rates? What might be the reasons for these higher rates?

3. Upon discussion of the findings and examination of the flowcharted processes, the laboratory manager noted a subtle change in clinic processes that probably was contributing to the problem. House staff had begun at some point to Multistix the

Table 9.1.   Average time to point-of-care screening with confidence intervals (in minutes)

Point-of-Care Training & Processing	Internal Medicine Clinic	Pediatrics Clinic	General Surgery Clinic	Orthopedic Surgery Clinic	Obstetrics Clinic	Gynecology Clinic	Specialty Clinic
Nurse	5.0 (4.0, 6.0)	4.25 (3.0, 5.5)	6.25 (5.0, 7.5)	6.0 (5.0, 7.0)	3.25 (2.75, 3.75)	3.0 (2.0, 4.0)	3.0 (2.0, 4.0)
House staff	10.0 (7.0, 13.0)	8.0 (6.0, 10.0)	12.13 (10.0, 14.25)	11.0 (9.0, 13.0)	6.5 (4.0, 9.0)	6.0 (4.0, 8.0)	7.5 (5.5, 9.5)

Table 9.2.   Random STAT processing of clean-catch/cath urine specimens (percentage of positive specimens for culture)

Collector	Internal Medicine Clinic	Pediatrics Clinic	General Surgery Clinic	Orthopedic Surgery Clinic	Obstetrics Clinic	Gynecology Clinic	Specialty Clinic
Nurse or patient	5.6	13.2	4.2	3.4	7.0	3.9	5.7
House staff or patient	4.2	12.1	3.4	5.2	6.8	4.2	6.2
Parent	—	27.5	11.7	9.0	—	25.2	—

Table 9.3.   Routine processing of clean-catch/cath specimens (percentage of positive specimens for culture)

Collector	Internal Medicine Clinic	Pediatrics Clinic	General Surgery Clinic	Orthopedic Surgery Clinic	Obstetrics Clinic	Gynecology Clinic	Specialty Clinic
Nurse or patient	5.7	12.4	5.1	4.1	7.2	4.1	5.2
House staff or patient	36.8	25.6	10.2	8.7	10.0	9.2	14.2
Parent	—	25.6	12.2	8.0	—	23.0	—

specimens in the original collection containers. Thus, what had been a clean-catch specimen could become a contaminated one when staff opened the container to perform the Multistix. What really should have been done was to pour off a small amount or *aliquot* of the specimen into another container, reseal the original container for the laboratory, and perform the Multistix on the aliquot container. This process would minimize the possibility of contaminating the original specimen. How would this change in process be represented in the flow charts presented in the case study?

Project Application

Students should consider using flow chart techniques in their projects.

Summary

The management of infectious disease is an organization-wide performance issue that involves every area of the facility and affects every employee, patient, and visitor. The ability of individuals to perform their jobs depends on how carefully IC is managed in the facility. Facility IC also affects the ability of patients to recover as rapidly as possible without complications. Means by which the impact of infection is limited in healthcare organizations include use of standard precautions, infection surveillance procedures, appropriate treatment regimens, and staff and patient screening.

References

29 CFR 1910.1030: OSHA regulation on bloodborne pathogens. 1992.

Centers for Disease Control and Prevention. 2010. http://www.cdc.gov/hai/.

Centers for Disease Control and Prevention. 2011. Hand hygiene guidelines fact sheet. http://www.paramounthealthcare.com/documents/safety/hand-hygiene-fact-sheet.pdf.

Directors of Health Promotion and Education. 2005. Addressing infectious disease threats. http://www.dhpe.org/infectintro.asp.

Dugdale, D., J. Vyas, and D. Zieve. 2011. Reportable diseases. Medline Plus. http://www.nlm.nih.gov/medlineplus/ency/article/001929.htm.

Jarvis WR, Edwards JR, Culver DH, Hughes JM, Horan T, Emori TG, Banerjee S, Tolson J, Henderson T, Gaynes RP. 1991. Nosocomial infection rates in adult and pediatric intensive care units in the United States. National Nosocomial Infections Surveillance System. The American Journal Of Medicine, 1991 Sep 16; Vol. 91 (3B), pp. 185S-191S; PMID: 1928163

Joint Commission. 2011a. National Patient Safety Goals. *Hospital Accreditation Standards*. Oakbrook Terrace, IL: Joint Commission Resources.

Joint Commission. 2011b. *Hospital Accreditation Standards*. Oakbrook Terrace, IL: Joint Commission Resources.

Klevens, R.M., J.R. Edwards, C.L. Richards, Jr., T.C. Horan, R.P. Gaynes, D.A. Pollock, and D.M. Cardo. 2007. Estimating health care–associated infections and deaths in U.S. hospitals, 2002. *Public Health Reports* 122:160–166.

Resources

ADAM. 2011. Medical encyclopedia. http://www.nlm.nih.gov/medlineplus/ency/article/001929.htm.

Arias, K.M. 2010. *Outbreak Investigation and Control in Health Care Settings*, 2nd ed. Sudbury, MA: Jones & Bartlett.

Atkinson, W., L.K. Pickering, B. Schwartz, B.G. Weniger, J.K. Islander, and J.C. Watson. 2002. http://www.cdc.gov/mmwr/preview/mmwrhtml/rr5102a1.htm.

Benneyan, J.C. 1998. Statistical quality control methods in infection control and hospital epidemiology, part I: Introduction and basic theory. *Infectious Control and Hospital Epidemiology* 19(3):194–214 (review).

Centers for Disease Control and Prevention. 2011. Healthcare-associated infections. http://www.cdc.gov/hai/.

Health Insurance Portability and Accountability Act of 1996. Public Law 104-191.

Joint Commission. 2011. National Patient Safety Goals. http://www.jointcommission.org/standards_information/npsgs.aspx.

Appendix to Chapter 9

Hand Hygiene Guidelines Fact Sheet

- Improved adherence to hand hygiene (i.e. hand washing or use of alcohol-based hand rubs) has been shown to terminate outbreaks in health care facilities, to reduce transmission of antimicrobial resistant organisms (e.g. methicillin resistant staphylococcus aureus) and reduce overall infection rates.

- CDC is releasing guidelines to improve adherence to hand hygiene in health care settings. In addition to traditional handwashing with soap and water, CDC is recommending the use of alcohol-based handrubs by health care personnel for patient care because they address some of the obstacles that health care professionals face when taking care of patients.

- Handwashing with soap and water remains a sensible strategy for hand hygiene in non-health care settings and is recommended by CDC and other experts.

- When health care personnel's hands are visibly soiled, they should wash with soap and water.

- The use of gloves does not eliminate the need for hand hygiene. Likewise, the use of hand hygiene does not eliminate the need for gloves. Gloves reduce hand contamination by 70 percent to 80 percent, prevent cross-contamination, and protect patients and health care personnel from infection. Handrubs should be used before and after each patient just as gloves should be changed before and after each patient.

- When using an alcohol-based handrub, apply product to palm of one hand and rub hands together, covering all surfaces of hands and fingers, until hands are dry. Note that the volume needed to reduce the number of bacteria on hands varies by product.

- Alcohol-based handrubs significantly reduce the number of microorganisms on skin, are fast acting, and cause less skin irritation.

- Health care personnel should avoid wearing artificial nails and keep natural nails less than one quarter of an inch long if they care for patients at high risk of acquiring infections (e.g. patients in intensive care units or in transplant units).

- When evaluating hand hygiene products for potential use in health care facilities, administrators or product selection committees should consider the relative efficacy of antiseptic agents against various pathogens and the acceptability of hand hygiene products by personnel. Characteristics of a product that can affect acceptance and therefore usage include its smell, consistency, color and the effect of dryness on hands.

- As part of these recommendations, CDC is asking health care facilities to develop and implement a system for measuring improvements in adherence to these hand hygiene recommendations. Some of the suggested performance indicators include: periodic monitoring of hand hygiene adherence and providing feedback to personnel regarding their performance, monitoring the volume of alcohol-based handrub used/1000 patient days, monitoring adherence to policies dealing with wearing artificial nails, and focused assessment of the adequacy of health care personnel hand hygiene when outbreaks of infection occur.

- Allergic contact dermatitis due to alcohol hand rubs is very uncommon. However, with increasing use of such products by health care personnel, it is likely that true allergic reactions to such products will occasionally be encountered.

- Alcohol-based hand rubs take less time to use than traditional hand washing. In an eight-hour shift, an estimated one hour of an ICU nurse's time will be saved by using an alcohol-based handrub.

- These guidelines should not be construed to legalize product claims that are not allowed by an FDA product approval by FDA's Over-the-Counter Drug Review. The recommendations are not intended to apply to consumer use of the products discussed.

CDC protects people's health and safety by preventing and controlling diseases and injuries; enhances health decisions by providing credible information on critical health issues; and promotes healthy living through strong partnerships with local, national, and international organizations.

Source: CDC 2011.

Chapter 10
Decreasing Risk Exposure

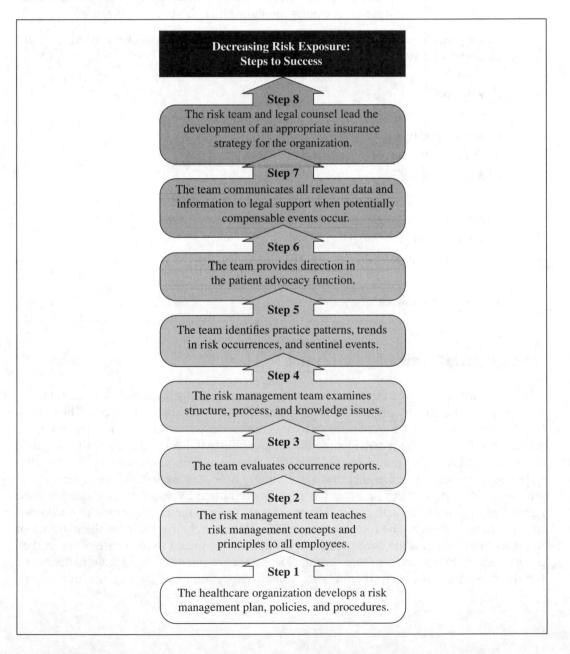

Decreasing Risk Exposure:
Steps to Success

Step 8
The risk team and legal counsel lead the development of an appropriate insurance strategy for the organization.

Step 7
The team communicates all relevant data and information to legal support when potentially compensable events occur.

Step 6
The team provides direction in the patient advocacy function.

Step 5
The team identifies practice patterns, trends in risk occurrences, and sentinel events.

Step 4
The risk management team examines structure, process, and knowledge issues.

Step 3
The team evaluates occurrence reports.

Step 2
The risk management team teaches risk management concepts and principles to all employees.

Step 1
The healthcare organization develops a risk management plan, policies, and procedures.

Learning Objectives

- To describe the importance of managing risk exposure in today's healthcare organization

- To explain the importance of using occurrence reporting to decrease risk exposure

- To define the concept of a sentinel event

- To describe how sentinel events can point to important opportunities to improve safety in healthcare organizations

- To explain how risk managers use their skills in patient advocacy to lessen the impact that potentially compensable events can have on healthcare organizations

- To emphasize the importance of National Patient Safety Goals for healthcare organizations and strategies for proactive risk reduction activities

Key Terms

Cause-and-effect diagram

Failure mode and effects analysis (FMEA)

Fishbone diagram

Incident report

Medication error

Occurrence report

Potentially compensable events (PCEs)

Risk

Root-cause analysis

Background and Significance

It is important to recognize that patients, residents, and clients have very special relationships with the healthcare organizations that provide their healthcare services. Those relationships are built on a set of mutual and very complex expectations of each other, which, when not valued by either participant in the relationship, can lead to unanticipated negative occurrences that neither really desires. For the patients, residents, and clients, the expectations are based on a set of rights that are willingly accorded by healthcare organizations with ethics-based practices and that have become codified by federal mandates for most healthcare organizations in the United States. An example of the rights commonly accorded in acute care settings can be found in figure 10.1. Note that the list includes the majority of important issues that acute care patients and their families need to be aware of when they accept care from providers in that setting. The rights are intended to educate patients and family members and to help them frame realistic expectations of the organization and its

Figure 10.1.   Example of patient rights in an acute care facility

As a patient in our organization you have the right to the following:

- Reasonable access to care and continuity of care, to the best of our ability, up to and including transfer.

- Necessary healthcare services to the best of our ability. If treatment, referral, or transfer is requested or recommended, you will be informed of risks, benefits, and alternatives. You will not be transferred until the other institution agrees to accept you.

- Care that is considerate and respectful of your personal values and beliefs.

- Privacy protection. The hospital, your physician, and others caring for you will protect your privacy as much as possible.

- Information and participation in care decisions.

- The name of the person in charge of your care.

- Complete information regarding your care and current information concerning diagnosis, treatment options, and expected outlook in terms you are able to understand. Your Medical Record is available upon request. Information can be made available to a designee on your behalf.

- Answers to ethical questions that arise in the course of your care, including issues of conflict resolution, formulating advance directives, withholding resuscitation, foregoing or withdrawal of life-sustaining treatment, participation in investigative studies or trials, and end-of-life care. This includes information about outcomes of care to include unanticipated outcomes and your right to exclude any or all family members from participating in your healthcare decisions.

- Opportunities to request or refuse treatment.

- Choice to consent to or decline to take part in research affecting your care. If you choose not to take part, you will receive the most effective care the hospital otherwise provides. If you do choose to participate, you have the right to full informed consent.

- Information about realistic care alternatives when hospital care is no longer appropriate.

- Prompt notification of your admission to a family member and your physician.

- Expert reasonable safety insofar as the hospital's practices and environment allow.

- Freedom from all forms of abuse or harassment.

- Freedom from restraints (or seclusion) of any form that are not medically necessary or are used as a means of coercion, discipline, convenience, or retaliation.

- Privacy and security to the extent consistent with adequate medical care and confidentiality of all records, except as otherwise provided by law or third-party payment contract.

- An itemized explanation of charges, regardless of source of payment.

- Disclosure about how the hospital's rules and regulations apply to your conduct.

- Reasonable response to requests for services customarily rendered by the facility and consistent with treatment.

- Recognition of advance healthcare decisions in case you are unable to communicate your wishes.

- Information about pain and pain-relief measures. Our staff will respond quickly to your pain-relief needs with state-of-the-art pain management.

- Treatment without discrimination regardless of race, color, religion, sex, national origin, source of payment, political belief, or handicap, including services for hearing and speech impairment.

- Access to patient representative to express grievances and suggestions to the organization with the assurance that grievances will be reviewed with resolution.

(Continued on next page)

Figure 10.1. *(Continued)*

- Information necessary to provide informed consent prior to any procedure and/or treatment. You may designate a decision maker in the event you are incapable of understanding a proposed treatment or to communicate your wishes regarding care.

- Access to protective services, which include assistance relative to guardianship and advocacy services, conservatorship, and child or adult protective services.

- Access to pastoral care and other spiritual services if you so desire.

- Effective communication including services for the hearing and speech impaired, without cost.

- Transfer to another health facility. The transfer is to be conducted in accordance with the Emergency Medical Treatment and Active Labor Act (EMTALA). The transfer must be initiated either by the legally responsible person acting on your behalf or by physician order with the appropriate certification. All benefits and risks of transfer will be explained and outlined in writing to you or your designated representative.

Source: MountainStar Family of Hospitals 2008.

providers. And, conversely, they help providers remember to focus on their responsibilities that form the common basis of the provider-patient relationship in this country. Figure 10.2 shows an example of a resident's rights form for a long-term nursing facility. Patients also have responsibilities, as illustrated by the example from an acute care facility in figure 10.3.

Other rights existing in the relationship that are not stated in the federal mandate but are implicit when an organization holds itself available to patients as a provider include assertions that care is provided concurrent with that common in community practice; that all providers employed by or affiliated with the organization are credentialed, licensed, or certified as required by common practice or state licensing laws; and that the basic intent and vision of the organization is to effect outcomes deemed positive for patients, residents, or clients through the care processes employed in the organization.

For the most part, these expectations are met. However, sometimes this is not the case. The risk of unanticipated negative occurrences is inherent in noncompliance with any of the issues discussed above or listed in figures 10.1, 10.2, and 10.3.

The very nature of healthcare organizations makes them susceptible to risk. **Risk** is defined as an exposure to the chance of injury or financial loss and its associated liability. Claims associated with risk result from physical or psychological incidents that may adversely affect patients, visitors, or employees. Every day, employees in healthcare organizations work with equipment and substances that are dangerous even when used appropriately. Clinical laboratories perform analyses using chemicals that can cause burns. Radiological instruments deliver high doses of radiation. Hospital pharmacies package and deliver medications that may be harmful to patients when not administered precisely or in the correct dosages. Those involved in patient care are surrounded by numerous conditions and situations that could potentially cause injury.

Patients may also contribute to their own health risks through noncompliance with basic good-health practices. They may continue to smoke or overeat in spite of education about these risks to health. Some patients in the hospital setting may refuse to wait for assistance before getting out of bed to use the bathroom, or they may refuse to sleep with side rails on their beds and risk dangerous falls. Patients' personal belongings may

Figure 10.2. Example of resident rights in a long-term nursing facility

RESIDENT RIGHTS

As a resident of this facility, you have the right to a dignified existence and to communicate with individuals and representatives of choice. The facility will protect and promote your rights as designated below.

Exercise of Rights–

- You have the right and freedom to exercise your rights as a resident of this facility and as a citizen or resident of the United States without fear of discrimination, restraint, interference, coercion or reprisal.
- If you are unable to act in your own behalf, your rights are exercised by the person appointed under state law to act in your behalf.

Notice of Rights and Services–

- You will be informed of your rights and of all rules and regulations governing resident conduct and responsibilities both orally and in writing.
- You have the right to inspect and purchase photocopies of your records.
- You have the right to be fully informed of your total health status.
- You have the right to refuse medication or treatment and the right to refuse to participate in experimental research.
- You have the right to formulate an advance directive in accordance with facility policy and applicable state law.
- You must be informed of Medicare and Medicaid benefits both orally and in writing, including how to receive refunds.
- You must be informed of facility services and charges and any changes to benefits or charges.
- The facility must inform you of procedures for protecting personal funds.
- You must be informed of your physician, his or her specialty, and ways of contacting him or her.
- The facility must consult with you and notify your physician and interested family member of any significant change in your condition or treatment, or of any decision to transfer or discharge.
- The facility must notify you and interested family member of a room or roommate change.
- You have the right to refuse room changes requested by the facility.
- The facility must periodically record and update the address and telephone number of your legal representative or interested family member.
- The facility must notify you and interested family member of changes in your rights.
- The facility must post the names, addresses and telephone numbers of all pertinent state client advocacy groups. If you deem necessary, you may file a complaint with the state survey and certification agency concerning resident abuse, neglect, misappropriation of resident property, and non-adherence to advance directive requirements.

Protection of Funds–

- You may manage your own financial affairs. You are not required to deposit personal funds with the facility.
- The facility must manage your deposited funds with your best interests in mind. Your money must not be commingled with facility funds.
- The facility will provide you with an individualized financial report quarterly and upon your request.
- Any remaining estate will be conveyed to your named successor.
- All funds held by the facility will be protected by a security bond.
- The facility must not charge you for any items or services you do not request or which are included in your Medicare or Medicaid payment. The facility must tell you what the charge will be for any of these requested items or services.

CFS 1-3 © 1992 Briggs Corporation, Des Moines, IA 50306
R203 To order, phone 1-800-247-2343 www.BriggsCorp.com PRINTED IN U.S.A.

(Continued on next page)

Figure 10.2. *(Continued)*

Free Choice–
- You may choose your own personal physician.
- You must be informed of and may participate in planning your care and treatment and any changes in your care and treatment.

Privacy–
- You have the right of privacy over your personal and clinical records.
- Your privacy will include: personal care, medical treatments, telephone use, visits, letters, and meetings of family and resident groups.
- You may approve or refuse the release of your records except in the event of a transfer or legal situation.

Grievances–
- You may voice grievances concerning your care without fear of discrimination or reprisal.
- You may expect prompt efforts for the resolution of grievances.

Examination of Survey Results–
- You may examine survey results and the plan of correction. These, or a notice of their location, will be posted in a readily accessible place.
- You may contact client advocate agencies and receive information from them.

Work–
- You have the right to perform or refuse to perform services for the facility.
- All services performed must be well documented in the care plan to include nature of the work and compensation.

Mail–
- You have the right to send and promptly receive your mail unopened and have access to writing supplies you have requested.

Access and Visitation Rights–
- You have the right to receive or deny visitors.
- You have the right and the facility must provide access to visit with any relevant agency of the state or any entity providing health, social, legal or other services.

Telephone–
- You have the right to use the telephone in private.

Personal Property–
- You can retain and use personal possessions as space permits.

Married Couples–
- A married couple may share a room.

Self-Administration of Drugs–
- You may self-administer drugs if determined safe by the interdisciplinary care team.

Figure 10.2. *(Continued)*

ADMISSION, TRANSFER AND DISCHARGE RIGHTS

Transfer and Discharge–
- You may not be transferred or discharged unless your needs cannot be met, your safety is endangered, or services are no longer required.
- Notice of and reason(s) for transfer or discharge must be provided to you in an understandable manner.
- Notice of transfer or discharge must be given to you 30 days prior, except in cases of health and safety needs.
- The transfer or discharge notice must include the name, address and telephone number of the appropriate, responsible advocacy agency.
- A facility must provide you sufficient preparation and orientation to ensure a safe transfer or discharge.

Notice of Bed-Hold Policy and Readmission–
- You and a family member must receive written notice of state and facility bed-hold policies before and at the time of a transfer which specifies the duration of the policy, if applicable.
- The facility must follow a written policy for readmittance if the bed-hold period is exceeded.

Equal Access to Quality Care–
- The facility must use identical policies regarding transfer, discharge and services for all residents regardless of payer source.
- The facility may determine charges for a non-Medicaid resident as long as written notice was provided at the time of admission.

Admission Policy–
- The facility must not require a third party guarantee of payment or accept any gifts as a condition of admission or continued stay.
- The facility cannot require you to waive your right to receive or apply for Medicare or Medicaid benefits.
- The facility may obtain a contract from someone who has legal financial access for payment without incurring your personal liability for payment.
- The facility may charge a Medicaid-eligible resident for items and services requested that are not covered in the state plan.
- The facility may only accept contributions if they are not solicited or offered as a condition of admission or continued stay.

RESIDENT BEHAVIOR AND FACILITY PRACTICES

Restraints–
- The facility must not use physical restraints or psychoactive drugs for discipline or convenience or when they are not required to treat medical symptoms.

Abuse–
- You have the right to be free from verbal, sexual, physical or mental abuse, corporal punishment and involuntary seclusion.

Staff Treatment–
- The facility must implement procedures that protect you from abuse, neglect or mistreatment, and misappropriation of your property.
- In the event of an alleged violation involving your treatment, the facility is required to report it to the appropriate officials.
- All alleged violations must be promptly and thoroughly investigated and the results reported to appropriate agencies. Corrective action must be taken.

(Continued on next page)

Figure 10.2. *(Continued)*

Quality of Life–
- The facility must care for you in a manner and environment that enhances or promotes your quality of life.

Dignity–
- The facility will treat you with dignity and respect in full recognition of your individuality.

Self Determination–
- You may choose your own activities, schedules and health care and any other aspect significant to and affecting your life within the facility.
- You may interact with visitors of your choice or with members of the community both inside or outside of the facility.

Participation in Resident and Family Groups–
- You may organize or participate in groups of choice.
- Families have the right to visit with other families.
- The facility must provide a private space for group meetings.
- Staff or visitors may attend meetings at the group's invitation.
- The facility will provide a staff person to assist and follow up with the group's written requests.
- The facility must listen to and act upon requests or concerns of the group.

Participation in Other Activities–
- You have the right to participate in activities of choice that do not interfere with the rights of other residents.

Accommodation of Needs–
- You have the right to receive services with reasonable accommodations to individual needs and preferences.
- You will be notified of room or roommate changes.
- You have the right to make choices about aspects of your life in the facility that are important to you.

Activities–
- The facility must provide a program of activities designed to meet your needs and interests.

Social Services–
- The facility must provide social services to attain or maintain your highest level of well-being.

Environment–
- The facility must provide a safe, clean, comfortable, home-like environment, allowing you the opportunity to use your personal belongings to the extent possible.
- The facility will provide housekeeping and maintenance services.
- The facility will assure you have clean bath and bed linens and that they are in good repair.
- The facility will provide you with private closet space as space permits.
- The facility will provide you with adequate and comfortable lighting and sound levels.
- The facility will provide you with comfortable and safe temperature levels.

Source: Reprinted with permission of Briggs' Corporation, Des Moines, Iowa 50306, (800) 247-2343.

Figure 10.3.   Example of patient responsibilities in an acute care facility

- Provide information: Provide an accurate medical history of your condition to your physician. You have the responsibility to provide, to the best of your knowledge, accurate and complete information about present complaints, past illnesses, hospitalizations, medications, and other matters relating to your health. You have the responsibility to report unexpected changes in your condition to the responsible practitioner. You are also responsible for reporting whether or not you clearly comprehend a contemplated course of action and what is expected of you.

- Follow the hospital's rules and regulations: You are responsible for following hospital rules and regulations affecting patient care and conduct.

- Follow your treatment plan: You are responsible for following the agreed upon treatment plan recommended by the practitioner primarily responsible for your care.

- Provide accurate financial information: You are responsible to provide accurate financial information, so that appropriate billing may be made to the person responsible for payment of services, and for assuring that the financial obligations of your healthcare are fulfilled as promptly as possible.

- Show respect and consideration: You are responsible for being considerate of the rights of other patients and hospital personnel and for assisting in the control of noise, smoking, and the number of visitors. Please be respectful of the property of others and of the hospital.

- Your role in promoting safe healthcare:
    - Please ask if you have questions about your health or safety.
    - We remind you to look for an identification badge to be worn by all healthcare providers.
    - Please adhere to the hospital's No Smoking policy.

Source: MountainStar Family of Hospitals 2008.

disappear due to theft or negligence. Confused or sedated patients may pull out their own intravenous lines and expose nursing staff to bloodborne pathogens. Patient care settings are places of complex and intense interactions that carry many potential opportunities for injury to patients, staff, and visitors. There also are the unintended consequences of treatment to consider. Patients do not always respond to therapy as planned. The surgeon's knife sometimes nicks contiguous structures. The possibility of unintended injury is everywhere in healthcare organizations.

In 1999, the Institute of Medicine (IOM) published a report on medical errors in healthcare titled *To Err Is Human: Building a Safer Health System*, which sent shock waves through the American healthcare industry. The IOM reported that "at least 44,000 people, and perhaps as many as 98,000 people, die in hospitals each year as a result of medical errors that could have been prevented" (Kohn et al. 1999). Since the IOM's report, both the government and the private sector have begun to focus on safety issues in healthcare. The Clinton administration issued an executive order instructing government agencies that conduct or oversee healthcare programs to create a task force to find new strategies for reducing errors, and Congress appropriated $50 million to support efforts targeted at reducing medical errors. In response to these initiatives, the Patient Safety Improvement Act of 2003 was introduced to create a new system for voluntary reporting of medical errors. On July 29, 2005, President George W. Bush signed into law the Patient Safety and Quality Improvement Act of 2005. The focus of the act is to provide federal protection across healthcare settings to promote cultures of safety by encouraging thorough reviews of errors and by developing effective solutions to prevent their recurrence. The goal is to provide full federal privilege to patient safety information that is sent to a patient safety organization. There are many patient safety organizations, each with its own specific focus on creating better, safer healthcare. The act was designed to make healthcare information available to resources that can help develop and implement changes in medical errors that will save lives.

In addition, state licensing agencies mandate that healthcare organizations report adverse medical events that result in death and serious harm. In the private sector, businesses buying insurance coverage for their employees are being encouraged to make safety a prime concern in their contracting decisions, and patients and their families are being urged to take a proactive role in reducing medical errors by participating in safety initiatives established by healthcare providers.

In this atmosphere of complexity, danger, chance, and emotion, risk managers work to accomplish their professional objectives. Risk managers seek to manage organizations' risk exposure and improve processes so that the threat of injury and its associated liability is minimized. Occurrences involving liability for injury or property loss are called **potentially compensable events** (PCEs).

Patients and clients come to healthcare organizations expecting improved physical and emotional health benefits for themselves and their family members. Employees come to work intending to provide the best-quality healthcare they can deliver. Because everyone comes to the healthcare setting with the best intentions, negative occurrences can result in anger and guilt. Generally, faulty systems, ineffective processes, and conditions that lead people to make mistakes or fail to prevent them cause errors in healthcare. Such occurrences present healthcare organizations with opportunities for reducing errors and improving patient safety. The cornerstone of patient safety for healthcare organizations is to foster an environment that acknowledges the unintentional nature of human error and emphasizes how organizations can learn from their mistakes.

Decreasing Risk Exposure: Steps to Success

Most people think of risk management as the process of working through a malpractice suit. Although that is sometimes the case, risk managers are more often trying to identify organizational conditions that increase risk exposure *before* occurrences involving injury happen. Identification before injury allows the organization to be proactive in improving care processes prior to incurring the exposure. Most healthcare organizations use an incident or occurrence reporting system to collect and report data. The system is set up to track all different types of incidents and rate them anywhere from "no harm" to "severe harm or death." This performance improvement (PI) process is reported monthly to the leadership team and quarterly to the governing board. There is usually an assigned risk manager or team depending on the size of the organization. This team is involved in investigating incidents and is usually directed by legal support from the healthcare facility or a contracted agency. Some risk management teams also are active in the patient advocacy program. They help track patient grievances and many times act as an intermediary between the patient and the organization to resolve conflicts that, if left unaddressed, could lead to incidents. The goal of the risk management team is to spot patterns in incidents and, through an intense investigative process, identify problems or concerns. They work through the PI council to address the patterns and problems identified and to develop interventions to resolve the problems.

Most recently, any healthcare organization's patient safety program must include proactive error-reduction activities to meet Joint Commission (2011) accreditation criteria. In other words, healthcare organizations are to identify and address underlying system problems that may result in adverse patient incidents. Most healthcare organizations are integrating these proactive error-reduction activities into their PI plans and goals. All healthcare settings are required to identify high-risk processes in which a failure of some type could jeopardize the safety of individuals to whom they provide services. The standards further require that, at any given time, a healthcare organization perform an ongoing intense analysis of at least one high-risk process by utilizing methods such as **failure mode and effects analysis** (FMEA), a technique that promotes systems thinking (Joint Commission 2011). FMEA includes defining high-risk processes using flow charts; identifying potential failure points in current processes; and scoring each potential failure by considering factors such as the frequency of failure, potential harm, and the likelihood that the failure will be detected before it reaches the patient. Potential failures with the highest criticality score become the focus of process redesign.

The Joint Commission established the following goals with regard to an organization's sentinel event policy:

- To have a positive impact in improving care, treatment, and services and preventing sentinel events

- To focus the attention of an organization that has experienced a sentinel event on understanding the causes that underlie the event and on changing the organization's systems and processes to reduce the probability of such an event in the future on underlying causes and risk reduction

- To increase the general knowledge about sentinel events, their causes, and strategies for prevention

- To maintain the confidence of the public and accredited organizations in the accreditation process (Joint Commission 2011, SE1)

The Joint Commission defines a sentinel event as an unexpected occurrence involving death or serious physical or psychological injury, or the risk thereof. Serious injury specifically includes loss of limb or function. The phrase "or the risk thereof" includes any process variation for which a recurrence would carry a significant chance of a serious adverse outcome. The following events are called "sentinel" because they signal the need for immediate investigation and response:

- Suicide of any patient receiving care, treatment, and services in a staffed round-the-clock care setting or within 72 hours of discharge

- Unanticipated death of a full-term infant

- Abduction of any patient receiving care, treatment, or services

- Discharge of an infant to the wrong family

- Rape committed against anyone in a facility: patient, resident, client, staff member, etc.

- Hemolytic transfusion reaction involving administration of blood or blood products having major blood group incompatibilities

- Surgery on a wrong patient or wrong body part

- Unintended retention of a foreign object in a patient after surgery or other procedure

- Severe neonatal hyperbilirubinemia (bilirubin >30 milligrams/deciliter)

- Prolonged fluoroscopy with cumulative dose >1500 rads to a single field or any delivery of radiotherapy to the wrong body region or 25 percent above the planned radiotherapy dose (Joint Commission 2011, SE1–SE5)

An organization also should include near misses in its definition of events that require intense investigation. *Near misses* include occurrences that do not necessarily affect an outcome, but if they were to recur they would carry significant chance of being a serious adverse event. Near misses fall under the definition of a sentinel event but are not reviewable by the Joint Commission under its current sentinel event policy. Near misses are a valuable tool for evaluation of processes and procedures, especially in high-risk or high-volume areas of facilities.

The Joint Commission (1998) established a "Sentinel Event Alert" notification and has currently identified in its Sentinel Event database 35 high-risk issues such as high-alert medication and bedrail deaths and injuries in addition to the occurrences noted above. (A complete list is available on the Joint Commission Web site at http://www.jointcommission. org.) The publication includes detailed assessment of the problems with recommendations for changes to be implemented to prevent a sentinel event. Three major categories of data elements in this database include sentinel event data, root-cause data, and risk reduction data. Other initiatives related to patient safety and proactive error reduction include the Joint Commission's National Patient Safety Goals (NPSGs) (Croteau 2005). In 2003, the Joint Commission initially established six goals to help accredited organizations address specific areas of concern in relation to patient safety. The Sentinel Event Advisory Group determined these goals from the Sentinel Event Alerts. Each year, the goals are reevaluated and published for survey by midyear. Since 2009, the NPSGs have been accorded an entire chapter of the accreditation standards manuals. A small number of specific requirements for each of the goals will be identified for survey for each goal. Some of the patient safety goals may continue, while others may be adopted as standards of care or changed because of emerging new priorities and areas of focus in other chapters of the accreditation standards. All accredited organizations must implement the goals and associated recommendations that are relevant to the services their organization provides. Please see chapter 8 and figure 8.3 for initial discussion of this topic.

These goals and recommendations are the results of lessons learned from organizations that have experienced a sentinel event. Lessons learned are the findings from a **root-cause analysis** that determined process issues and new solutions to prevent sentinel events from occurring. Additional information on sentinel events and associated root-cause analysis is addressed in step 5.

Step 1: The Healthcare Organization Develops a Risk Management Plan, Policies, and Procedures

The risk manager leads the development of risk management policies and procedures for the organization. The risk manager also helps the organization define and prioritize its own self-assessed risk factors for the population it serves. Policies and procedures in the risk management area include a policy describing the organization's insurance strategy, procedures outlining its claims-tracking and negotiation system, and procedures outlining how its databases are maintained and risk management reports are developed. Risk managers also routinely review the operational policies and procedures of all departments to ensure that they have been designed in ways that reduce, rather than increase, the possibility of risk exposure. Risk management procedures also define requirements for occurrence reporting and reporting to insurers, licensing agencies, public health departments, governing bodies, the National Practitioner Data Bank, and other accrediting and regulatory agencies. In addition, risk managers review all policies and procedures approved in the organization to ensure that none of the activities will expose the organization to risk. Currently, ensuring compliance with all requirements for the NPSGs has become a major component of the risk manager's job.

Step 2: The Risk Management Team Teaches Risk Management Concepts and Principles to All Employees

In conjunction with staff development coordinators, risk managers develop educational activities for employees, including the governing board. Examples of such activities include hand-washing techniques, needle safety protocol, NPSGs including universal protocol, fall-risk prevention, surgical fire prevention, behavior treatment protocols, seclusion and restraint procedures, and incident documentation and reporting. Educational topics are based on data derived from risk management reports. Program attendance is documented in each employee's personnel file, and competency testing for comprehension and retention is performed.

Step 3: The Team Evaluates Occurrence Reports

The risk manager's principal tool for capturing the facts about PCEs is the **occurrence report,** sometimes called the **incident report.** Effective occurrence reports carefully structure the collection of data, information, and facts in a relatively simple format. An excellent example of an occurrence report is provided in figure 10.4. Note that this example captures information about the persons involved. It records information about the date and the time of day that the employees involved were working. Page 2 of the

Figure 10.4. Sample occurrence report

Med Rec #: *00-05-45*
Name: *Jackson, Julia*
Date of Birth: *06-22-23*
Street: *6401 Fremont Ave*
City: *Western City, CA*

Risk Management use only: _____

Patient ID/Name of individual involved.
Use addressograph for patient.

INSTRUCTIONS: (1) Fill out the first page of the Incident Report Form. (2) Select the type of incident from the bottom of page 2. (3) Fill out all appropriate sections as directed. The report must be dated and filled out by the end of the shift in which the incident occurred or was discovered. **DO NOT COPY THIS FORM.** Please print; this report must be legible. **Please fill out all applicable parts of this form.** Upon completion of this form, route it to your Nurse Manager or Supervisor. Do not leave this form in the patient's chart.

Date of incident: *05/29/03*   Time (2400 Clock): *1645*   Hospital Unit: *Med/Surg*

What day of the week did it occur?

Sun	[√]	Thurs	[ ]
Mon	[ ]	Fri	[ ]
Tues	[ ]	Sat	[ ]
Wed	[ ]		

Did the incident occur during:
Day 0701–1500 [ ]
Evening 1501–2300 [√]
Night 2301–0700 [ ]

Employee involved worked a(n):
8 Hour shift [√]
10 Hour shift [ ]
12 Hour shift [ ]
Double shift [ ]
Other _____

Where did the incident occur? *patient room*

Description of incident. Include follow-up care given (i.e., vital signs, x-ray, laboratory tests, etc.).
Pt. developed a macular rash over trunk and extremities after 10 mg dose of Compazine given for postop nausea. Compazine stopped and Benadryl given IM.

IMMEDIATE EFFECT OF THE INCIDENT: *Severe macular rash over trunk*

Involved Person Data

Date of Admission: *05/29/03*
What sex is the person?
Male [ ]
Female [√]

What is the person's age? _____

Inpatient [√]
Outpatient [ ]
Student [ ]
Employee [ ]
Visitor [ ]
Volunteer [ ]
Other: _____

Current Diagnosis/Reason for visit: *Bowel Obstruction*

Is the involved person aware of the incident?   Yes [√]   No [ ]
Is the family aware of incident?   Yes [ ]   No [√]

Figure 10.4. *(Continued)*

DO NOT COPY

**** **PLEASE PRINT** ****

Person preparing report (signature): *Gwen Nelson. R.N.* Print: *Gwen Nelson, R.N.*

Name of individual witnessing incident (print): *Bob Patterson, R.N.*

Dept/Address: *Med/Surg Team Leader*

Name of employee involved in incident: *Gwen Nelson, R.N.* Dept/Address: *Med/Surg*

Name of employee discovering incident: *Gwen Nelson, R.N.* Dept/Address: *Med/Surg*

**** **STAFF TO NOTIFY ATTENDING PHYSICIAN AND/OR DESIGNATED RESIDENT/NURSE PRACTITIONER OF INCIDENT** ****

I notified Dr./NP: *Jeff Cook* at: *1650* (time).

M.D./NP responded ☐ in person ☑ by phone at: *1705* (time).

Was the attending physician notified?

Yes [√] Date: *05 / 29 / 03* Time: *1650*

No [ ] Why not? _____

Examining Physician/Nurse Practitioner statement regarding condition/outcome of person involved:

Pt. was examined by me at 1700 hours. Trunk and extremities show a macular rash on them. One dose of Benadryl given IM to pt. and rash began to subside. Compazine stopped.

Examining MD/NP signature: *Tom Lander. M.D. House Staff*

Examining MD/NP name (print): *Tom Lander, M.D.*

Date: *05 / 29 / 03* Time: *1700* Clinical Service: *Medicine*

CHOOSE THE TYPE OF INCIDENT YOU ARE REPORTING. Use the index below to locate the type of incident you are reporting, go to that section, and mark the appropriate box(es). THERE MAY BE MORE THAN ONE ITEM APPLICABLE IN A SECTION. CHECK BOX(ES) IN APPROPRIATE SECTIONS.

Medication/IV Incident	Page 3, Section 1	Patient Behavioral Incident	Page 5, Section 6
Blood/Blood Incident	Page 3, Section 2	Safety Incident	Page 5, Section 9
Burns	Page 5, Section 7	Security Incident	Page 5, Section 8
Equipment Incident	Page 5, Section 10	Surgery Incident	Page 5, Section 4
Falls	Page 4, Section 3	Treatment/Procedure Incident	Page 5, Section 5
Fire Incident	Page 5, Section 11		

CONFIDENTIAL: This material is prepared pursuant to Code Annotated, §26-25-1, et seq., and 58-12-43 (7, 8, and 9), for the purpose of evaluating healthcare rendered by hospitals or physicians and is NOT PART of the medical record.

(Continued on next page)

Figure 10.4. *(Continued)*

SECTION 1 MEDICATION/IV INCIDENT

1A. TYPE OF MEDICATION

Fill in specific medication/solution on the adjacent line.

Analgesic _____
Anesthetic agent _____
Antibiotic _____
Anticoagulant _____
Anticonvulsant _____
Antidepressant _____
Antiemetic___*Compazine*_____
Antihistamine _____
Antineoplastic _____
Bronchodilator _____
Cardiovascular _____
Contrast media _____
Diuretic _____
Immunizations _____
Immunosuppressive _____
Insulin _____
Intralipids _____
Investigational drug _____
IV solution _____
Laxative_____
Narcotic_____
Oxytocics _____
Psychotherapeutic _____
Radionuclides _____
Sedative/tranquilizer _____
TPN _____
Vasodilator _____
Vasopressor _____
Vitamin _____
Other _____

1B. TYPE OF MEDICATION OR IV INCIDENT

Adverse reaction . . . . [ ] 1B01
Allergic/contraindication. . . . . [ ] 1B02
Delayed stat order . . . . [ ] 1B03
Improper order (MD/NP) . . . . [ ] 1B04
Incompatible additive . . . . [ ] 1B05
Incorrect additive . . . . [ ] 1B06
Incorrect dosage . . . . [ ] 1B07
Incorrect drug . . . . [ ] 1B08
Incorrect narcotic count . . . . [ ] 1B09
Incorrect patient . . . . [ ] 1B10
Incorrect rate of flow . . . . [ ] 1B11
Incorrect route. . . . . [ ] 1B12
Incorrect schedule . . . . [ ] 1B13
Incorrect solution/type . . . . [ ] 1B14
Incorrect time . . . . [ ] 1B15
Incorrect volume. . . . . [ ] 1B16
Infiltration . . . . [ ] 1B17
Given before culture taken . . . . [ ] 1B18
Medication given before lab
     results returned . . . . [ ] 1B19
Medication missing from cart. . . . . [ ] 1B20

Not documented . . . . [ ] 1B21
Not prescribed. . . . . [ ] 1B22
Omitted . . . . [ ] 1B23
Outdated . . . . [ ] 1B24
Out-of-sequence . . . . [ ] 1B25
Patient took unprescribed medication. . . . . [ ] 1B26
Repeat administration . . . . [ ] 1B27
Transcription error . . . . [ ] 1B28
Other_____   1B29

1C. ROUTE OF MEDICATION ORDERED:

IM. . . . . [ ] 1C01
IV . . . . [ ] 1C02
PO . . . . [ ] 1C03
Other___*Suppository*_____   1C04

1D. MEDICATION DISPENSING INCIDENT

Meds not sent/delayed from pharmacy. . . . . . . [ ] 1D01
Incorrectly labeled . . . . [ ] 1D02
Incorrect dose . . . . [ ] 1D03
Incorrect drug sent . . . . [ ] 1D04
Incorrect IV additive . . . . [ ] 1D05
Incorrect IV fluid . . . . [ ] 1D06
Incorrect route (IV, PO, IM, PR) . . . . [ ] 1D07
Mislabeled. . . . . [ ] 1D08
Other_____   1D09

SECTION 2
BLOOD/BLOOD COMPONENT INCIDENT

2A. BLOOD/BLOOD COMPONENT TYPE

Albumin. . . . . [ ] 2A01
Cryoprecipitate . . . . [ ] 2A02
Factor VIII (AHF). . . . . [ ] 2A03
Factor IX (Konyne) . . . . [ ] 2A04
Fresh frozen plasma. [ ] 2A05
Packed red blood cells (PRBC) . . . . [ ] 2A06
Plasmanate®. . . . . [ ] 2A07
Platelets. . . . . [ ] 2A08
RhoGAM®. . . . . [ ] 2A09
Washed red blood cells (WRBC) . . . . [ ] 2A10
Whole blood . . . . [ ] 2A11
Other_____   2A12

2B. TYPE OF BLOOD/BLOOD COMPONENT
INCIDENT

Crossmatch problem . . . . [ ] 2B01
Improper unit verification. . . . . [ ] 2B02
Inappropriate IV fluids administered
     with blood components. . . . . [ ] 2B03
Inappropriate documentation . . . . [ ] 2B04
Inappropriate storage. [ ] 2B05
Incomplete patient ID. . . . . [ ] 2B06
Incorrect patient . . . . [ ] 2B07
Incorrect rate. . . . . [ ] 2B08
Incorrect type . . . . [ ] 2B09
Incorrect volume. . . . . [ ] 2B10
Patient refused . . . . [ ] 2B11
Other_____   2B12

Figure 10.4. *(Continued)*

DO NOT COPY

SECTION 3
FALLS

3A. FALL CODE STATUS OF PATIENT
Attended................................. [ ] 3A01
Unattended.............................. [ ] 3A02

3B. LOCATION OF FALL
Bathroom in patient's room............... [ ] 3B01
Bathroom (other location)................ [ ] 3B02
Elevator................................. [ ] 3B03
Examining/treatment room................. [ ] 3B04
Hallway/corridor......................... [ ] 3B05
Nursing station.......................... [ ] 3B06
Parking lot.............................. [ ] 3B07
Patient's room........................... [ ] 3B08
Recreation area.......................... [ ] 3B09
Shower/tub room.......................... [ ] 3B10
Stairs................................... [ ] 3B11
Waiting room............................. [ ] 3B12
Walkway/sidewalk......................... [ ] 3B13
Other_____   3B14

3C. FALL OCCURRED IN CONJUNCTION WITH:
Bedside commode.......................... [ ] 3C01
Chair.................................... [ ] 3C02
Due to toy............................... [ ] 3C03
During transfer.......................... [ ] 3C04
Exam table............................... [ ] 3C05
Fainting/dizzy........................... [ ] 3C06
Fall/slip................................ [ ] 3C07
From bed................................. [ ] 3C08
Improperly locked device................. [ ] 3C09
Recreational activity.................... [ ] 3C10
Scales................................... [ ] 3C11
Stretcher................................ [ ] 3C12
Table.................................... [ ] 3C13
Tripped.................................. [ ] 3C14
While ambulating unattended.............. [ ] 3C15
While ambulating with assist............. [ ] 3C16
While entering or leaving bed............ [ ] 3C17
While using ambulatory device............ [ ] 3C18
Other_____   3C19

3D. PATIENT ACTIVITY PRIVILEGES
    (As per medical order)
Ambulate with assistance................. [ ] 3D01
Ambulate with walker..................... [ ] 3D02
Ambulate without assistance.............. [ ] 3D03
Bathroom privileges with assistance...... [ ] 3D04
Bathroom privileges without assistance... [ ] 3D05
Bedrest.................................. [ ] 3D06
Up Ad lib................................ [ ] 3D07
Up in chair/wheelchair................... [ ] 3D08
Other_____   3D09

3E. PATIENT MENTAL CONDITION AT THE
    TIME OF THE FALL
Confused/poor judgment................... [ ] 3E01
Language barrier......................... [ ] 3E02
Oriented................................. [ ] 3E03
Unconscious.............................. [ ] 3E04
Uncooperative............................ [ ] 3E05
Unresponsive/medicated................... [ ] 3E06
Other_____

3F. PATIENT'S CALL LIGHT WAS:
On....................................... [ ] 3F01
Off...................................... [ ] 3F02
Not within reach......................... [ ] 3F03
Patient unable to use.................... [ ] 3F04
Not applicable........................... [ ] 3F05

3G. POSITION OF BED
High..................................... [ ] 3G01
Low...................................... [ ] 3G02
Intermediate............................. [ ] 3G03
Not applicable........................... [ ] 3G04

3H. BED ALARM
On....................................... [ ] 3H01
Off...................................... [ ] 3H02
Not applicable........................... [ ] 3H03

3I. POSITION OF SIDE RAILS
(At the time of the fall)

Half Rails	[ ] 3I01	Full Rails	[ ] 3I06
1 Up	[ ] 3I02	1 Up	[ ] 3I07
2 Up	[ ] 3I03	2 Up	[ ] 3I08
3 Up	[ ] 3I04		
4 Up	[ ] 3I05		

Not applicable   [ ] 3I09

3J. PATIENT RESTRAINTS
Removed by patient....................... [ ] 3J01
Restraints intact........................ [ ] 3J02
Not applicable........................... [ ] 3J03
Other_____   3J04

3K. CONDITION OF AREA WHERE FALL
    OCCURRED
Normal/dry............................... [ ] 3K01
Wet floor................................ [ ] 3K02
Ice condition............................ [ ] 3K03
Other_____   3K04

3L. FALLS IN CONJUNCTION
    WITH MEDICATION
Narcotic or sedative received by patient
in the past 12 hours?.................... [ ] 3L01
When was the last dose? _____ 3L02
What was the drug? _____   3L03
What was the route of administration?_____ 3L04

CONFIDENTIAL: This material is prepared pursuant to Code Annotated, §26-25-1, et seq., and 58-12-43 (7, 8, and 9), for the purpose
of evaluating healthcare rendered by hospitals or physicians and is NOT PART of the medical record.

(Continued on next page)

Figure 10.4. *(Continued)*

DO NOT COPY

SECTION 4
SURGERY INCIDENT

Anesthesia occurrence . . . . [ ] 0401
Contamination . . . . [ ] 0402
Incorrect needle count . . . . [ ] 0403
Incorrect sponge count . . . . [ ] 0404
Informed consent absent . . . . [ ] 0405
Informed consent incorrect . . . . [ ] 0406
Instrument lost/broken . . . . [ ] 0407
Retained foreign body . . . . [ ] 0408
Other_____   0409

SECTION 5
TREATMENT/PROCEDURE INCIDENT

Adverse reaction . . . . [ ] 0501
Allergic response . . . . [ ] 0502
Application/removal of cast/splint. . . . . [ ] 0503
Cancellation of procedures . . . . [ ] 0504
Catheter or tube related . . . . [ ] 0505
Delay . . . . [ ] 0506
Dietary problem . . . . [ ] 0507
Dressing/wound occurrence. . . . . [ ] 0508
Informed consent absent . . . . [ ] 0509
Informed consent incorrect . . . . [ ] 0510
Injection site. . . . . [ ] 0511
Invasive procedure/placement . . . . [ ] 0512
Mislabeled specimen . . . . [ ] 0513
Missing specimen . . . . [ ] 0514
Not documented. . . . .[ ] 0515
Omitted . . . . [ ] 0516
Patient/site identification . . . . [ ] 0517
Positioning. . . . . [ ] 0518
Prep problem . . . . [ ] 0519
Repeat procedure. . . . . [ ] 0520
Reporting of test results. . . . . [ ] 0521
Thermoregulation problem . . . . [ ] 0522
Transcription error. [ ] 0523
Transfer/moving of patient . . . . [ ] 0524
Other_____   0525

SECTION 6
PATIENT BEHAVIORAL INCIDENT

Attempted AWOL . . . . [ ] 0601
AWOL . . . . [ ] 0602
Inappropriate sexual behavior . . . . [ ] 0603
Injured by other patient . . . . [ ] 0604
Patient altercation . . . . [ ] 0605
Self-inflicted injury . . . . [ ] 0606
Suicide gesture. . . . . [ ] 0607
Other_____   0608

SECTION 7
BURNS

Chemical . . . . [ ] 0701
Electrical . . . . [ ] 0702
Inhalation. . . . . [ ] 0703
Radioactive . . . . [ ] 0704
Thermal . . . . [ ] 0705

SECTION 8
SECURITY INCIDENT

Bomb threat . . . . [ ] 0801
Breaking and entering . . . . [ ] 0802
Drug theft . . . . [ ] 0803
Secure area key loss/missing. . . . . [ ] 0804
Major theft (over $250) . . . . [ ] 0805
   Amount:_____
Minor theft. . . . . [ ] 0806
   Amount:_____
Personal property damage/loss . . . . [ ] 0807
   Amount:_____
Hospital property damage . . . . [ ] 0808
   Amount:_____
Other_____

SECTION 9
SAFETY INCIDENT (patients and visitors only)

Body fluid exposure. . . . .[ ] 0901
Chemical exposure. [ ] 0902
Chemotherapy spill . . . . [ ] 0903
Drug exposure . . . . [ ] 0904
Hazardous material spill . . . . [ ] 0905
Needlestick . . . . [ ] 0906
Other_____   0907

SECTION 10
EQUIPMENT INCIDENT

Disconnected . . . . [ ] 1001
Electrical problem . . . . [ ] 1002
Improper use . . . . [ ] 1003
Malfunction/defect. [ ] 1004
Mechanical problem . . . . [ ] 1005
Not available . . . . [ ] 1006
Electrical shock . . . . [ ] 1007
Electrical spark . . . . [ ] 1008
Struck by . . . . [ ] 1009
Wrong equipment . . . . [ ] 1010
Tampered with
   By patient . . . . [ ] 1011
   Non-patient . . . . [ ] 1012
Other_____   1013

SECTION 11
FIRE INCIDENT

Equipment caused . . . . [ ] 1101
Cigarette caused. . . . . [ ] 1102
Laser caused . . . . [ ] 1103
Other_____   1104

CONFIDENTIAL: This material is prepared pursuant to Code Annotated, §26-25-1, et seq., and 58-12-43 (7, 8, and 9), for the purpose of evaluating healthcare rendered by hospitals or physicians and is NOT PART of the medical record.

Figure 10.4. *(Continued)*

DO NOT COPY

**EMPLOYEES DO NOT COMPLETE BELOW,
FOR NURSE MANAGER/SUPERVISOR USE ONLY.**

Recommendations and/or corrective actions based on review of report and discussion with employee:

NURSE MANAGER/SUPERVISOR Follow-Up [Check appropriate box(es)/Corrective action]

Policy/Procedure:

Evaluate . . . . [ ] 1201	**Discussed with:**	
Recommend change. . . . . [ ] 1202	Physician. . . . . [ ] 1209
Changed . . . . [ ] 1203	Staff . . . . [ ] 1210
No action taken . . . . [ ] 1204	Patient. . . . . [ ] 1211
Noncompliance . . . . [ ] 1205	Other. . . . . [ ] 1212
Inadequate . . . . [ ] 1206	
Needs enforcement . . . . [ ] 1207	Date: _____
Review with involved individual(s). . . . [ ] 1208	Time: _____

Describe specific follow-up actions taken (if applicable include names of depts). _____
_____
_____

SIGN AND DATE: (Indicates review of report)

1. Quality Management/Risk Management _____ ___/___/___

2. Nurse Manager/Supervisor (as applicable) _____ ___/___/___

3. Department Head/DON (as applicable) _____ ___/___/___

4. QM Coordinator (as applicable)_____ ___/___/___

5. Other: Title_____ Name _____ ___/___/___

BIOENGINEERING USE ONLY

Manufacturer contacted	[ ] 1301
Manufacturer instructions followed.	[ ] 1302
Needs enforcement of policy/procedure	[ ] 1303
Include instructions in staff education and training	[ ] 1304
Preventative maintenance or biomedical evaluation of equipment ordered . . .	[ ] 1305
Recommend repair or replacement.	[ ] 1306
Removed from service	[ ] 1307
Other _____	[ ] 1308

RISK MANAGEMENT USE ONLY

IMMEDIATE EFFECT OF THE INCIDENT

Alteration in skin integrity . . . . [ ] 1401	Patient discomfort/inconvenience. . . . . . [ ] 1411
Birth related injury . . . . [ ] 1402	Psycho/social trauma . . . . [ ] 1412
Breach of confidentiality . . . . [ ] 1403	Reproductive injury or loss . . . . [ ] 1413
Death. . . . . [ ] 1404	Sensory impairment . . . . [ ] 1414
Disability . . . . [ ] 1405	Severe internal injuries. . . . . [ ] 1415
Disfigurement. . . . . [ ] 1406	Substantial disability. . . . . [ ] 1416
Drug/blood reaction. . . . . [ ] 1407	Unanticipated neuro deficit . . . . [ ] 1417
Fluid imbalance . . . . [ ] 1408	Unanticipated systemic deficit . . . . [ ] 1418
Neuro deficit . . . . [ ] 1409	Indeterminate . . . . [ ] 1419
Orthopedic injury . . . . [ ] 1410	None . . . . [ ] 1420
	Other_____ [ ] 1421

Description_____

CONFIDENTIAL: This material is prepared pursuant to Code Annotated, §26-25-1, et seq., and 58-12-43 (7, 8, and 9), for the purpose of evaluating healthcare rendered by hospitals or physicians and is NOT PART of the medical record.

report gathers information about the witnesses to the incident and gives the results of the patient's contact with and examination by a physician or nurse-practitioner. Pages 3, 4, and 5 of this example gather information regarding specific aspects of the most common incidents that occur in healthcare. For example, in section 7, the report collects data on the type of burn. All data collected in these incident-specific sections are coded for easy checking and entry into a database management system for incident tracking.

Following completion by individuals in the department or facility area where the incident occurred, the occurrence report is sent to the risk manager. The risk manager reviews policy, procedure, and other aspects of the occurrence, and involves management and administrative staff as necessary. After the cause analysis and revision of policy, "recommendations and/or corrective actions based on review" of the incident are documented on page 6 of the report. This would include actions regarding policies and procedures, the outcome for the injured individual, contacts with manufacturers, and retraining of personnel.

The second important document for managing risk exposure is the patient's health record. Every response to an incident that relates to a patient must be documented in the patient's health record. If a case of injury should result in a malpractice suit or other legal action, this documentation becomes crucial. The clinicians involved in an incident must be certain that all appropriate clinical documentation regarding the occurrence is added to the health record as well as documented on the occurrence report.

Occurrence reports are generally not open to view by the plaintiff's attorney. Thus, to communicate the care given the patient in its entirety, and especially regarding an occurrence, the health record must be documented carefully because it will be used to portray the events to the public. The risk manager must develop a careful balance while overseeing the documentation of a PCE. Complete details on all persons involved, actions taken, and condition and responses of the patient should be recorded on the occurrence record. However, in the patient's health record, the details should be limited to those documenting care given to the patient. No details about how or what contributed to the occurrence should be recorded. No mention should be made in the patient's health record of an incident or occurrence report having been completed (figure 10.5). The documentation of a **medication error** in the sample occurrence report is a good example. The Joint Commission has implemented a new patient-right standard related to disclosing outcomes. The standard does not require that the organization inform the patient that an incident has occurred and has been reported. However, it does require that all patients be informed of any outcomes, unanticipated or otherwise, from an error such as a decrease in medication dosage due to a reaction from an ordered medication or a medical intervention initiated because of the original error. For instance, suppose a patient received an inaccurate dose of Lasix®, causing an excess of fluid depletion from the body and concomitant light-headedness requiring oxygen. The initial error may be a medication error caused by the prescriber or a dosing error caused by the personnel giving the medication. It also may simply be the patient's adverse reaction to the particular medication. Generally, the patient is not informed that an incident report has been completed. The patient will be informed that due to a reaction from the medication, he or she will need oxygen for a period of time.

Figure 10.5.   Sample progress note in a patient's record

PROGRESS NOTES	Med Rec# 00-05-45 Jackson, Julia

DATE & TIME	NOTES MUST BE DATED AND TIMED
5/29/03 1650	Patient developed a macular rash over entire trunk and extremities after 10 mg of Compazine given for nausea. Dr. Cook and house staff notified. Gwen Nelson, R.N.
5/29/03 1700	Called to pt. for rash on trunk & extremities. Pt. examined, adverse reaction to Compazine most likely. Patient to receive 20 mg of Benadryl IM now. If nausea continues, Dramamine 50 mg IV prn. T. Lander, M.D.
5/29/03 1700	Dr. Lander examined patient and ordered Benadryl 20 mg IM. Patient injected IM 20 mg of Benadryl. Gwen Nelson, R.N.
5/29/03 1810	Rash is subsiding and nausea less. Gwen Nelson, R.N.

PROGRESS NOTES

Step 4: The Risk Management Team Examines Structure, Process, and Knowledge Issues

As department members and PI teams begin to identify customers and review performance, issues in organizational structures, processes, outcomes, and knowledge may become apparent. Commonly, these issues are documented in department or team communications to a PI or leadership council. (See the discussion of documentation recommendations in chapter 6.) Risk managers are members of the council and routinely review communications from the departments and teams for this purpose. Issues, in turn, should be documented in risk-management databases so that corrective action may be initiated if and when they meet a performance threshold (the level above which the occurrence is not occurring by chance and cannot be tolerated). If it becomes apparent that members of the organization do not have an appropriate understanding of procedure or policy, the risk manager may have to initiate training sessions to educate staff regarding the issue.

Step 5: The Team Identifies Practice Patterns, Trends in Risk Occurrences, and Sentinel Events

Using aggregate data summarized from the occurrence report discussed in step 3, the risk manager attempts to identify trends in risk occurrences within the organization. A Joint Commission (http://www.jointcommission.org/sentinelevents/sentineleventalert/) notification called "Sentinel Event Alert" features aggregate data related to root causes and risk reduction strategies for sentinel events that occur with significant frequency. These lessons learned from frequently occurring sentinel events form the basis for error-prevention advice to organizations. For instance, if there were an increase in blood transfusion reactions, the manager might request a focused review by blood bank personnel to be sure that typing and grouping procedures are being followed appropriately. If there were an increase in occurrence reports documenting patients' falls on a particular nursing unit, the risk manager might ask the nurse manager on that unit to be sure that staff understand how to identify a patient at risk for falls, that assessments for fall risks are completed, and that appropriate preventive measures are instituted with identified patients.

Another important PI activity that contributes to the risk manager's databases is the credentialing of physicians and the validation of nurses' and other clinicians' licenses to practice. (See chapter 13 for additional information on competency and credentialing.) Committees of the medical staff and other disciplines standardize monitoring of clinicians' practice patterns and outcomes. Documentation of these reviews is analyzed by these committees, disciplines, and the risk manager to identify clinicians who may be practicing outside their scope of licensure or who may benefit from additional education regarding policy, procedure, or the current standard of practice in the region where the healthcare organization does business. A critical area of liability for a healthcare organization is the process of verifying staff clinical competency and practitioners working outside their scope of licensure or approved privileges. Malpractice claims against a provider would be in favor of the plaintiff if unfavorable information related to competency or privileging is revealed during the discovery process of a lawsuit.

Step 6: The Team Provides Direction in the Patient Advocacy Function

The first major objective of a proactive risk management program is to minimize the organization's exposure to risk or legal action. The second major objective is to minimize the economic impact of indemnity and expense payments related to claims. The economic impact of a quality risk program should be measured by the development of goodwill and the satisfaction of its customers. Historically, this second objective has been a function of risk management and is known as *patient advocacy*. Some healthcare organizations have removed this responsibility from the risk manager and established a separate patient advocate service that works with the risk manager on complaints specific to PCEs.

The objective of patient advocacy is to support the patient through difficult interactions with the healthcare organization. The Joint Commission (2011) defines an *advocate* as "a person who represents the rights and interests of another individual as though they were the person's own, in order to realize the rights to which the individual is entitled, obtain needed services, and remove barriers to meeting the individual's needs." Most businesses can be somewhat bureaucratic, and healthcare organizations are no exception. Add the confusion, complexity, danger, and chance of PCEs, and the patient may feel shunned and isolated by the organization at a time of great personal strife. The patient needs to express his or her anger to lessen it and needs someone in the organization to validate his or her right to feel it. All licensed healthcare organizations are required to inform patients of their rights to initiate a complaint or grievance and to have their complaints reviewed and, if possible, resolved.

The risk manager as patient advocate must be sure that the patient knows the facts associated with an occurrence. The patient advocate must accept responsibility for the occurrence in the customer's eyes when the organization's employees were responsible for the situation during which the incident occurred. If the organization's employees were not responsible for the situation but the customer believes that they were, the patient advocate should continue to serve a neutral role in resolving the situation. The challenge for the patient advocate is to investigate the complaint and address the issues specific to the event in such a way as to avoid legal action against the organization. Sometimes just listening to the patient's concerns, offering an apology, or negotiating monetary compensation can resolve the complaint without any further legal action against the organization.

Step 7: The Team Communicates All Relevant Data and Information to Legal Support When PCEs Occur

Inevitably, some claims of liability involve formal legal action. The facility's attorneys, the representatives of the facility's insurance company, and the plaintiff's attorneys then become involved.

The risk manager should continue to function as the organization's representative in such legal environments. He or she coordinates all requests for information by *subpoena duces tecum* from attorneys or from the courts. The risk manager explains the organization's perspective to attorneys regarding the completion of interrogatories and coordinates the appearance of employees at depositions or at trial. He or she remains open to negotiation of an appropriate settlement to conclude the action before it goes to trial.

The risk manager is responsible for communicating all relevant data and information to the organization's insurer as soon as possible after a PCE is recognized. The risk management department routinely provides the organization's insurance company with copies of the occurrence reports for all PCEs. The timeliness and efficiency of such communications are extremely important if PCEs are to be resolved rapidly and without litigation. Subsequently, the risk manager must keep the insurer apprised of important communications with the customer or the customer's attorneys. Insurance company representatives must have complete information to make appropriate resolution decisions.

Step 8: The Risk Team and Legal Counsel Lead the Development of an Appropriate Insurance Strategy for the Organization

In addition to transmitting information regarding PCEs, the risk manager also takes the lead in designing an insurance strategy that meets the needs of the healthcare organization. To be effective in this area, the risk manager must have an in-depth knowledge of the organization's services, facilities, equipment, procedures, and staff capabilities.

The insurance strategy is developed with reference to the healthcare service lines of the organization. For example, the perinatal service is one of the service lines that has the greatest inherent risk of liability. Numerous complications can occur during a woman's pregnancy, labor, and delivery, and many of these complications cannot be foreseen. The fact that the organization provides perinatal services would be taken into consideration by the organization's management and insurer.

Real-Life Example

At Community Hospital of the West, Dr. Low, an obstetrician, delivered Mrs. Yu's infant with relatively little difficulty. However, when the placenta was delivered, a rush of blood appeared at the patient's cervical os. Dr. Low attempted to explore the patient's uterus to see whether there were still pieces of the placenta inside that were causing the bleeding, but there was so much blood that she could not adequately explore the uterus. After several minutes of trying to deal with the situation, she realized that the bleeding did not appear to be abating even though the uterus was contracting appropriately. Dr. Low decided to take Mrs. Yu to surgery to perform an exploratory laparotomy and possible emergency hysterectomy. The physician knew that if she could not stop the bleeding, the patient's life would be in danger. She packed the uterus as tightly as possible, instructed nursing staff to find blood for a transfusion, covered the patient with a sheet, placed the patient on oxygen, and began wheeling the patient's gurney to the elevator.

Community Hospital of the West is a major tertiary care facility in a large US city. It has always provided obstetrical delivery and neonatal services in the north wing of the second floor of the facility. Delivery rooms were developed in this wing. Surgical services and the operating rooms were developed in the north wing on the third floor. When patients required cesarean section deliveries or other surgical treatment, they had to be transferred from the delivery rooms on the second floor to the operating rooms on the third floor.

Dr. Low and the obstetrical nurses assisting her waited for approximately one minute before an elevator arrived. Most of the hospital staff found the elevators very slow and had commented on this many times over the years. Dr. Low, the nurse, and Mrs. Yu arrived in about another minute and a half on the third floor, and they rushed into an operating room. Crash induction of anesthesia was begun. As the operating room staff tried to get a line in to start the blood transfusion and Dr. Low began to remove the packing from the uterus, a massive amount of blood gushed from the organ. The patient's heart went into ventricular fibrillation, and despite emergency resuscitative efforts, Mrs. Yu died.

Because the death occurred during a surgical procedure, it was reportable to the county coroner's office. The coroner accepted the case and performed an autopsy. Mrs. Yu was found to have an anomalous uterine artery that had been opened upon delivery of the placenta, and she bled to death.

QI Toolbox Techniques

The death of a patient as discussed in the real-life example is always classified as a sentinel event. In such cases, the Joint Commission requires the organization to do a root-cause analysis of the event to discover what processes in the organization led to the occurrence. There is always the possibility that unusual and unexpected events will occur. No one really could have known that Mrs. Yu's uterus was anomalous in its blood supply. Does that mean that Mrs. Yu's death was truly inadvertent? Could the death of this patient have been averted despite the anomaly in her anatomy?

The toolbox technique used most often in root-cause analysis is the **cause-and-effect** or **fishbone diagram.** This technique structures the root-cause inquiry and ensures that the investigators examine the situation from all perspectives. As figure 10.6 shows, the fish

Figure 10.6.   Sample cause-and-effect diagram

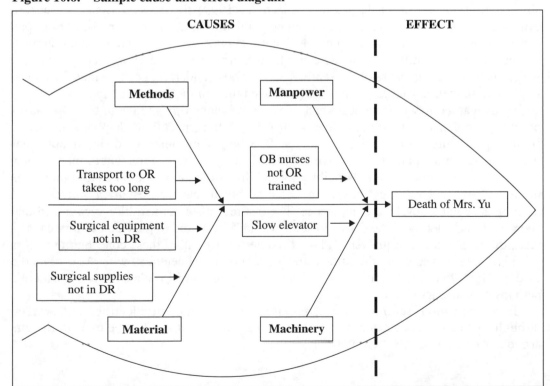

bones delineate the causes of the situation (the effect is at the head of the fish) as classified in four categories. In the structure shown, the categories all begin with the letter *M*. This design was intended to make it easier to remember the categories as "the four *M*s": *Manpower*, *Material*, *Methods*, and *Machinery*. Other approaches use other names for the categories, for example, *People*, *Policies*, *Procedures*, and *Equipment*.

- *Manpower* examines influences of the human worker on the situation. In the case of Mrs. Yu's death, a human worker influence was the obstetrical nurses' lack of training in surgical procedures. This lack of training meant that surgical procedures could not be performed in the delivery room.

- *Material* examines the influences of supplies and equipment on the situation. In the real-life example, surgical supplies and equipment were not available to Dr. Low in the delivery room, so she could not perform the necessary exploratory procedure there.

- *Methods* examines influences of policies and procedures on the situation. In Mrs. Yu's case, it was the policy of the institution to take all obstetrical cases requiring surgical delivery or other surgical procedures to the operating room on the third floor of the hospital. This policy caused a fairly long period of time to elapse during transport, and in this situation led to the patient's death from blood loss.

- *Machinery* examines influences of machines or other major pieces of equipment on the situation. In this case, the slowness of the elevator in the hospital contributed to the delay in effective treatment.

In root-cause analysis, it is important to continue to ask the question *Why*? until the absolute root cause has been discovered. Omachonu (1999) discusses proximate versus root causes. *Proximate causes* are those that can be pointed to directly. In the real-life example, a proximate cause was the inability of the obstetrical nurses to assist in emergency surgical procedures. However, that proximate cause has, in turn, many underlying causes, some of which may be the root cause of the sentinel event. Those underlying causes must be identified, because their existence is what really allowed the sentinel event to happen.

Investigators of Mrs. Yu's death had to ask *Why*? many times to get to the root causes of all the problems contributing to that occurrence. With respect to the lack of expertise in surgical procedures of obstetrical nursing staff, asking *Why*? uncovered significant negative attitudes on the part of all involved. Obstetrical nurses were reluctant to take on new responsibilities. Nursing administration was unwilling to commit the funds to train nurses in new expertise. Obstetrical physicians were skeptical that the obstetrical nurses could develop acceptable levels of competence. The institution's administration recognized that significant remodeling of the delivery suites would be required to provide the surgical services there. If root-cause analysis had not been performed, all of these contributing factors would have remained under the surface and would not have been dealt with. As is often the case, many different situations came together at the same time to contribute to a patient's perhaps unnecessary death.

In any situation, several levels of proximate causes must be identified and worked through to finally uncover the root causes. Repeatedly asking *Why*? helps investigators arrive at root causes. (See figure 10.7.)

Figure 10.7. Sample root-cause analysis

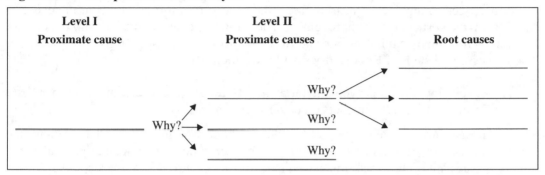

After the investigation and root-cause analysis of the factors that contributed to Mrs. Yu's death, administrators at Community Hospital of the West recognized that the current configuration of the delivery suite in the facility had directly contributed to a patient's death. In a situation in which her anomalous uterine anatomy presented the care team with dangerous and unexpected consequences, she need not have died. If the exploratory laparotomy and possible emergency hysterectomy procedures could have been performed in the delivery room, Mrs. Yu's life probably could have been saved.

The administrators recognized that every transport of a patient from the delivery room to the operating rooms exposed the patient to unnecessary risk. The time wasted in transport in this case had proved fatal. The administrators undertook reconfiguration of the system to prevent the recurrence of this situation. The delivery rooms were rapidly remodeled and equipped with all the supplies and equipment necessary to support the performance of surgical procedures. Obstetrical nurses were retrained to assist on surgical procedures so that these procedures could be performed in the delivery room just as they would be performed in the operating rooms. Following that episode, all cesarean sections and other emergency procedures were performed without requiring the patient to be transported to an operating room.

Robust Process Improvement

In preparing to revise Joint Commission publications and processes to be released for 2009, Commission leadership carefully examined the performance of healthcare organizations in improving patient care and, in particular, dealing with the patient safety issues for which the Commission had begun the NPSG initiatives. Findings of this evaluation revealed less than stellar performance on the part of the industry in dealing with these issues. It was apparently realized that part of the problem was the ability of organizations to carry through on improvement initiatives using previously disseminated improvement processes. Commission officials found the industry as a whole had not developed very reliable responses (in the statistical sense of being able to maintain improvements on the same issue continuously over time).

In response, the Joint Commission has begun to focus attention on this issue with its presentation of "Robust Process Improvement." This initiative first recognizes that root-cause analysis often ends up being somewhat superficial when actually put into action in a healthcare organization. It often does not effectively direct investigation and, as currently practiced, often does not assemble all the necessary information about the event to best inform the best course of improvement. There is also no way in the industry to compile learning across many similar events and over time to inform best practices for everyone. The five essential steps of Robust Process Improvement are:

1. specifying the improvement target [that] requires participants to narrow the issue . . . to its core impacts on patient care and safety;

2. measuring the size of the problem with current data, identifying the absolute frequency of occurrence over recent periods of time and remembering that these issues are often so risk-intensive that even one occurrence is unacceptable;

3. identifying the SPECIFIC causes for the occurrence from all vantage points: leadership, personnel policy, standardized procedures, information systems and technology, communication pathways, management and supervision philosophies and processes, teamwork and coordination, staffing patterns and levels, equipment, care environment, and individuals;

4. targeting interventions to the most important, modifiable causes; [and]

5. embedding interventions into routine work processes (Chassin 2008).

To assist organizations in maintaining the gains made through Robust Process Improvement, the Commission also intends during the second decade of the 21st century to become a clearinghouse to facilitate more rapid and widespread development and adoption of proven solutions to problems and errors with which many or most healthcare organizations are trying to deal, particularly in the areas identified by the NPSGs.

Case Study

Derek Johnson, MD, has been an anesthesiologist at Community Hospital of the West for 15 years. He is 45 years old. The physician is board certified to perform all kinds of anesthesia procedures, including every type of surgical procedure and obstetrical anesthetic procedure. His colleagues have noticed for some time that he has become more and more haggard looking, but they ascribe this to the hectic work schedule that anesthesiologists often must maintain.

One day, Dr. Johnson was admitted to the intensive care unit at Community Hospital of the West. The news quickly spread through the organization. He was suffering from a compromised immune system and was close to dying from septicemia that had developed from abscesses in his arm as a result of injections. Some of the operating room (OR) nurses discussed the situation on dinner break. They speculated that Dr. Johnson was a drug addict. The anesthesiologists provided morphine to patients from a lockbox to which only the anesthesiologists had keys. They were not required to account for narcotics beyond signing out dosages from the lockbox on a clipboard that hung beside it. Some of the OR nurses had noticed over the past six months to a year that Dr. Johnson's patients invariably received morphine for pain as recorded on the clipboard. In many cases, the patients clearly did not need it. For most, there was no documentation in their medical charts of morphine administration.

One of the nurses reported that three months earlier she had cornered the chief of the anesthesia service and told him of Dr. Johnson's narcotics irregularities. Not wanting to challenge or accuse a fellow physician, the chief said indignantly that there must be some other explanation and terminated the conversation. The nurse did not discuss the problem with anyone else—not the director of surgical services, the chief of surgery, the director of nursing, or an administrator. The possibility of personal addiction among healthcare workers is a job-related issue. Individuals who have access to pain medication and who frequently medicate others to help relieve pain can become caught in an addictive cycle themselves, especially when system processes fail to hold professionals accountable for narcotic use or abuse in the provision of patient care. Most agencies offer employees access to confidential counseling. Unfortunately, many times those who have problems with alcohol or drugs are unable to see their problem and justify their use in a variety of ways. In addition, many employees are untrained about the signs and symptoms of addiction. It is unfortunate that the facility did not have a mechanism in place for confidentially reporting the suspected abuse. It may have been possible to offer the physician a professional intervention that could have saved him physically and mentally from such severe trauma.

Case Study Questions

1. Besides basic human weakness, what other reasons are evident for Dr. Johnson's narcotics problem?

2. Does Community Hospital of the West bear any responsibility for Dr. Johnson's predicament?

3. What are the root causes of this situation? Build a cause-and-effect diagram on the basis of the findings in this case study.

4. What is the likely response of the hospital's governing body to this situation?

5. Discuss a situation that you have experienced as a visitor to a healthcare facility. How was the incident handled? Was a patient advocate involved? Did the incident have a good outcome?

Project Application

Students should consider using a cause-and-effect diagram or findings from a root-cause analysis in their storyboard projects.

Summary

Healthcare facilities can be dangerous places. Employees in healthcare organizations must be continuously aware of situations that might result in injury to patients, visitors, or staff. To help manage the dangerous work setting, healthcare organizations use occurrence reporting systems that track and document incidents. Healthcare organizations are experiencing greater scrutiny and regulation from external supervisory agencies to proactively identify and monitor potential areas of high risk. Greater data collection in all areas of healthcare has led to more defined disease-specific care standards, NPSGs, and improved processes for eliminating errors in care.

Risk managers carefully review their organizations' policies and procedures and assess their staffs' ability to execute them. Risk managers also maintain open channels of communication with any person injured in a facility until a satisfactory resolution of the claim or litigation has been reached. Finally, risk managers provide information to the organizations' insurers and represent their organizations at all formal meetings and legal proceedings related to injury claims.

References

Chassin, M.R. 2008. Hospital executive briefings: Current challenges in safety and quality. Presentation to the Joint Commission, September.

Croteau, R.J. 2005. National Patient Safety Goals. Joint Commission on Accreditation of Healthcare Organizations Conference.

Joint Commission on Accreditation of Healthcare Organizations. 1998. Sentinel events: Approaches to error reduction and prevention. *Joint Commission Journal of Quality Improvement* 24(4):175–186.

Joint Commission. 2011. *Hospital Accreditation Standards*. Oakbrook Terrace, IL: Joint Commission Resources.

Kohn, L.T., J.M. Corrigan, and M.S. Donaldson, eds. 1999. Committee on Quality of Health in America, Institute of Medicine. *To Err Is Human: Building a Safer Health System*. Washington, DC: National Academy Press.

MountainStar Family of Hospitals. 2008. Your Patient Rights & Responsibilities.

Omachonu, V.K. 1999. *Healthcare Performance Improvement*. Norcross, GA: Engineering and Management Press.

Patient Safety and Quality Improvement Act of 2005. Public Law 109-41.

Resources

ASHRM and R. Carroll. 2009. *Risk Management Handbook for Health Care Organizations*. San Francisco: Jossey-Bass.

Spath, P.L., ed. 2000. *Error Reduction in Health Care: A Systems Approach to Patient Safety*. San Francisco: Jossey-Bass.

Spath, P.L. 2002. Target: Patient safety. *Journal of AHIMA* 73(3):26–33.

Wakefield, D.S., B.J. Wakefield, T. Uden-Holmon, T. Borders, M. Blegen, and T. Vaughn. 1999. Understanding why medication administration errors may not be reported. *American Journal of Medical Quality* 14(2):81–88.

Youngberg, B.J., ed. 1999. *Essentials of Hospital Risk Management*. Gaithersburg, MD: Aspen Publishers.

Chapter 11
Building a Safe Medication Management System

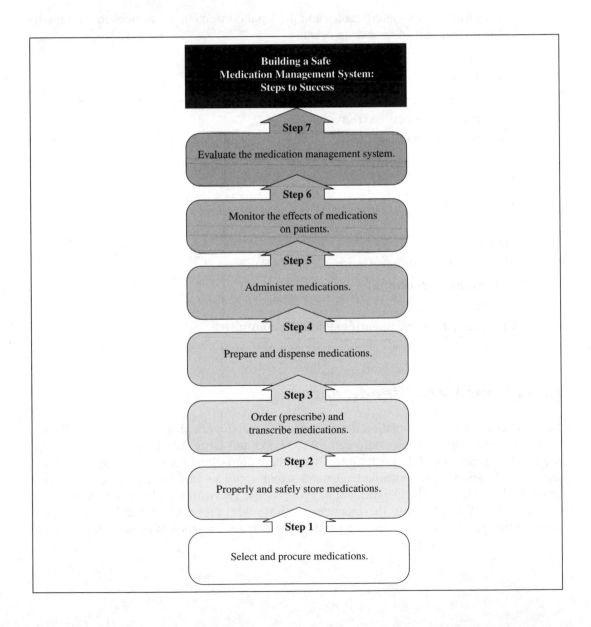

Building a Safe
Medication Management System:
Steps to Success

Step 7

Evaluate the medication management system.

Step 6

Monitor the effects of medications on patients.

Step 5

Administer medications.

Step 4

Prepare and dispense medications.

Step 3

Order (prescribe) and transcribe medications.

Step 2

Properly and safely store medications.

Step 1

Select and procure medications.

Learning Objectives

- To identify how health policy, national initiatives, the private sector, and professional advocacy all contribute to the design of safe medication management systems

- To recognize the important functions included in a safe and effective medication management system

- To use the failure mode and effects analysis (FMEA) tool as a proactive risk reduction strategy in anticipating medication system failures

- To become familiar with the process of monitoring and reporting medication errors and adverse drug events

- To describe patient safety issues and the legal consequences associated with medication errors and adverse drug events

Key Terms

Adverse drug events (ADEs)

Adverse drug reaction (ADR)

Brand name

Diversion

Drug pedigree

Formulary

Generic

Medication administration record (MAR)

Medication reconciliation

Near miss

Pharmacy and therapeutics (P and T) committee

Background and Significance

Federal laws provide a foundation for the state laws that govern pharmacy practice. In addition to the specific drug laws enforced by the Food and Drug Administration (FDA) and the Drug Enforcement Administration (DEA), there are federal laws regulating the licensing of medications and controlled substances that apply to various aspects of pharmacy practice. In each state, the Department of Professional Licensing (DOPL) or its equivalent is responsible for regulating the practices of those who prescribe and dispense medication. There are instances in regulating pharmacy practice in which state law may be more stringent than federal law or vice versa. These regulations have been developed to protect the patient and to provide for minimum standards of practice. The rules and regulations that govern pharmacy practice are continually evaluated and updated as new technologies, new medications, and new protocols are developed and adopted.

In the United States, drug regulation is performed by the FDA. FDA activity is a major factor in the nation's public health and safety. Before a drug can be marketed, testing must show that it is safe and effective for its intended use. Once marketed, the drugs are monitored by the FDA to make sure that they work as intended and that there are no serious negative (adverse) effects from their use. If drugs that are marketed are found to have significant adverse effects, the FDA can recall them (take them off the market). Bringing a new drug to market is a long and difficult process in which the vast majority of research does not produce a successful drug. Thousands of chemical combinations must be tried to find one that might work as hoped. Once a potentially useful drug is created, it must undergo an extensive testing and approval process before it can be made available to the public. In the United States, the length of time from the beginning of development through testing and ultimate FDA approval is often more than 10 years.

The sheer number of available drugs; their different names and costs; multiple prescriptions from different physicians; and the potential for system errors in the ordering, preparing, dispensing, and administration of medications are among the many factors that make using prescription drugs a complex area filled with many risks. More than a decade has passed since the publication of a landmark study in which Leape et al. (1995) identified system failures as fundamental to errors that cause **adverse drug events (ADEs)**. That study found that 39 percent of errors occurred in prescriber ordering and 38 percent in nurse administration. The most common type of errors were dosing errors, which occurred more than three times as frequently as any other error, and which most commonly included wrong-dose errors and errors in drug choice. More important, Leape and colleagues identified lack of knowledge about the drug as the most common proximal cause of drug errors, accounting for 22 percent of ADEs. Of particular concern to health professionals involved in the medication-use process was a later study in 1995 by Bates et al. that showed that adverse medical events originate more frequently from errors and accidents in the processes of prescribing, ordering, dispensing, administration, and monitoring of medication than from any other sources.

Since the much-publicized report by the Institute of Medicine (IOM) in 1999, *To Err Is Human: Building a Safer Health System*, numerous initiatives have emerged to address the problems associated with medical errors. The IOM itself orchestrated the drive to improve safety and quality in US healthcare by publishing a series of reports on various problems associated with the healthcare delivery system (Kohn et al. 1999).

The Agency for Healthcare Research and Quality (AHRQ) of the Department of Health and Human Services (HHS) has provided grants in excess of $50 million to sponsor studies aimed at learning more about how errors occur, how technology can be used most effectively, and how processes of care can be improved. Technologies such as computerized prescriber order entry (CPOE), bedside scanning using bar code technology, electronic health records, e-prescribing, "smart" infusion devices, and automated storage and distribution devices that record information at the point of care hold great promise, especially if the data being captured are analyzed using standard terminology and translated into quality improvement at all levels.

The Leapfrog Group was founded in 2000 by the Business Roundtable (a national association of Fortune 500 chief executive officers). Mobilizing the purchasing power of 150 large employers, the group's intent was to leverage its influence to initiate and advance safety improvements in healthcare, thereby giving consumers information to make more informed healthcare choices. The Leapfrog Group advocates a variety of quality improvement standards, including CPOE and evidence-based medicine.

Since 2000, the Joint Commission has engaged in significant efforts to redesign standards and survey processes to better reflect national initiatives aimed at quality improvement and patient safety. The Joint Commission made medication management a top priority by increasing the stringency of its standards and aligning them with a survey process that uses a tracer methodology (see chapter 15 for a full discussion of tracer methodology) to track the care, treatment, and services that patients receive. Using this tracer activity allows surveyors to assess how staff from various disciplines work together and communicate across services to provide safe, high-quality care. Medication reconciliation is a National Patient Safety Goal (NPSG) (Joint Commission 2011a) aimed at addressing a major cause of medication-related sentinel events and medication errors due to a lack of information. (See chapter 8 for a full discussion on NPSGs.) This goal encourages disciplines including physicians, nurses, and pharmacists, as well as the patient and family, to work together to safely prescribe medications and assess for potential allergic or adverse drug reactions. **Medication reconciliation** is the process of identifying the most accurate list of all medications a patient is currently taking (including prescription and nonprescription drugs, vitamins, herbal agents, and nutritional supplements) and then comparing (reconciling) the list against the physician's admission, transfer, and discharge orders at each transition point along the patient's continuum of care. For example, when a patient is transferred from one organization to another, the complete and reconciled list of medications is communicated to the next provider of service, and the communication is documented. Alternatively, when the patient leaves the organization's care and goes directly to his or her home, the complete and reconciled list of medications is provided to the patient's known primary care provider, the original referring provider, or a known next provider of service, or it may be provided directly to the patient.

The list of organizations involved in patient safety efforts continues to grow. Research on the nature, frequency, and preventability of adverse medical events has begun to bear fruit as health insurance payers and companies grow more insistent that providers demonstrate they are implementing strategies for patients' safety.

Building a Safe and Effective Medication Management System: Steps to Success

The medication management system is complex and involves many processes (figure 11.1). Medications are typically prescribed by physicians, dispensed by pharmacists, and administered by nurses. All efforts in the design and implementation of a medication management

Figure 11.1.   Steps in medication management

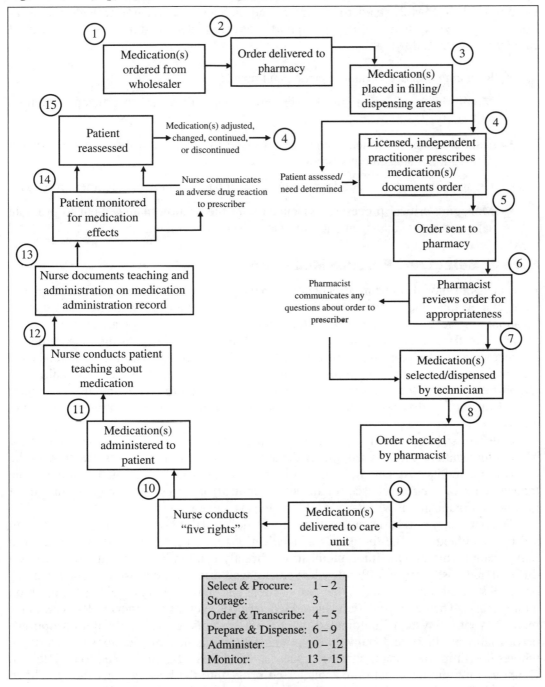

system must be collaborative and multidisciplinary to be fully effective. The Joint Commission (2011b, MM-2) standards define a well-planned and well-implemented medication management system as one that supports patient safety and improves the quality of care by doing the following:

- Reducing practice variation, errors, and misuse

- Monitoring medication management processes with regard to efficiency, quality, and safety

- Standardizing equipment and processes across the organization to improve the medication management system

- Using evidence-based good practices to develop medication management processes

- Managing critical processes associated with medication management to promote safe medication management throughout the organization

Step 1: Select and Procure Medications

Pharmacies in most healthcare organizations have processes in place to select, purchase, store, and evaluate medications. The list of medications maintained in the healthcare organization is generally referred to as a **formulary** and includes medications selected by members of the healthcare team—those involved in ordering, dispensing, or administering medications or monitoring their use. The formulary is composed of medications used for commonly occurring conditions or diagnoses treated in the healthcare organization. Organizations accredited by the Joint Commission are required to maintain a formulary and document that they review it at least annually for a medication's continued safety and efficacy.

Criteria used to determine an organization's formulary may include indications for when a medication is to be used, the medication's effectiveness, risks associated with the medication, and its cost. Due in large part to the costs associated with medication use, the management of drug purchases (or inventory control) is an essential process that most healthcare organizations will have to address to stay solvent.

The pharmacy purchases medications from a licensed drug wholesaler or directly from a drug manufacturer. The thousands of medications that a pharmacy stocks come from many manufacturers. Obtaining medications directly from individual manufacturers is a difficult and costly process. Wholesalers stock inventories of the most used medications, obtain less used medications as they are needed, and make frequent deliveries, often on a daily basis. They also provide value-added services such as emergency delivery, automated inventory systems, automated purchasing systems, generic substitution options, private label products, and many other options. Obtaining most medications from a single wholesaler simplifies the purchasing process and reduces a facility's need to maintain it. Counteracting the introduction of counterfeit drugs into the US drug distribution chain, the FDA, through the Prescription Drug Amendment (2007), established requirements related to the distribution of prescription drugs. Manufacturers, wholesalers, repackagers, and pharmacies must maintain a record (known as a **drug pedigree**) of the chain of custody of the drug as it moves through the supply chain from manufacturer to pharmacy. For the pharmacy, this includes establishing a relationship with a single wholesaler (FDA 2007).

Step 2: Properly and Safely Store Medications

Medications stored in the pharmacy and in patient care areas are tightly controlled, and policies clearly delineate who has access to these storage areas. Federal and state laws require all medications be stored in a manner that prevents access by unauthorized individuals. These same laws require that controlled medications (medications classified as narcotics) be maintained in double-locked storage. Tracking and recordkeeping in the purchasing, prescribing, and dispensing of controlled medication are more regulated than that for noncontrolled medications because of their potential for abuse and diversion. Automated storage and dispensing devices are new technologies being used to control unauthorized access to medications.

Medications approved for use in an organization are routinely stored under conditions suitable for product stability as recommended by the drug manufacturer. This includes storing medications at certain temperatures—for example, room temperature (68°–77°F), refrigeration (36°–46°F), or freezing (4°–14°F)—in refrigerators designated "medication only." A schedule to inventory all medications stored in the facility to check for "out-dates" or expired medications also should be considered when addressing policies related to product stability. Additional storage considerations related to product stability and safety include storing medications for external use separately from medications for internal use and storing extremely flammable products in a specially designed area.

Each healthcare organization must determine whether a patient's own medications may be used and how they will be stored, controlled, and administered. These medications, if allowed, can be administered only in response to orders that permit their administration, and only after they have been evaluated and identified as correct. Some organizations may prohibit patients from using their own medications if the medication is on the facility's formulary and available for use. An organization may allow a patient's use of his or her own medication when it is a nonformulary medication or when an alternative is not available. The organization must define its responsibilities for the safe use and proper storage of these medications.

Several NPSGs involving proper and safe storage of medications have become Joint Commission accreditation requirements in recent years. For example, an organization must select and require at least an annual review of a list of look-alike or sound-alike drugs used in the facility; ensure medications and the chemicals used to prepare medications are accurately labeled with contents, expiration dates, and warnings; limit or standardize the number of drug concentrations available in the organization; remove concentrated electrolytes from care units or areas; and maintain medications in patient care areas in the most ready-to-administer forms available from the manufacturer (unit doses prepackaged by the pharmacy). Each of these standards evolved from findings noted in root-cause analyses conducted when a related sentinel event or near miss occurred in a healthcare organization. These NPSGs have evolved as "best practices" (in the industry) for controlling medication-related adverse events. For a full discussion of NPSGs, see chapter 8.

Ensuring proper and safe storage of medications requires periodically inspecting all medication storage areas (including areas where emergency medications and supplies are kept and where sample medications are used) to confirm controls are in place and working. Inspections should focus on storage conditions (for example, refrigeration and protection from light), security (especially for controlled substances), removal of expired and other unusable medications, identification of hazardous conditions, and labeling errors. Findings from inspections should be documented, communicated to appropriate stakeholders in the organization, and corrected as appropriate.

Step 3: Order (Prescribe) and Transcribe Medications

Many medication errors occur while communicating or transcribing medication orders. A clear understanding and communication among staff involved in the medication process are essential. The healthcare organization is responsible for taking steps to reduce the potential for error or misinterpretation when orders are written or verbally communicated. To reinforce the skills and judgments needed for safe medication ordering, organizations often provide training and orientation to providers involved in this step of medication use management.

The required elements of how orders are written or communicated must be specified in policies and procedures. State and federal laws require medication orders to include the patient's name, medication, strength, route, rate, and frequency. Medication orders should clearly state administration times or time intervals between doses. The organization has to be very clear about which abbreviations are *not acceptable to use* when writing or communicating medication orders. The Joint Commission (2011c) has a published list of abbreviations classified as "Do Not Use" that healthcare organizations cannot use in writing or communicating medication orders. (See figure 11.2.) Organization policy should also define whether or when the diagnosis, condition, or indication for use is included on a medication order. Some organizations require an indication for use or special precautions when ordering medications to be taken "as needed," or for medications specified as confusing or high risk (for example, those with look-alike, sound-alike names).

During surveys with the Joint Commission, an organization's staff may be asked to discuss efforts made to minimize the use of verbal medication orders. Policies should define when verbal (orally transmitted) orders are acceptable to use and how "read-back" requirements are met. A current Joint Commission standard (2011b, PC 02.01.03) requires the person taking the verbal order to read it back to the prescriber to confirm the order was transcribed correctly. Some organizations prohibit verbal orders for nonurgent, high-risk medications or for high-risk patients. The Joint Commission (2011c) has defined several types of orders to consider and address in organization policy as "acceptable to use"; these are listed in figure 11.3. Additional policy considerations specific to ordering medications may include determining when **generic** or **brand name** medications are acceptable or required as part of a medication order; when weight-based dosing for pediatric populations is required; and what actions to take when medication orders are incomplete, illegible, or unclear.

Figure 11.2.   The Joint Commission's "Do Not Use" abbreviations

Official "Do Not Use" List[1]		
Do Not Use	**Potential Problem**	**Use Instead**
U (unit)	Mistaken for "0" (zero), the number "4" (four) or "cc"	Write "unit"
IU (International Unit)	Mistaken for "IV" (intravenous) or the number 10 (ten)	Write "International Unit"
Q.D., QD, q.d., qd (daily) Q.O.D., QOD, q.o.d, qod (every other day)	Mistaken for each other Period after the "Q" mistaken for "I" and the "O" mistaken for "I"	Write "daily" Write "every other day"
Trailing zero (X.0 mg)* Lack of leading zero (.X mg)	Decimal point is missed	Write "X mg" Write "0.X mg"
MS MSO4 and MgSO4	Can mean "morphine sulfate" or "magnesium sulfate" Confused for one another	Write "morphine sulfate" Write "magnesium sulfate"

[1]Applies to all orders and all medication-related documentation that is handwritten (including free-text computer entry) or on preprinted forms.

*Exception: A "trailing zero" may be used only where required to demonstrate the level of precision of the value being reported, such as for laboratory results, imaging studies that report size of lesions, or catheter/tube sizes. It may not be used in medication orders or other medication-related documentation.

Additional Abbreviations, Acronyms, and Symbols (For *possible* future inclusion in the Official "Do Not Use" List)		
Do Not Use	**Potential Problem**	**Use Instead**
> (greater than) < (less than)	Misinterpreted as the number "7" (seven) or the letter "L" Confused for one another	Write "greater than" Write "less than"
Abbreviations for drug names	Misinterpreted due to similar abbreviations for multiple drugs	Write drug names in full
Apothecary units	Unfamiliar to many practitioners Confused with metric units	Use metric units
@	Mistaken for the number "2" (two)	Write "at"
cc	Mistaken for U (units) when poorly written	Write "mL" or "milliliters"
µg	Mistaken for mg (milligrams) resulting in one thousand-fold overdose	Write "mcg" or "micrograms"

Source: Joint Commission 2011c.

Figure 11.3.   **Organization policy defines whether these types of orders are acceptable to use**

- "As needed" (PRN) orders–orders acted upon based on the occurrence of a specific indication or symptom

- Standing orders–written instruction to administer a medication without a prescription to a person in circumstances specified in instructions

- Hold orders–instructions to temporarily suspend (place medication orders on hold) under specified conditions and to alert users at specified times while a medication is on hold

- Automatic stop orders–a date or time to discontinue a medication

- Resume orders–restart an order that was previously held (a blanket statement for reinstatement of previous orders for medications is not acceptable)

- Titrating orders–orders in which the dose is either progressively increased or decreased in response to the patient's status

- Taper orders–orders in which the dose is decreased by a particular amount with each dosing interval

- Range orders–orders in which the dose or dosing interval varies over a prescribed range, depending on the situation or patient's status

- Orders for compounded drugs or drug mixtures not commercially available

- Orders for medication-related devices (for example, nebulizers and catheters)

- Orders for investigational medications

- Orders for herbal products

- Orders for medications at discharge or transfer

Source: Joint Commission 2011b.

Step 4: Prepare and Dispense Medications

Joint Commission (2011b, MM 05.01.01) standards specify that before a medication can be prepared and dispensed, a pharmacist must review each prescription or medication order for appropriateness. No medication or patient care area is exempt from this requirement. For example, the standard applies to preprinted labor and delivery orders, orders for respiratory therapy medications, orders for emergency department patients awaiting transfer to an inpatient room, and orders for preoperative patients in an ambulatory surgery unit. However, there are exceptions to the (pharmacist) review requirement: if a licensed independent practitioner (LIP) controls the ordering, preparation, and administration of the medication; in urgent situations when the delay would harm the patient; or when the pharmacy is not open 24 hours a day, 7 days a week. In the last two instances, the pharmacist is required to conduct (and document) a retrospective review of all orders during this period as soon as the pharmacy reopens. The Joint Commission (2011b, MM 05.01.01) further defines minimum criteria to use when the pharmacist reviews each medication order. (See figure 11.4.) A number of studies that have evolved into regulatory requirements and standards of practice over the years have shown that pharmacist intervention can reduce costs and improve patient safety. Increased pharmacist involvement in the review of patient allergies, laboratory test results, and medication orders for appropriateness has been shown to significantly reduce ADEs. Types of errors prevented by pharmacist review include prescribing errors (inappropriate

Figure 11.4. The Joint Commission's minimum criteria for pharmacist reviews

Pharmacist-required review elements for each prescription or medication order
- The appropriateness of the drug, dose, frequency, and route of administration
- Therapeutic duplication
- Real or potential allergies or sensitivities
- Real or potential interactions between the prescription and other medications or food
- Current or potential impact as evidenced by laboratory values
- Other contraindications
- Variation from organizational criteria for use
- Other relevant medication-related issues or concerns such as legibility of the medication order

Source: Joint Commission 2011c.

dose, nonformulary agent, and medication errors related to transfer), administration errors (inappropriate timing of dose, transcription errors, missed doses, extra doses given, and doses administered after discontinuation), pharmacy errors (inappropriate dose recommendations, incomplete dispensing instructions), and discharge errors. Pharmacists providing patient education can help reduce errors that may occur after discharge because the patient does not understand how to take a medication. At a minimum, any concerns, issues, or questions a pharmacist may have in reviewing a medication order are clarified with the individual prescriber *before* dispensing the medication.

Activities associated with medication preparation and dispensing pose one of the greatest opportunities for error within the pharmacy. Preparation includes the selection, compounding (sterile or nonsterile), packaging, and labeling of the medication. For each of these steps it is critical that technical and professional staff understand the importance of following appropriate procedures and double-checking their work. Selecting the incorrect medication is the most common type of error that other healthcare professionals and the general public associate with the pharmacy. Safeguards must be instituted to ensure that the appropriate medication is selected 100 percent of the time. Practices such as separating look-alike and sound-alike medications and using bar-coded storage technology have improved medication selection safety.

Product selection is only the first step in the preparation phase. A large percentage of medications require further manipulation or labeling. Compounding for sterile and nonsterile medications often requires calculations to determine the amounts of medications and other ingredients to be used. All sterile compounding is performed in a clean environment, so pharmacy personnel need to be trained in aseptic technique and product handling. In particular, antineoplastic (cancer) agents require even greater safeguards because of their caustic nature and potential for harm.

The order delivery process also has the potential for error. As with selecting and compounding, standard safeguards can be employed to decrease the likelihood of errors in order delivery. Standardizing medication labeling and ensuring medications are delivered to the correct patient care unit and stored in a secure, patient-specific area labeled with the patient's name will help minimize errors.

Step 5: Administer Medications

In many healthcare organizations, medication administration is the step in the process that has the fewest safeguards, because it typically relies on a single healthcare professional to perform it correctly; there are generally no double-checks prior to administration. An NPSG, however, requires that the healthcare organization use at least two patient identifiers prior to administering medications as a safety precaution to ensure patients receive the correct medication. Hospitals also require a second check for certain medications, such as insulin, chemotherapy drugs, and other high-alert or high-risk drugs, prior to administering. Identifying ways that the patient, along with family members, can be involved in his or her own care is an important patient safety strategy (and NPSG). The patient can be an important source of information about aspects of his or her care and treatment.

One of the most effective ways to prevent administration errors is to provide all medications used within the organization in ready-to-administer form (for example, the unit dose system). All medications should remain intact in labeled packaging until the point of administration. Maintaining an accurate **medication administration record (MAR)**, which is the record used to document each dose of medication administered to a patient, is critical. Procedures must be in place to periodically review the accuracy of the MAR, particularly with respect to controlled substances like narcotics.

The "five rights" of medication administration (right patient, right drug, right dose, right route, and right time) should be observed at all times. This practice should be monitored periodically for validation as well. The pharmacy should provide appropriate administration instructions (for example, "take with food") for each medication. A pharmacist should be readily available to answer questions related to a particular drug or its administration. Pharmacists also should participate in the design of a medication administration course for nursing staff and other healthcare professionals responsible for drug administration.

Automated bedside point-of-care (BPOC) scanning is a relatively new process that uses bar code technology to guarantee that the five rights are followed. Using a handheld scanner, the nurse scans his or her own badge and the medication to be administered and then scans the patient's bar-coded identification bracelet. Because the system is electronically integrated with the MAR, it will alert the nurse if an error is detected (for example, wrong patient, wrong administration time, or wrong medication). These systems are now considered to be "best practice" because of their ability to reduce medication errors associated with drug administration by 65 to 86 percent.

Step 6: Monitor the Effects of Medications on Patients

Monitoring the effects of medications on patients helps ensure that medication therapy is appropriate, and minimizes the occurrence of an ADE. Each patient's response to his or her medication is monitored according to his or her clinical needs. Monitoring a medication's effect on a patient includes gathering the patient's own perceptions about side effects and, when appropriate, perceived efficacy, and referring to information from the patient's health record, relevant lab results, clinical response, and medication profile. A healthcare organization should have a well-defined process for monitoring a patient's response to the first dose(s) of a medication.

The most widely recognized and studied adverse event involving drug therapy is an **adverse drug reaction (ADR)**. The World Health Organization (WHO) (1970) defines an ADR as "any response that is noxious, unintended, and undesired and that occurs at doses normally used in man for prophylaxis, diagnosis, or therapy." Healthcare organizations using medication therapy as a treatment intervention need to have processes in place to respond to actual or potential ADRs. Reporting requirements may include external reporting to the United States Pharmacopoeia (USP), the FDA, or the Institute for Safe Medication Practices (ISMP). Internal reporting requirements should be incorporated into the organization's performance improvement (PI) program and integrated into the activities of the Pharmacy and Therapeutics Committee.

High-risk or high-alert drugs are those drugs involved in a high percentage of medication errors and sentinel events and medications that carry a higher risk for abuse, errors, or other adverse outcomes. Lists of high-risk and high-alert drugs available from resources such as the ISMP and the USP are developed by the organization based on its unique utilization patterns of drugs and its own internal data about medication errors and sentinel events. Examples of high-risk drugs include investigational drugs, controlled medications, medications not on the approved FDA list, medications with a narrow therapeutic range, psychotherapeutic medications, and look-alike or sound-alike medications that arc new to the market or new to the hospital.

The National Coordinating Council for Medication Error Reporting and Prevention (NCC MERP) (2011) has developed a widely used taxonomy for error reporting. The taxonomy provides a logical framework for the development of internal error-reporting programs as well as a means to classify and analyze medication errors.

Step 7: Evaluate the Medication Management System

The key to an effective medication management system is having mechanisms for reporting potential and actual medication-related errors and a process to improve patient safety based on this information. Today, most care settings have an organization-wide PI process to identify and analyze medical errors, medication errors, and near misses. A **near miss** can be described in the following way: If the error had not been identified, could it have caused patient harm? Many organizations treat near misses in the same way that they treat sentinel events, using error-reduction tools such as root-cause analysis or failure mode and effects analysis in an effort to prevent future occurrences. Reporting such adverse events should be nonpunitive, and each report should be reviewed and investigated.

The **pharmacy and therapeutics (P and T) committee** has a key role in multidisciplinary safety improvement activities; its importance cannot be understated. By design, the P and T committee consists of pharmacists, physicians, nurses, hospital administrators, and other healthcare professionals. The committee should have a leadership role in the organization's medication safety efforts. Improvement initiatives should be a major part of every P and T agenda.

Many hospitals have established a medication safety committee that is often a subcommittee of the P and T committee. The medication safety committee reviews and evaluates current literature, national error reports, internal reports, and hospital processes to assist with recommendations for improvement. Membership on this committee also should be multidisciplinary and should include representatives from the hospital's risk management and quality departments. In some hospitals, this committee is charged with forming risk-reduction teams and developing auditing systems to investigate patterns of medication errors. From these findings, they identify and recommend system-based changes.

One very important aspect of medication management in healthcare facilities is the monitoring of the use and administration of controlled substances because of the prominent utilization of these medications in treatment of patients of all kinds. Inpatient acute care settings utilize various types of pain control medications, outpatient clinic settings may distribute narcotics for outpatient control of pain issues, and substance-abuse treatment settings may distribute psychotropics and synthetic opiates to their clients. Any of these uses and settings can be at risk of diversion. **Diversion** is the removal of a medication from its usual stream of preparation, dispensing, and administration by personnel involved in those steps in order to use or sell the medication in nonhealthcare settings. An individual might take the medication for personal use, to sell on the street, to sell directly to a user as a dealer, or to sell to others who will redistribute for the diverting individual. Documentation of the preparation, dispensing, and administration may still be entered in information systems or health records as though the medication were given as ordered. Therefore, the work of all staff involved in the medication processes must be regularly monitored specifically to ensure that all policies and procedures are being followed to the letter and that every dose of medication can be accounted for through all steps of the process. When carelessness or infractions in following policy and procedure are identified, the individual involved must be counseled and must undergo disciplinary action. The organization must also determine whether to report the individual to law enforcement and licensing or credentialing agencies. State licensure is usually revoked for infractions of these policies, and professional discipline is instituted per the certifying agency. If the individual involved is diverting for personal use, the organization may have to be further involved as an employer to assist the individual in habilitation of substance-abuse issues.

QI Toolbox Techniques

There are two proven approaches to error analysis and reduction that are used by the healthcare industry and are standard requirements of the Joint Commission. The first approach, root-cause analysis (RCA), is a (reactive) retrospective tool used to analyze the true cause of error. The second approach, failure mode and effects analysis (FMEA), is a (proactive) prospective tool useful in analyzing potential problems when introducing new systems or equipment or when looking anew at an existing process. Both tools are used frequently in analyzing potential or real medication errors. Each of us, in fact, uses RCA and FMEA every day. Manasse and Thompson (2005) provide straightforward examples to understanding both tools:

> In using RCA, suppose, for example, you turn on a light switch and nothing happens. The room remains dark. The problem is evident: The light does not go on. Your job is to find out why. There may be many reasons: The bulb might need to be replaced, the switch might be broken, the wiring

might need to be repaired, the wall receptacle may not be working, or the circuit breaker may have tripped. You search until you determine why your light did not go on. In doing so, you perform a root-cause analysis. Once you determine the root cause, you can fix the problem.

FMEA is equally easy to understand. Assume you are about to take a vacation. In planning your time away from home, you probably consider what might go wrong. What is the chance of rain? If you run out of money, how would you access your banking account? If you are visiting a location where Montezuma's revenge may strike, how likely is that to occur, and what should you take with you just in case? These are all examples of anticipating a problem (error) that might occur, determining the relative risk that it may occur, and planning how to prevent it or minimize its impact. In short, you have conducted a FMEA: a failure mode (it might rain) and effects (you would have to stay inside to keep dry if you didn't have the proper rain gear) analysis.

Organizations are increasingly using RCA as one step of a proactive risk reduction effort combined with FMEA. One step of an FMEA involves identifying the root causes of failures (failure mode).

Real-Life Example: The Thalidomide Lesson

In 1962, a new sleeping pill containing the drug thalidomide was found to cause severe birth defects when used by pregnant women. This included lost limbs and other major deformities that affected thousands of children in Europe, where the drug had been widely used. In the United States, the drug was not yet approved for marketing and was only being used in tests. However, the nature of the defects and the number of children affected created a public demand in the United States for tighter drug regulations that resulted in the Kefauver-Harris Amendment. From then on, manufacturers were required to provide proof of both safety and effectiveness of a drug before they could market it. Later studies found thalidomide to be safe and effective in treating multiple myeloma, and it is now approved for that use.

Case Study

In the medication reconciliation process a healthcare organization needs to identify the most current list of medications that a patient is taking, both prescription and nonprescription. The reconciliation process involves multiple levels of the care team, including nursing, pharmacy, attending physician, and the house staff. In figures 11.5 through 11.8 you will find printouts from the pharmacy system that show an example of the medication reconciliation process. During this hospitalization, the patient was admitted to the nursing unit 4E. Her attending physician began the medication reconciliation process by documenting all medications this patient is currently taking on the Physician Medication Reconciliation List in figure 11.5. Then in figure 11.6, the house staff, pharmacist, and nursing staff verify the list of medications for the patient prior to her transfer to the nursing unit 4B. At the time of this transfer all orders for medications are re-sent to the pharmacy system. In figure 11.7, the house staff, pharmacist, and nursing staff verify the list of medications for the patient prior to her transfer to the nursing unit 4D with subsequent transmission of these orders to

Figure 11.5. Example of physician medication reconciliation list

Community Hospital of the West Physician Medication Reconciliation List		
Patient Name: Jan Smith DOB: 7/25/1995 MRN: 45-89-65 Primary Care Physician: David Jones, MD Account #: 41125468		
Allergies: No Allergy Information	Location: 4E	Date: 1/23/11

Order Date	Medication
1/23/11	See ICU Electrolyte Ordersheet For C 0.87-0.99 Infuse at 2GM/HR Calcium Gluconate 2000 MG Sodium Chloride 0.9% 50 ML
1/23/11	See ICU Electrolyte Ordersheet For C 0.75-0.86 Infuse at 2GM/HR Calcium Gluconate 3000 MG Sodium Chloride 0.9% 100 ML
1/23/11	See ICU Electrolyte Ordersheet For C <0.75 Infuse at 2GM/HR Calcium Gluconate 4000 MG Sodium Chloride 0.9% 100 ML
1/23/11	Fentanyl Citrate 25-50 MCG IV Q15Min PRN Pain
1/23/11	Hydromorphone HCL 1MG/ML 0.2-0.6 MG IV Q 1 HR PRN Pain Hold for RR<8 or Sedation
1/23/11	Mag Sulfate 2GM In NS 50ML 2-6 GM IV See ICU Electrolyte Ordersheet
1/23/11	Naloxone Hydrochloride 0.4MG IV PRN
1/23/11	Ondansetron Hydrochloride 4MG IV Q 6 Hours PRN Nausea/Vomiting
1/23/11	Potassium Chloride 10 MEQ IV See ICU Electrolyte Ordersheet K 3.3-3.5 40 MEQ, 3.0-3.2 50 MEQ, <3.0 Notify House Staff, Infuse at 10 MEQ/HR
1/23/11	Potassium Chloride 40 MEQ PO ICU Lytes sliding scale K 3.3-3.5 MEQ PO/NG
1/23/11	Potassium Chloride 50 MEQ PO ICU Lytes sliding scale K 3.0-3.2 PO/NG
1/23/11	Propofol 1 Infusion IV 10-100 MCG/KG/Min Titrate as directed
Sign below to indicate a medication reconciliation has been performed. Signature: _____*David Jones, MD*_____ MD # __4528__ Date: ____1/23/11____	

Figure 11.6.   Example of first physician transfer order reconciliation

<table>
<tr><td colspan="4" align="center">**Community Hospital of the West**
Physician Transfer Orders
Transmit to Inpatient Pharmacy</td></tr>
<tr><td colspan="4">Patient Name: Jan Smith
DOB: 7/25/1995
MRN: 45-89-65
Primary Care Physician: David Jones, MD
Account #: 41125468</td></tr>
<tr><td colspan="4">*Initial EACH medication in the appropriate column to indicate continue or discontinue.</td></tr>
<tr><td colspan="4">Allergies: No Allergy Information   Location: 4E   Date: 1/25/11</td></tr>
<tr><td>**Order Date**</td><td>**Medication**</td><td>**Cont**</td><td>**D/C**</td></tr>
<tr><td>1/23/11</td><td>See ICU Electrolyte Ordersheet For C 0.87-0.99
Infuse at 2GM/HR
Calcium Gluconate 2000 MG
Sodium Chloride 0.9% 50 ML</td><td></td><td>*JB*</td></tr>
<tr><td>1/23/11</td><td>See ICU Electrolyte Ordersheet For C 0.75-0.86
Infuse at 2GM/HR
Calcium Gluconate 3000 MG
Sodium Chloride 0.9% 100 ML</td><td></td><td>*JB*</td></tr>
<tr><td>1/23/11</td><td>See ICU Electrolyte Ordersheet For C <0.75
Infuse at 2GM/HR
Calcium Gluconate 4000 MG
Sodium Chloride 0.9% 100 ML</td><td></td><td>*JB*</td></tr>
<tr><td>1/23/11</td><td>Cefazolin Sodium 1000 MG IV
Every 8 HRS</td><td>*JB*</td><td></td></tr>
<tr><td>1/24/11</td><td>Diphenhydramine HCL 25–50 MG IV
Q6 HRS PRN Itching</td><td>*JB*</td><td></td></tr>
<tr><td>1/24/11</td><td>(Dextrose 5% - 1/2NS-KCL 20 MEQ)
D5-1/2NS with KCL 20 MEQ 1000ML
Continuous Infusion Rate = 75 ML/HR</td><td>*JB*</td><td></td></tr>
<tr><td>1/23/11</td><td>(Lovenox)
Enoxaparin Sodium 30 MG SQ
Twice Daily Inject in Abdominal area</td><td>*JB*</td><td></td></tr>
<tr><td>1/23/11</td><td>(Sublimaze (Generic))
Fentanyl citrate 25-50 MCG IV
Q 15 MIN PRN Pain (ICU Orders)</td><td></td><td>*JB*</td></tr>
<tr><td>1/23/11</td><td>(Fentanyl Citrate)
Fentanyl Drip 10 MCG/ML Drip Rate: 25 MCG/HR
    Fentanyl Citrate   2500 MCG
    Sodium Chloride 0.9%   250 ML</td><td></td><td>*JB*</td></tr>
<tr><td>1/24/11</td><td>(Dilaudid)
Hydromorphone HCL 1MG/ML 0.2-0.6 MG IV
Q 1 HR PRN Pain   Hold for RR <8 or Sedation</td><td></td><td>*JB*</td></tr>
<tr><td>1/24/11</td><td>(Hydromorphone Hydrochloride)
Hydromorphone PCA 1 MG/ML 30 ML
Dose: 0.4 MG Lock Out: 10 Min
    Hydromorphone Hydrochloride 30 MG/3 ML
    Sodium Chloride 0.9%   30 ML</td><td>*JB*</td><td></td></tr>
</table>

(Continued on next page)

Figure 11.6. *(Continued)*

Orders continued for this patient
Patient Name: Jan Smith DOB: 7/25/1995 MRN: 45-89-65 Primary Care Physician: David Jones, MD Account #: 41125468

Order Date	Medication	Cont	D/C
1/23/11	(Mag Sulfate 2 GM in NS 50 ML) Mag Sulfate 2 GM in NS 50 ML 2-6 GM IV See ICU Electrolyte Ordersheet		JB
1/23/11	(Naloxone HCL) Naloxone Hydrochloride 0.4 MG IV PRN	JB	
1/23/11	(Naloxone HCL) Naloxone Hydrochloride 0.1 MG IV While on PCA PRN RR <8 per Min or Sedation Scale >=5 Repeat dose Q1-2 Min X3 PRN		JB
1/23/11	(Zofran) Ondansetron Hydrochloride 4 MG IV Q 6 Hours PRN Nausea/Vomiting	JB	
1/23/11	(Potassium Chloride) Potassium Chloride 10 MEQ IV See ICU Electrolyte Ordersheet K 3.3-3.5 40 MEQ, 3.0-3.2 50 MEQ, <3.0 Notify House Staff, Infuse at 10 MEQ/HR		JB
1/23/11	(Potassium Chloride) Potassium Chloride 40 MEQ PO ICU Sliding Scale K 3.3-3.5 40 MEQ, PO/NG		JB
1/23/11	(Potassium Chloride) Potassium Chloride 50 MEQ PO ICU Sliding Scale 3.0-3.2 MEQ, PO/NG		JB
1/23/11	(Diprivan) Propofol 1 Infusion IV 10-100 MCG/KG/Min Titrate as Directed		JB

1/23/11	(Sodium Phosphate)
	See ICU Electrolyte Ordersheet Infuse over 4 hours
	PRN Phos 1.6-1.9
	  Sodium Phosphate 15 MML
	  Sodium Chloride 0.9% 250 ML
			JB

1/23/11	(Sodium Phosphate)
	See ICU Electrolyte Ordersheet Infuse over 4 hours
	PRN Phos <1.6
	  Sodium Phosphate 30 MML
	  Sodium Chloride 0.9% 250 ML
			JB

Signature: *Jared Briggs, MD*   MD # 87962 Date/Time: 1/25/11 0700
RN Signature: *June Anderson, RN*   ID: 587   Date/Time: 1/25/11 0830

Figure 11.7.   Example of second physician transfer order reconciliation

Community Hospital of the West **Physician Transfer Orders** Transmit to Inpatient Pharmacy	

Patient Name: Jan Smith
DOB: 7/25/1995
MRN: 45-89-65
Primary Care Physician: David Jones, MD
Account #: 41125468

*Initial EACH medication in the appropriate column to indicate continue or discontinue.

Allergies: No Allergy Information	Location: 4B	Date: 1/30/11

Order Date	Medication	Cont	D/C
1/25/11	Diphenhydramine HCL 25–50 MG IV Q6 HRS PRN Itching	*DN*	
1/25/11	(Dextrose 5% - 1/2NS-KCL 20 MEQ) D5-1/2NS with KCL 20 MEQ 1000ML IVF Continuous Infusion Rate = 100 ML/HR	*DN*	
1/27/11	(Lovenox) Enoxaparin Sodium 90 MG SQ Every 12 Hours (For PE)	*DN*	
1/30/11	(Neurotin) Gabapentin 400 MG PO Three Times A Day	*DN*	
1/27/11	(Dilaudid) Hydromorphone HCL 1MG/ML 0.4 MG IV Q 2 HR PRN Severe Breakthrough pain while on PCA	*DN*	

1/27/11	(Hydromorphone Hydrochloride)
	Hydromorphone PCA 1 MG/ML 30 ML
	Dose: 0.2 MG Lock Out: 10 Min
	    Hydromorphone Hydrochloride 30 MG/3 ML
	    Sodium Chloride 0.9% 30 ML
		DN	

1/27/11	(Naloxone HCL) Naloxone Hydrochloride 0.1 MG IV While on PCA PRN RR <8 per Min or Sedation Scale >=5 Repeat dose Q1-2 Min X3 PRN	*DN*	
1/27/11	(Zofran) Ondansetron Hydrochloride 4 MG IV Q 6 Hours PRN Nausea/Vomiting	*DN*	

Signature: ___*Darren Nelson, MD*___   MD # 98750 Date/Time: _1/30/11 1135_

RN Signature: ___*Louise Sullivan, RN*___   ID: _451_   Date/Time: _1/30/11 2000_

Figure 11.8.   NPSGs related to medication management

The Joint Commission on Accreditation of Hospitals	
National Patient Safety Goal 8	Accurately and completely reconcile medications across the continuum of care
NPSG.08.01.01	A process exists for comparing the patient's current medications with those ordered for the patient while under the care of the hospital.
NPSG.08.02.01	When a patient is referred to or transferred from one hospital [or unit] to another, the complete and reconciled list of medications is communicated to the next provider of service, and the communication is documented. Alternatively, when a patient leaves the hospital's care to go directly to his or her home, the complete and reconciled list of medications is provided to the patient's known primary care provider, the original referring provider, or a known next provider of service.
NPSG.08.03.01	When a patient leaves the hospital's care, a complete and reconciled list of the patient's medications is provided directly to the patient, and, as needed, the family, and the list is explained to the patient and/or family.
NPSG.08.04.01	In settings where medications are used minimally, or prescribed for a short duration, modified medication reconciliation processes are performed.

Source: Joint Commission 2011a, NPSG 14–18.

the pharmacy system. Note in this example that at each point of transfer all medications are verified by the patient's physician, nurse, and the pharmacist. This process is an effort to minimize the potential for medication errors.

1. What documentation on the medication list for the nursing unit 4E to 4B indicates the double-checks by the pharmacy?

2. How would you evaluate this medication reconciliation process in regard to the Joint Commission standards for Medication Management as presented in figure 11.8?

Summary

Medication use is one of the most regulated functions in healthcare. Medication errors and ADEs are the leading causes of medical errors reported in healthcare. A comprehensive medication management system addresses processes related to medication selection, ordering, preparation, administration, and monitoring for effects. Tools used to proactively analyze potential medication errors and reactively analyze actual medication errors include FMEA and RCA. Monitoring medication errors is one way to effectively address medication management system improvements.

References

Bates, D.W., D.J. Cullen, N. Laird, L.A. Petersen, S.D. Small, D. Servi, G. Laffel, B.J. Sweitzer, B.F. Shea, and R. Hallisey. 1995. Incidence of adverse drug events and potential adverse drug events: Implications for prevention. *JAMA* 279:1200–1205.

Food and Drug Administration. 2007. http://www.fda.gov.

Joint Commission. 2011a. National Patient Safety Goals. *2011 Hospital Accreditation Standards*. Oakbrook Terrace, IL: Joint Commission Resources.

Joint Commission. 2011b. Medication management. *2011 Hospital Accreditation Standards*. Oakbrook Terrace, IL: Joint Commission Resources.

Joint Commission. 2011c. The Official "Do Not Use" List. http://www.jointcommission.org/assets/1/18/Official_Do%20Not%20Use_List_%206_10.pdf.

Kohn, L.T., J.M. Corrigan, and M.S. Donaldson, eds. 1999. Committee on Quality of Health in America, Institute of Medicine. *To Err Is Human: Building a Safer Health System*. Washington, DC: National Academy Press.

Leape, L.L., D.W. Bates, D.J. Cullen, J. Cooper, H.J. Demonaco, T. Gallivan, R. Hallisey, J. Ives, N. Laird, and G. Laffel. 1995. Systems analysis of adverse drug events. *JAMA* 274:35–43.

Manasse, H.R., and K.K. Thompson. 2005. *Medication Safety: A Guide for Health Care Facilities*. Bethesda, MD: American Society of Health-System Pharmacists.

National Coordinating Council for Medication Error Reporting and Prevention (NCC MERP). 2011. http://www.nccmerp.org/councilRecs.html.

Prescription Drug Amendment of 2007. Public Law 110-85.

World Health Organization. 1970. International drug monitoring: The role of the hospital—a WHO report. *Drug Intelligence & Clinical Pharmacy* 4:101–110.

Resources

Ash, J.S., P.N. Gorman, V. Seshadri, and W.R. Hersh. 2004. Computerized prescriber order entry in U.S. hospitals: Results of a 2002 survey. *Journal of the American Medical Informatics Association* 11(2):95–99.

Committee on Quality of Health Care in America; Institute of Medicine. 2001. *Crossing the Quality Chasm: A New Health System for the 21st Century*. Washington, DC: National Academy Press.

Chapter 12
Managing the Environment of Care

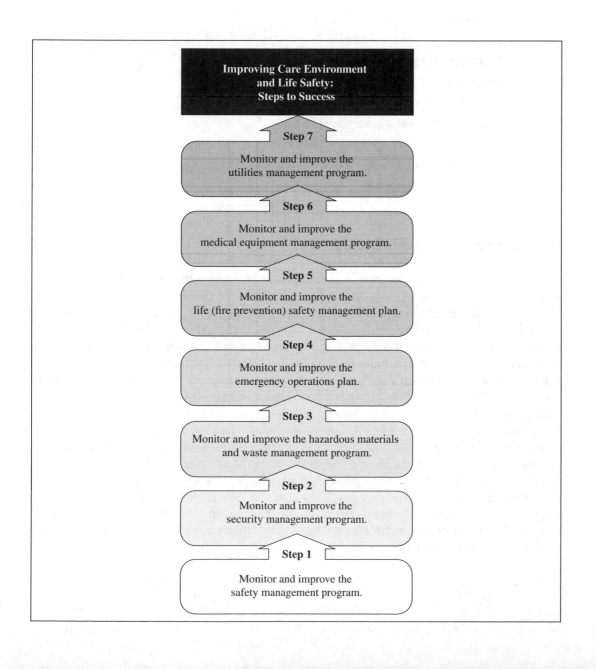

Learning Objectives

- To describe the seven programs and plans that are key elements in a healthcare organization's environment of care
- To identify the relationship between the Joint Commission Environment of Care (EOC) standards and the National Incident Management System (NIMS) in the development of an emergency operations plan
- To describe a risk assessment and a hazard vulnerability analysis
- To describe the safety monitoring process

Key Terms

All hazards approach

Emergency

Emergency operations plan (EOP)

Hazard vulnerability analysis (HVA)

Material safety data sheets (MSDSs)

National Incident Management System (NIMS)

Total program approach

Background and Significance

The goal of managing the care environment in any healthcare organization is to provide a safe, functional, supportive, and effective environment for patients, staff, and visitors. By their nature, healthcare organizations have the potential to be dangerous environments. They house complex equipment, hazardous materials, toxic and flammable chemicals, infectious materials, and medical devices that can injure patients, visitors, and staff when inappropriately managed. Also of major importance, healthcare organizations need to be prepared for catastrophic emergencies such as natural, human-caused, or technology-caused events and the handling of an influx of injured individuals. Additionally, healthcare workers provide care to all individuals and attendant lifestyles, and family relationships or other visitor issues may spill over into the healthcare environment. These same issues in the lives of the healthcare worker may affect the work area. Violence in the workplace is a threat that must be assessed and managed. Because of these and other safety issues, healthcare organizations must continuously monitor and evaluate their patient environments and the safety and security of the individuals receiving or providing care services. Developing plans to manage the healthcare environment, educating staff regarding their role in supporting a safe environment, monitoring and assessing performance, and making improvements based on these findings are all critical functions that contribute to effectively managing the environment of care.

Improving the Environment of Care: Steps to Success

The Joint Commission requires a varying number of safety functions and plans, depending on the type of license or services provided by an organization. This chapter will review all seven safety programs required by the Joint Commission for an acute care hospital. The standards require the assessment of safety features for patients, staff, and visitors. The environment of care (EOC) includes the safety, security, and comfort of staff, patients, and visitors. For the purposes of safety, a visitor is defined as anyone in the healthcare organization who is not an employee. In addition to patients and patient families and other guests, this includes independent contract physicians, nursing students, agency personnel, and vendors. A quality program emphasizes clinical care and patient well-being, as do the Joint Commission patient safety standards. The patient safety standards, as they relate to the EOC, are discussed later in this chapter.

The seven written safety standards or plans for the EOC cover the following areas (Joint Commission 2011a):

- Safety management

- Security management

- Hazardous materials and waste management

- Emergency management

- Life safety management

- Medical equipment management

- Utilities management

This chapter discusses the scope, goals, and objectives of each program or plan. Common to each plan is an orientation and education program for personnel, with their specific roles and responsibilities defined, as well as an annual evaluation of each plan's objectives, scope, performance, and effectiveness.

Step 1: Monitor and Improve the Safety Management Program

The safety management program is the overall plan for the EOC. It demonstrates the master plan and outlines the design of the safety functions for the organization. The safety committee oversees all safety programs, including:

- Designating an individual or individuals to develop, implement, and monitor the safety management activities

- Designating an individual or individuals to intervene whenever conditions immediately threaten life or health or threaten damage to equipment or buildings

- Overseeing the worker safety program

- Conducting comprehensive, proactive risk assessments that evaluate potential adverse impact on buildings, grounds, equipment, occupants, and internal physical systems

- Establishing safety policies and procedures that are practiced and reviewed as frequently as necessary

- Responding to product medical/equipment/pharmaceutical safety recalls

- Ensuring that all grounds and equipment are maintained appropriately

The overall safety plan describes the risk assessment of the physical environment, the design of services that support the therapeutic and work environment, and the education and preparation of the staff to safely and securely serve the organization's patient population. The plan describes how to train staff on use of equipment and how to maintain an environment that is responsive to patient care needs, including responding to emergencies.

Additionally, the plan includes organizational goals for monitoring and maintaining the physical components of the EOC and for managing human activities. Reporting organizational incidents (reports of unusual occurrences, incident reports, security reports, and so forth) relevant to the safety programs is integral to each safety function. Each safety program is evaluated annually, and plans are updated or revised to address current regulatory compliance, policy, and procedural changes based on the organizational experiences and staff training needs.

Step 2: Monitor and Improve the Security Management Program

The security management program is designed to manage the physical and personal security of the patients served, staff, and individuals coming to the organization as well as the security of the building, equipment, supplies, and information.

The security management program is reflective of the security risk assessment conducted annually. Table 12.1 shows an example of a security risk assessment and program evaluation. Included in the risk assessment is the trending of the prior-year statistics of security incidents in the facility and on the grounds, including any workplace violence against employees. If possible, the assessment should include a police grid of crime in the areas or neighborhoods surrounding the facility. Neighborhood crime statistics may be available on Web sites, through local hospital or merchants security associations, or by calling local police precincts. Security risks determined by the assessment are evaluated, and processes, procedures, and education are designed and implemented to avoid those risks. Efficacy of the security plan is monitored, trended, and reported to the safety committee, administration, medical staff, and the board of trustees. Staff are educated and trained to report or respond to security events.

The security management program and security policies describe procedures to manage door access, visiting hours, and after-hours access to the facility; security in parking areas; high-risk patients, such as victims of crime or patients in police custody; high-profile patients or visitors; weapons in the facilities; suspicious individuals and disruptive visitors; Code Green (manpower) alerts; and the issuing of trespass notices, to name a few.

Security emergency response may address phone threats, use of panic alarms, abduction of babies or children, civil unrest, bomb threats, and hostage crises. In addressing

Table 12.1.   Security risk assessment and program evaluation

---

FACILITY DESCRIPTION

Name of facility: _____

Type of facility (e.g., acute care hospital): _____

City and State: _____

Location: _____ inner city   _____ suburban   _____ rural   ____university

Licensed beds: _____

Avg. beds occupied: _____

Number of buildings: _____

Total square footage occupied: _____

Number of parking garages: _____

Total number of surface parking lots: _____

Total number of parking spaces: _____

Emergency room services? ____ yes   _____ no

If yes, what level? _____

Birthing services? _____ yes   _____no

If yes, what is the annual number of births per year? _____

Psychiatry unit? _____ yes   _____ no

Local crime rate (as determined by police statistics): ____ high   ____ medium   ____ low

---

SECURITY DEPARTMENT DESCRIPTION

Special authority? _____ yes   _____ no

If yes, please describe: _____

_____

Weapons carried? _____ yes   _____ no

If yes, please describe: _____

_____

To what department and position does security report? _____

_____

Position	Number	FTEs
Director	_____	_____
Manager(s)	_____	_____
Coordinator(s)	_____	_____
Supervisor(s)	_____	_____
Officer(s)	_____	_____
Parking Officers	_____	_____
Secretary	_____	_____
Dispatch Coord.	_____	_____
Dispatch	_____	_____
Other	_____	_____
Copy Drive Record	_____	_____

(Continued on next page)

Table 12.1. *(Continued)*

SECURITY PROGRAM EVALUATION

Date of last internal program evaluation: _____

Date of last external program evaluation: _____

High Risk Areas/Departments	Vulnerability/Risk
_____	_____
_____	_____
_____	_____
_____	_____

List major vulnerabilities/risks identified, actions taken, and status (use additional sheets, if necessary):

Vulnerability/Risk	Actions Taken	Status
_____	_____	_____
_____	_____	_____
_____	_____	_____

SECURITY-RELATED STATISTICS			
Type of Incident	**Number**	**Increase from 2008**	**Value-Cost—N/A**
Homicide(s)			
Abduction(s)			
Abduction attempt(s)			
Arson(s)			
Rape(s)			
Other sexual assault(s)			
Robbery(s)—armed			
• Facility departments			
• Public areas (internal)			
• Public areas (grounds)			
• Parking lot(s)			
• Parking garage(s)			
Robbery(s)—unarmed			
• Facility departments			
• Public areas (internal)			
• Public areas (grounds)			
• Parking lot(s)			
• Parking garage(s)			
Auto theft(s)			

Table 12.1. *(Continued)*

Type of Incident	Number	Increase from 2008	Value-Cost—N/A
Auto break-ins			
Assaults(s)			
• Emergency room			
• Psychiatry			
• Patient care areas			
• Public areas (internal)			
• Public areas (grounds)			
• Parking lot(s)			
• Parking garage(s)			
Threats			
• Emergency room			
• Psychiatry			
• Patient care areas			
• Public areas (internal)			
• Public areas (grounds)			
• Parking lot(s)			
• Parking garage(s)			
Bombing(s)			
Bomb threat(s)			
Theft			
• Facility property			
• Patient property			
• Staff property			
• Visitor property			
• Contractor property			
Vandalism			
• Graffiti			
Fraud(s)			
Suicide(s)			
Unsecured doors			
Workplace violence			
Auto accidents			
Tickets issued			
Total number	_____	_____	
Total value			_____

(Continued on next page)

Table 12.1.   *(Continued)*

SPECIAL EVENTS	DATE	# PARTICIPANTS

BACKGROUND CHECKS	_____ yes	_____ no
DRUG SCREENING	_____ yes	_____ no

SECURITY RISK ASSESSMENT

Item	Yes	No	Comments
Is there a security plan for the entire organization?			
Is it reviewed and revised at least annually?			
Does it contain a mission statement that parallels the hospital mission?			
Is there a letter of authority from the CEO for the security director?			
Is the local geographic area deteriorating?			
Is crime in the area increasing?			
Is there a relationship between security and the state and local police?			
Do patients, staff, and visitors feel secure?			
Has the organization's patient mix changed since last year?			
Has security staffing increased, decreased, or stayed the same?			
Is the current staffing level adequate? If not, why?			
Can security resources be better utilized?			
Have security resources changed in relation to hospital resources?			
Have electronic security devices been installed, altering staffing needs?			
Are security staff competent to do their jobs? How do you know?			
Have security personnel performed to the expected level?			
Does security staff receive training and education as needed?			

Table 12.1.   *(Continued)*

Item	Yes	No	Comments
Are education and training effective? How do you know?			
How are employees made aware of their security roles?			
Do you know how to respond to a security incident (how to contact security and complete an incident report)?			
Is security addressed in the hospital's orientation program?			
Are security policies and procedures up to date?			
Do they accurately guide security staff on how to do their jobs?			
Is security addressed regularly by the safety committee?			
Does the safety committee make recommendations for security?			
Are security incidents tracked and analyzed as trends? Who does this?			
Are there performance standards in place that measure key aspects of the security program?			
Is security participating in any performance improvement projects?			
Has security improved, gotten worse, or stayed the same in the last year?			
Are security radios/pagers, etc., appropriate?			
Are there emergency phones/intercoms in place?			
Is there a security hot line?			
Is closed-circuit television appropriate, in place, functional, etc.?			
Are there alarms in place, with policies that explain them?			
Are patrol vehicles appropriate?			
Do officers carry protective weapons? Are they trained to do so?			
Do security personnel know and observe all applicable laws, standards, and guidelines?			
Do security staff participate in policy development?			
Are lighting levels appropriate throughout the facility?			
Are access control policies in place and adequate?			

(Continued on next page)

Table 12.1. *(Continued)*

Item	Yes	No	Comments
Are doors checked and secured appropriately?			
Does the facility design allow for hiding areas?			
What are the sensitive, high-risk areas?			
How were they determined to be high risk?			
What measures were taken to reduce this risk? Have they worked?			
Are there security policies for infant abduction, workplace violence, bomb threats, hostage situations, emergency preparedness, fires, VIPs, hazardous spills, weapons, theft, trespassing, identification, and visitation?			
Are these policies enforced?			

terrorist activities, plans may include handling of suspicious packages and mail or securing ventilation systems. If animal research is conducted at the facility, the research lab may be vulnerable to activist groups from the community, and security should address securing the labs and protecting personnel.

Security management is a technology-rich field, and an organization needs to describe the technology it uses in the plan or policies. The security office is usually responsible for issuing employee identification badges and keys or authorizing electronic card access to doors. It usually also is responsible for camera surveillance, and in many organizations, security works closely with telephone operators, dispatchers, or receptionists who may assist with monitoring cameras.

The security management program identifies security-sensitive areas in the hospital, for example, cash-handling areas (such as the cafeteria, pharmacy, gift shop, and admitting), registration or clinic areas where copays are collected, and the cashier's office (where all processing of events involving money are based). Other sensitive areas are the inpatient and outpatient pharmacies, where drugs and controlled substances are stored for dispensing. The emergency department can be a high-risk area for violence, as police may bring crime victims or perpetrators here for medical treatment. Gang violence may spill into the treatment area as rivals try to finish criminal activity that began on the streets.

Care providers in the nursery, pediatric units, and labor and delivery may be forced to handle domestic disputes or violence as divorced parents, estranged families, or unmarried parents carry their arguments into the healthcare organization. An abused child may need protection from the abuse perpetrator, or a child may be at risk from a parent faced with losing custody to a state family protection agency.

Security addresses the multiple forms of workplace violence that occur within the healthcare organization. A plan may coordinate activities with the human resources department, social work, employee assistance programs, or the senior leadership of an organization.

Most people think of violence as a physical assault or battery. However, workplace violence is a much broader problem, comprising any act in which a person is abused, threatened, intimidated, or assaulted in his or her employment. Workplace violence includes:

- *Threatening behavior*: Making menacing gestures such as shaking fists, destroying property, or throwing objects

- *Verbal* or *written threats*: Making a verbal threat to harm another individual or destroy property

- *Harassment*: Any behavior that demeans, embarrasses, humiliates, annoys, alarms, or verbally abuses a person and that is known or would be expected to be unwelcome. This includes words, gestures, intimidation, bullying, or other inappropriate activities.

- *Verbal abuse*: Swearing, insulting, or using condescending language

- *Physical attacks*: Hitting, shoving, pushing, or kicking

- *Employee to employee harassment*: Rumors, swearing, verbal abuse, pranks, arguments, or property damage

- *Domestic violence*: Domestic violence does not stay home when its victims go to work. It can follow them, resulting in violence in the workplace.

- *Stranger violence*: Violence perpetrated by clients, visitors, or complete strangers who come to the workplace

Security education should include defining workplace violence and training employees how to defuse potentially violent situations, how to protect against them, and what methods to use to alert security or other personnel. Employees experiencing domestic violence should be encouraged to notify security, their supervisor, or the human resources department. Support and backup can be provided to the employee, such as an escort to and from the car and surveillance of the facility and grounds for a stalker.

Security events should be trended and reported to the safety committee at least quarterly. (See table 12.2.) The prior year's security events are reviewed annually with the risk assessment. The evaluation and analysis of event trends and concerns determine the need for new security equipment, technology, and procedures, along with education for the staff if needed. The annual appraisal is submitted to the safety committee, medical staff, and board of trustees for recommendations and approval.

Step 3: Monitor and Improve the Hazardous Materials and Waste Management Program

Healthcare facilities manage toxic and hazardous materials and wastes by identifying chemicals and materials that need special handling and disposal. Organizations are required by regulations of the US Department of Labor, Occupational Safety and Health Administration (OSHA), to have a written hazards communication program and to educate and train staff about the unique hazards in the workplace.

Table 12.2. Security risk assessment and program evaluation

SAFETY MANAGEMENT	1st quarter	2nd quarter	3rd quarter	4th quarter	YTD	GOAL
WORKER SAFETY						
Total industrial accidents						
OSHA reportables						
Type of injury						
• Back injury						
• Needlestick total						
—Employees						
—Student/contract staff						
—# Avoidable						
—# Not avoidable						
• Blood fluid exposure						
• Chemical exposure						
• Repetitive motion injury						
• Patient related						
Productive hours						
Hours lost						
Rate						
Modified duty hours						
PPDs						100%
Safety inspections						1/yr nonpatient 2/yr clinical areas
SECURITY MANAGEMENT	**1st quarter**	**2nd quarter**	**3rd quarter**	**4th quarter**	**YTD**	**GOAL**
Security investigations						
Theft						

This material is prepared for the quality of the hospital and medical care rendered by hospitals and physicians. This document is confidential and, to the extent the law applies, is protected pursuant to Utah Annotated Code 26-25-1-5 and 58-13-4.

Table 12.2. (*Continued*)

SECURITY MANAGEMENT	1st quarter	2nd quarter	3rd quarter	4th quarter	YTD	GOAL
Unsecured doors						
Narcotic discrepancy						
Vehicle accidents						
Vandalism						
Suspicious individual/ trespass						
Code Pink/missing child						
Elopement						
Psych assists						
Visitor injury						
Missing patient belongings						
Calls to police						
Total helipad landings						
Night helipad landings						
EMERGENCY MANAGEMENT	1st quarter	2nd quarter	3rd quarter	4th quarter	YTD	GOALS
Disaster/Drills						2 drills/year Every 4 months
HAZARDOUS MATERIALS MANAGEMENT	1st quarter	2nd quarter	3rd quarter	4th quarter	YTD	GOALS
Inventory updated						Minimum annually
Number of hazmat spills						
Biohazard waste found in landfill						·
Air quality sampling						

(*Continued on next page*)

Table 12.2. (*Continued*)

LIFE SAFETY MANAGEMENT	1st quarter	2nd quarter	3rd quarter	4th quarter	YTD	GOALS
# Fire drills						1/shift/quarter
# Participants						
Staff demonstrate knowledge of fire safety						
Staff describe evacuation procedures						
Annual fire extinguisher inspection						
Monthly fire extinguisher inspection						
Fire alarm system inspections						
# Items listed in SOC						
EQUIPMENT MANAGEMENT	**1st quarter**	**2nd quarter**	**3rd quarter**	**4th quarter**	**YTD**	**GOAL**
Equipment PMs						
Equipment scheduled for PM						
% of PMs completed						
PMs not completed						
Malfunctioning equipment						
% of malfunctioning equipment						

This material is prepared for the quality of the hospital and medical care rendered by hospitals and physicians. This document is confidential and, to the extent the law applies, is protected pursuant to Utah Annotated Code 26-25-1-5 and 58-13–4.

Table 12.2. *(Continued)*

EQUIPMENT MANAGEMENT	1st quarter	2nd quarter	3rd quarter	4th quarter	YTD	GOAL
Abuse errors						
Unduplicated errors						
% of unduplicated errors						
Patient injured						
Alarm testing						
Alarm testing (%)						
UTILITIES MANAGEMENT	**1st quarter**	**2nd quarter**	**3rd quarter**	**4th quarter**	**YTD**	**GOAL**
Utility failures						
Emergency generator testing						
Medical gas testing (annually)						
RECALLS REQUIRING ACTION	**1st quarter**	**2nd quarter**	**3rd quarter**	**4th quarter**	**YTD**	**GOAL**
Equipment						
Medical devices						
Pharmaceuticals						
EDUCATION	**1st quarter**	**2nd quarter**	**3rd quarter**	**4th quarter**	**YTD**	**GOAL**

This material is prepared for the quality of the hospital and medical care rendered by hospitals and physicians. This document is confidential and, to the extent the law applies, is protected pursuant to Utah Annotated Code 26-25-1-5 and 58-13-4.

OSHA (1994) Hazard Communication Standard 1910.1200 is based on the premise that employees who may be exposed to hazardous chemicals in the workplace have a right to know about the hazards and how to protect themselves. For this reason, the Hazard Communication Standard is sometimes referred to as the Worker Right-to-Know Legislation, or more often just as the Right-to-Know Law.

The Hazard Communication Standard sets forth guidelines and requirements in six areas:

- *Chemical labeling provision*: Requires that all chemicals in the workplace be labeled. The label is to include the name of the chemical and warnings about any hazards the material may present.

- **Material safety data sheets (MSDSs)**: Documents that give detailed information about a material, including any associated hazards. MSDSs must be available to employees at locations where hazardous materials are used, and they must include the following information (see figure 12.1 for an example of an MSDS):

  —*Identity*: The name of the chemical (same name as that on the container's label)

  —*Hazardous ingredients*: Chemical names of all the substances that make up the particular hazardous material

  —*Physical and chemical characteristics*: Additional information such as the material's appearance, odor, boiling point, vapor pressure, vapor density, solubility in water, melting point, and evaporation rate

  —*Fire and explosion hazards*: Specifications and special instructions, such as conditions when the material might catch fire or explode and what should be done to deal with the hazard

  —*Reactivity*: Identifies certain conditions under which a reactive material becomes dangerous. Reactive materials can burn or explode when exposed to air or water or when mixed with other substances. This section provides information to help prevent exposure of such materials to these conditions.

  —*Health hazards*: Identifies how the hazardous material could harm a person, symptoms of exposure, and the emergency first-aid procedures to use in case of overexposure

  —*Precautions for safe handling and use*: Details instructions for safe handling of the substance, including how to store, move, and use the materials and what to do in case of a spill or leak

  —*Control measures*: Details the personal protective equipment to use when working with the material, lists safe work procedures, and explains how to clean up after working and before eating so that the material will not cause personal injury or contaminate food

  —*Special precautions*: Lists special handling, transportation, storage, and disposal precautions

Figure 12.1. Example of an MSDS

Clorox®—Clorox Germicidal Bleach
Material Safety Data Sheet
NSN: 793000F046054
Manufacturer's CAGE: 93098
Part No. Indicator: A
Part Number/Trade Name: Clorox Germicidal Bleach
General Information
Company's Name: Clorox Co. (Headquarters)
Company's Street: 1221 Broadway
Company's P.O. Box: 24305
Company's City: Oakland
Company's State: CA
Company's Country: United States
Company's Zip Code: 94612
Company's Emergency Ph #: (800) 446-1014
Company's Info Ph #: (510) 271-7000
Record No. For Safety Entry: 001
Total Safety Entries This Stk#: 001
Status: SE
Date MSDS Prepared: 01NOV92
Safety Data Review Date: 18JAN06
Preparer's Company: Clorox Co. (Headquarters)
Preparer's Street or P.O. Box: 1221 Broadway
Preparer's City: Oakland
Preparer's State: CA
Preparer's Zip Code: 94612
MSDS Serial Number: BYMMQ
Ingredients/Identity Information
Proprietary: NO
Ingredient: Sodium hypochlorite, hypochlorous acid sodium salt
Ingredient Sequence Number: 01
Percent: 5.25
NIOSH (RTECS) Number: NH3486300
CAS Number: 7681-52-9

(Continued on next page)

Figure 12.1.   *(Continued)*

Physical/Chemical Characteristics
Appearance and Odor: Clear, light yellow liquid w/chlorine odor
Boiling Point: 212°F
Specific Gravity: 1.085
Solubility In Water: Complete
pH: 11.4
Fire and Explosion Hazard Data
Special Fire Fighting Procedures: In a fire, cool containers to prevent rupture and release of sodium chlorate.
Unusual Fire And Expl Hazards: Nonflammable/explosive
Reactivity Data
Stability: Yes S
Materials To Avoid: Strong oxidizing agent, acids, ammonia
Hazardous Decomp Products: Hazardous gases, chlorine, and other chlorinated species
Hazardous Poly Occur: No
Health Hazard Data
Route of Entry—Inhalation: Yes
Route of Entry—Skin: No
Route of Entry—Ingestion: Yes
Health Hazard Acute and Chronic: Eyes: Corneal injury. Skin: Irritation. Inhalation: Exposure to vapor/mist may irritate nose, throat, and lungs. Prolonged contact w/metal may cause pitting/discoloration.
Carcinogenicity—NTP: No
Carcinogenicity—IARC: No
Carcinogenicity—OSHA: No
Explanation Carcinogenicity: None
Signs/Symptoms of Overexposure: Irritation, nausea, vomiting.
Medical Conditions Aggravated by Exposure: Heart conditions, chronic respiratory problems, asthma, chronic bronchitis/obstructive lung disease. Wash area w/water. Ingestion: Drink a glassful of water. Inhalation: Remove to fresh air. Obtain medical attention in all cases.
Precautions for Safe Handling and Use
Steps If Material Released/Spill: Small (< 5 GALLONS)/LARGE (> 5 GALLONS): Absorb, containerize, and landfill in accordance w/local regulations. Wash down residual to sanitary sewer. Pump material to waste drums and dispose.
Waste Disposal Method: Contact the sanitary treatment facility in advance to ensure ability to process washed-down material. Dispose of in accordance w/federal, state, and local regulations.
Precautions-Handling/Storing: Use general ventilation to minimize exposure to vapor/mist.
Other Precautions: Avoid contact w/eyes and skin and inhalation of vapor/mist. Keep out of reach of children.

Figure 12.1. *(Continued)*

Control Measures
Ventilation: General
Protective Gloves: Required
Eye Protection: Safety glasses
Work Hygienic Practices: Remove/launder contaminated clothing before reuse.

Transportation Data

Disposal Data

Label Data
Label Required: Yes
Label Status: G
Common Name: Clorox Germicidal Bleach
Special Hazard Precautions: Eyes: Corneal injury. Skin: Irritation. Inhalation: Exposure to vapor/mist may irritate nose, throat, and lungs. Prolonged contact w/metal may cause pitting/discoloration.
Signs/Symptoms of Overexposure: Irritation, nausea, vomiting.
Label Name: Clorox Co. (Headquarters)
Label Street: 1221 Broadway
Label P.O. Box: 24305
Label City: Oakland
Label State: CA
Label Zip Code: 94612
Label Country: United States
Label Emergency Number: (800) 446-1014

- *Hazard determination provision*: Requires an employer to identify and maintain an inventory of all hazardous chemicals used in the workplace

- *Written implementation program*: Requires an employer to have a written hazard communication program plan

- *Employee training*: Requires that employers train employees how to handle hazardous materials, how to use and interpret MSDSs, and how to understand hazardous materials labeling and information about the Hazard Communication Standard

- *Trade secrets provision*: Sets forth the conditions under which a manufacturer may withhold information about a material and the conditions when such information must be provided to a healthcare provider (OSHA 1994)

The Joint Commission surveys organizations to ensure compliance with the OSHA standard and requires a written safety management plan for hazardous materials and waste. A healthcare organization designs its plan to:

- Develop an inventory (figure 12.2) of all hazardous materials and wastes used, stored, or generated. This includes vapors and gases used in surgery and medical gases used throughout the facility.

- Specify how it will maintain safety information for employees in the form of MSDSs. This MSDS information may be maintained as hard copy or electronic means. Various contract service companies provide electronic or fax copies of MSDSs to organizations as needed.

- Develop policies and procedures for selecting, handling, storing, transporting, using, and disposing of the hazardous materials and waste.

- Manage the following materials, as described in the hazardous materials and waste plan or policy, as applicable:

  —Chemicals

  —Chemotherapy drugs

  —Radioactive materials

  —Infectious and regulated medical waste, including sharps

  —Vapors and medical gases

- Specify a spill assessment team to respond to spills, to determine level of response, and to exercise the authority to notify fire department personnel if required.

- Provide education and training to employees regarding the Hazard Communication Standard. Employees should know:

  —Where to obtain MSDSs

  —The policies for safe handling of hazardous materials and waste

  —The procedures to follow in the event of an actual or suspected exposure to hazardous materials or waste

  —The health hazards of mishandling such materials and procedures for reporting exposure

  —How to define significant spills that require specialized handling and small spills that can be handled by staff in the department

  —How to clear spilled material from exposed areas and whether protective equipment must be worn or special precautions must be taken in the course of cleaning up and disposing of spilled materials

The plan also should specify supervisors' responsibility to provide adequate and appropriate space, containers, and personal protective equipment for the safe handling and

Figure 12.2. Hazardous materials inventory

Department: Product Name	Chemotherapy Drugs Manufacturer	Class	Hazardous Type Haz	Materials Inventory Spill Response	Quantity
				If fire, SCBA required. Call fire department.	
Cytarabine (ARA-c) 2 gm	Bedford 55390-0134-01				10
Dactinomycin (Cosmegen®) 0.5 mg/mL vial	Ovation Pharmaceuticals				8
Daunorubicin 20 mg/4 mL vial	Bedford 55390-0108-10				10
Docetaxel Taxotere® 80 mg/2 mL	Sanofi-Adventis 00075-8001-80				
Docetaxel (Taxotere) 20 mg/0.5 mL	Sanofi-Adventis 00075-8001-80				
Doxorubicin (Adriamycin®) 200 mg/100 mL	Bedford 55390-0238-01			Small spills—Wipe liquids with spill pad. Wipe solids with wet spill pad/sheet. Clean using detergent/water. Large spills—Cover liquid with spill pads/pillows, etc. Cover powder with damp cloth/spill sheet. Clean using detergents/water. Treat cloth, clothes, contaminated materials as hazardous materials. Incinerate.	
Etoposide (VePesid VP-16) 1 gm/50 mL	Bedford 55390-93-01				6
Fludarabine Phosphate (Fludara®) 50 mg vial	Berlex Labs 0015-511-06				4
Fluorouracil® 500 mg/10 mL (50 mg/mL)	Valeant Pharmaceuticals 63323-0117-10				10
Gemcitabine HCL (Gemzar®) 1 gm	Eli Lilly & Co 0002-7502-01				Order as needed
Hydroxyurea 500 mg capsule	Bristol Labs 00003-0830-50				100
Imiglucerase (Cerezyme) 400 units 200 units	Genzyme 58468-4663-01				
Idarubicin Hydrochloride 5 mg/5 mL	Pharmacia Upjohn				3
Ifosfamide (Ifex®) 3 gm/60 mL	GensiaSicor 00703-4100-68				4 boxes

storage of hazardous materials and wastes. Supervisors are to ensure that employees receive appropriate training on the hazardous materials and wastes in their work area, know how to obtain an MSDS, and know how to report hazardous material or waste spills or exposure.

Step 4: Monitor and Improve the Emergency Operations Plan

"An **emergency**, a natural or man-made event that significantly disrupts the environment of care (for example, damage to the organization's building[s] and grounds due to severe winds, storms, or earthquakes); that significantly disrupts care, treatment, and services (for example, loss of utilities such as power, water, or telephones as a result of floods, civil disturbances, accidents, or emergencies within the organization or in its community); or that results in sudden, significantly changed, or increased demands for the organization's services (for example, bioterrorist attack, building collapse, plane crash in the community). Some emergencies are called 'disasters' or 'potential injury creating events' (PICEs)" (Joint Commission 2011a).

Terrorist activity, such as the September 11, 2001 attacks in New York City and Washington, DC, and the natural disasters of hurricanes Katrina and Rita in 2005 have focused the nation's attention on emergency preparedness and the ability of the community, including hospitals, to respond. Response may consist of handling a large influx of patients or the need to evacuate patients from hospitals and extended care facilities to safer sites, as occurred in New Orleans and Port Arthur.

In response to these catastrophic emergencies, the **National Incident Management System (NIMS)** has evolved to include standardization or a **total program approach** for disaster/emergency management and business continuity programs in the private and public sectors. This standardization has required healthcare organizations to reevaluate their emergency operations plans (EOPs), and the Joint Commission to redefine standards that address six critical areas of emergency management with a focus that includes a linkage to community resources. Since 2008, the Joint Commission standards have included the following six critical areas that need to be addressed in a healthcare organization's EOP:

Communication—In the event that community infrastructure is damaged and/or a healthcare organization's power or facilities experience debilitation, communication pathways are likely to fail. The healthcare organization must develop a plan to maintain communication pathways both within the organization and to critical community resources.

Resources and assets—A solid understanding of the scope and availability of a healthcare organization's resources and assets during an emergency is important. Materials and supplies, vendor and community services, as well as state and federal programs, are some of the essential resources that hospitals must know how to access in times of crisis in order to ensure patient safety and sustain care, treatment, and services.

Safety and security—The safety and security of patients is the prime responsibility of the healthcare organization during an emergency. As emergency situations develop and parameters of operability shift, organizations must provide a safe and secure environment for their patients and staff.

Staff responsibilities—During an emergency, the probability that staff responsibilities will change is high. As new risks develop along with changing conditions, staff will need to adapt to their roles to meet new demands on their ability to care for patients. If staff cannot anticipate how they may be called to perform during an emergency, the likelihood that the organization will not sustain itself during an emergency increases.

Utilities management—A healthcare organization is dependent on the uninterrupted function of its utilities during an emergency. The supply of key utilities, such as power or potable water, ventilation, and fuel, must not be disrupted or adverse events may occur as a result.

Patient clinical and support activities—The clinical needs of patients during an emergency are of prime importance. The organization must have clear, reasonable plans in place to address the needs of patients during extreme conditions when the infrastructure and resources are taxed.

When a healthcare organization has a sound understanding of their response to these six critical areas of emergency management, they have developed an **all hazards approach** that supports a level of preparedness sufficient to address a range of emergencies, regardless of the cause (Joint Commission 2011a).

The Joint Commission further requires organizations to conduct an annual **hazard vulnerability analysis (HVA)** to identify potential hazards, threats, and adverse events and then assess their impact on the care, treatment, and services that must be sustained during an emergency. A sample HVA form is included in table 12.3. Once the top hazard vulnerabilities are identified, situational plans need to be developed for events such as utility failures, earthquakes, hurricanes, floods, tornadoes, and airline disasters. Emergency preparedness planning should be systematic and comprehensive. Planning should include activities that mitigate, prepare, respond, and provide recovery information from an emergency event. Table 12.4 illustrates these planning activities.

Emergency planning begins with an HVA to determine the types of disasters that the organization may face. Disasters may be technological, man-made, or natural. A good starting point for gathering information is the state health department Web site, which usually includes an analysis of the state's potential risk sites, such as earthen dams, industrial sites with hazardous or toxic chemicals, and the type and frequency of past natural disasters. An HVA may be found by county in some larger states, and the county Web sites will provide emergency preparedness for their locale.

The group conducting the HVA also should assess the organizational experience of the prior year (and longer, if available) taken from the safety monitoring and trending data. Events emanating from within the organization, such as security events, utility failures, information systems failures, hazardous material spills or exposures, or findings from disaster drill critiques, will provide direction as to which situational plans should be written or revised.

The organization's disaster coordinator should be involved with the county or state emergency management committees to provide another mechanism to obtain information regarding local concerns and to coordinate disaster response with local healthcare facilities and emergency response agencies. The Joint Commission (2011a) requires "cooperative planning amongst organizations that . . . provide services to a contiguous geographical area." When developing the EOP, the healthcare organization communicates its needs and vulnerabilities to community emergency response agencies and identifies the capabilities of the community in meeting the organization's needs.

An important element of emergency planning is the implementation of an incident command structure that can link and coordinate with community authorities and their

Table 12.3. Hospital hazard vulnerability assessment tool

TECHNOLOGIC EVENTS

Event	PROBABILITY	SEVERITY = (MAGNITUDE – MITIGATION)						RISK
		HUMAN IMPACT	PROPERTY IMPACT	BUSINESS IMPACT	PREPAREDNESS	INTERNAL RESPONSE	EXTERNAL RESPONSE	
	Likelihood this will occur	Possibility of death or injury	Physical losses and damages	Interruption of services	Preplanning	Time, effectiveness, resources	Community/ mutual aid staff and supplies	Relative threat*
SCORE	0 = N/A 1 = Low 2 = Moderate 3 = High	0 = N/A 1 = Low 2 = Moderate 3 = High	0 = N/A 1 = Low 2 = Moderate 3 = High	0 = N/A 1 = Low 2 = Moderate 3 = High	0 = N/A 1 = High 2 = Moderate 3 = Low or none	0 = N/A 1 = High 2 = Moderate 3 = Low or none	0 = N/A 1 = High 2 = Moderate 3 = Low or none	0–100%
Electrical Failure								
Generator Failure								
Transportation Failure								
Fuel Shortage								
Natural Gas Failure								
Water Failure								
Sewer Failure								
Steam Failure								
Fire Alarm Failure								
Communications Failure								
Medical Gas Failure								
Medical Vacuum Failure								
HVAC Failure								
Information Systems Failure								
Fire, Internal								
Flood, Internal								
Hazmat Exposure, Internal								
Supply Shortage								
Structural Damage								
AVERAGE SCORE								

*Threat increases with percentage.

RISK = PROBABILITY × SEVERITY

0.15   0.39   0.38

Table 12.3. *(Continued)*

HAZARDOUS MATERIALS

Event	PROBABILITY	SEVERITY = (MAGNITUDE – MITIGATION)						RISK
	Likelihood this will occur	HUMAN IMPACT	PROPERTY IMPACT	BUSINESS IMPACT	PREPAREDNESS	INTERNAL RESPONSE	EXTERNAL RESPONSE	Relative threat*
		Possibility of death or injury	Physical losses and damages	Interruption of services	Preplanning	Time, effectiveness, resources	Community/ mutual aid staff and supplies	
SCORE	0 = N/A 1 = Low 2 = Moderate 3 = High	0 = N/A 1 = Low 2 = Moderate 3 = High	0 = N/A 1 = Low 2 = Moderate 3 = High	0 = N/A 1 = Low 2 = Moderate 3 = High	0 = N/A 1 = High 2 = Moderate 3 = Low or none	0 = N/A 1 = High 2 = Moderate 3 = Low or none	0 = N/A 1 = High 2 = Moderate 3 = Low or none	0–100%
Mass Casualty Hazmat Incident (From historic events at your MC with ≥ 5 victims)								
Small Casualty Hazmat Incident (From historic events at your MC with < 5 victims)								
Chemical Exposure, External								
Small–Medium-Sized Internal Spill								
Large Internal Spill								
Terrorism, Chemical								
Radiologic Exposure, Internal								
Radiologic Exposure, External								
Terrorism, Radiologic								
AVERAGE SCORE								

*Threat increases with percentage.

RISK = PROBABILITY × SEVERITY

0.21   0.37   0.57

(Continued on next page)

Table 12.3. (*Continued*)

HUMAN EVENTS

Event	PROBABILITY	SEVERITY = (MAGNITUDE – MITIGATION)						RISK
		HUMAN IMPACT	PROPERTY IMPACT	BUSINESS IMPACT	PREPAREDNESS	INTERNAL RESPONSE	EXTERNAL RESPONSE	
	Likelihood this will occur	Possibility of death or injury	Physical losses and damages	Interruption of services	Preplanning	Time, effectiveness, resources	Community/ mutual aid staff and supplies	Relative threat*
SCORE	0 = N/A 1 = Low 2 = Moderate 3 = High	0 = N/A 1 = Low 2 = Moderate 3 = High	0 = N/A 1 = Low 2 = Moderate 3 = High	0 = N/A 1 = Low 2 = Moderate 3 = High	0 = N/A 1 = High 2 = Moderate 3 = Low or none	0 = N/A 1 = High 2 = Moderate 3 = Low or none	0 = N/A 1 = High 2 = Moderate 3 = Low or none	0–100%
Mass Casualty Incident (Trauma)								
Mass Casualty Incident (Medical/Infectious)								
Terrorism, Biological								
VIP Situation								
Infant Abduction								
Hostage Situation								
Civil Disturbance								
Labor Action								
Forensic Admission								
Bomb Threat								
AVERAGE SCORE								

*Threat increases with percentage.

RISK = PROBABILITY × SEVERITY

0.21   0.47   0.44

Table 12.3. *(Continued)*

NATURALLY OCCURRING EVENTS

Event	PROBABILITY	SEVERITY = (MAGNITUDE – MITIGATION)						RISK
		HUMAN IMPACT	PROPERTY IMPACT	BUSINESS IMPACT	PREPAREDNESS	INTERNAL RESPONSE	EXTERNAL RESPONSE	
SCORE	Likelihood this will occur	Possibility of death or injury	Physical losses and damages	Interruption of services	Preplanning	Time, effectiveness, resources	Community/ mutual aid staff and supplies	Relative threat*
	0 = N/A 1 = Low 2 = Moderate 3 = High	0 = N/A 1 = Low 2 = Moderate 3 = High	0 = N/A 1 = Low 2 = Moderate 3 = High	0 = N/A 1 = Low 2 = Moderate 3 = High	0 = N/A 1 = High 2 = Moderate 3 = Low or none	0 = N/A 1 = High 2 = Moderate 3 = Low or none	0 = N/A 1 = High 2 = Moderate 3 = Low or none	0–100%
Hurricane								
Tornado								
Severe Thunderstorm								
Snowfall								
Blizzard								
Ice Storm								
Earthquake								
Tidal Wave								
Temperature Extremes								
Drought								
Flood, External								
Wild Fire								
Landslide								
Dam Inundation								
Volcano								
Epidemic								
AVERAGE SCORE								

*Threat increases with percentage.

RISK = PROBABILITY × SEVERITY

0.03   0.21   0.16

Source: Adapted from http://www.hazmatforhealthcare.org. Reprinted with permission from Mitch Saruwatari, national threat assessment manager, Kaiser Permanente, and Paul Penn, EnMagine.

Table 12.4. Hazard vulnerability planning activities

Hazard	Mitigation (long-term)	Preparedness (to respond)	Response (to emergency)	Recovery (short and long term)
	Definition: Any activities that actually eliminate or reduce the occurrence of a disaster, including long-term activities that reduce the effects of unavoidable disasters.	Definition: Preparedness activities are necessary to the extent that mitigation measures cannot prevent disasters. Preparedness measures also seek to enhance disaster response operations.	Definition: Generally, responses are designed to provide emergency assistance for casualties. Responses also seek to reduce the probability of secondary damage and to speed recovery operations.	Definition: Recovery continues until all systems return to normal or better. Short-term recovery returns vital life support systems to minimum operating standards. Long-term recovery may continue for a number of years after a disaster. Recovery's purpose is to return life to normal.
Earthquake	• Secure moveable objects that may cause injury • Fasten shelves • Take pictures off walls • Place heavy objects on low shelves • Store sufficient fuel, medical supplies, pharmaceutical supplies, food, and water to sustain patients and staff for a short period of time • Prepare 72-hour kits for offices • Adhere to building codes • Store hazardous chemicals in appropriate cabinets • Contract/make arrangements with a building inspector • Educate staff	• Have utility schematics available • Encourage staff preparedness at home through provision of home disaster information	• Protect self • Protect patients • Activate plan • Conserve resources • Unplug nonessential equipment • Review need for rotating staff	• Have building inspection • Return utilities to normal • Assess and repair structural damage • Replace equipment • Restock supplies • Evaluate economic impact • Activate Incident Stress Debriefing Team
Hazardous Materials Facility	• Store hazardous chemicals appropriately • Educate staff on handling hazardous chemicals • Review possible alternative to hazardous chemicals • Routine removal for disposal • Lock hazmat disposal storage • Use nonsparking tools	• Have spill kits on hand • Use MSDS hotline number to obtain MSDS, as needed • Know chemical inventory in department • Train appropriate staff on use of ETO sniffer	• Secure area of spill • Evacuate if necessary • Notify security x2222 • Notify fire department, if appropriate	• Dispose of waste properly • Evaluate cause of spill • Replenish spill kit/ supplies

Table 12.4.   *(Continued)*

Information Systems	• Back up systems nightly • Maintain hard copies of business records off-site • Maintain updated virus protection • Create policy regarding not using CDs/flash drives from home • Move computer towers off floors			
Flood				
Power Failure				

Figure 12.3.   Incident command structure for a small healthcare organization

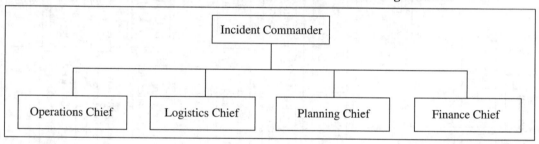

incident command structures. National initiatives require standardization of incident command structure and nomenclature at all levels of response: emergency medical services, fire and police, hospitals, and city and state emergency management agencies.

The incident command structure is used in each type of emergency event and is as elaborate or simple as the size of the organization or event requires. In other words, it is an all-hazards command structure. Two examples of incident command structures are shown in figures 12.3 and 12.4. Figure 12.3 shows an incident command structure for a small organization, and figure 12.4 shows one for a larger, more complex organization.

The basic **emergency operations plan (EOP)** describes the management of space, supplies, staff, and security (see figure 12.5) and describes the following processes in detail:

- Assignment of authority for notifying staff, notifying and communicating with external authorities, communicating with patients and their families, and communicating with the community when emergency response measures are initiated

- Setup of command center and identification of individuals to serve in the incident command structure

- Assignment of staff to cover all essential functions

Figure 12.4.   Incident command structure for a large healthcare organization

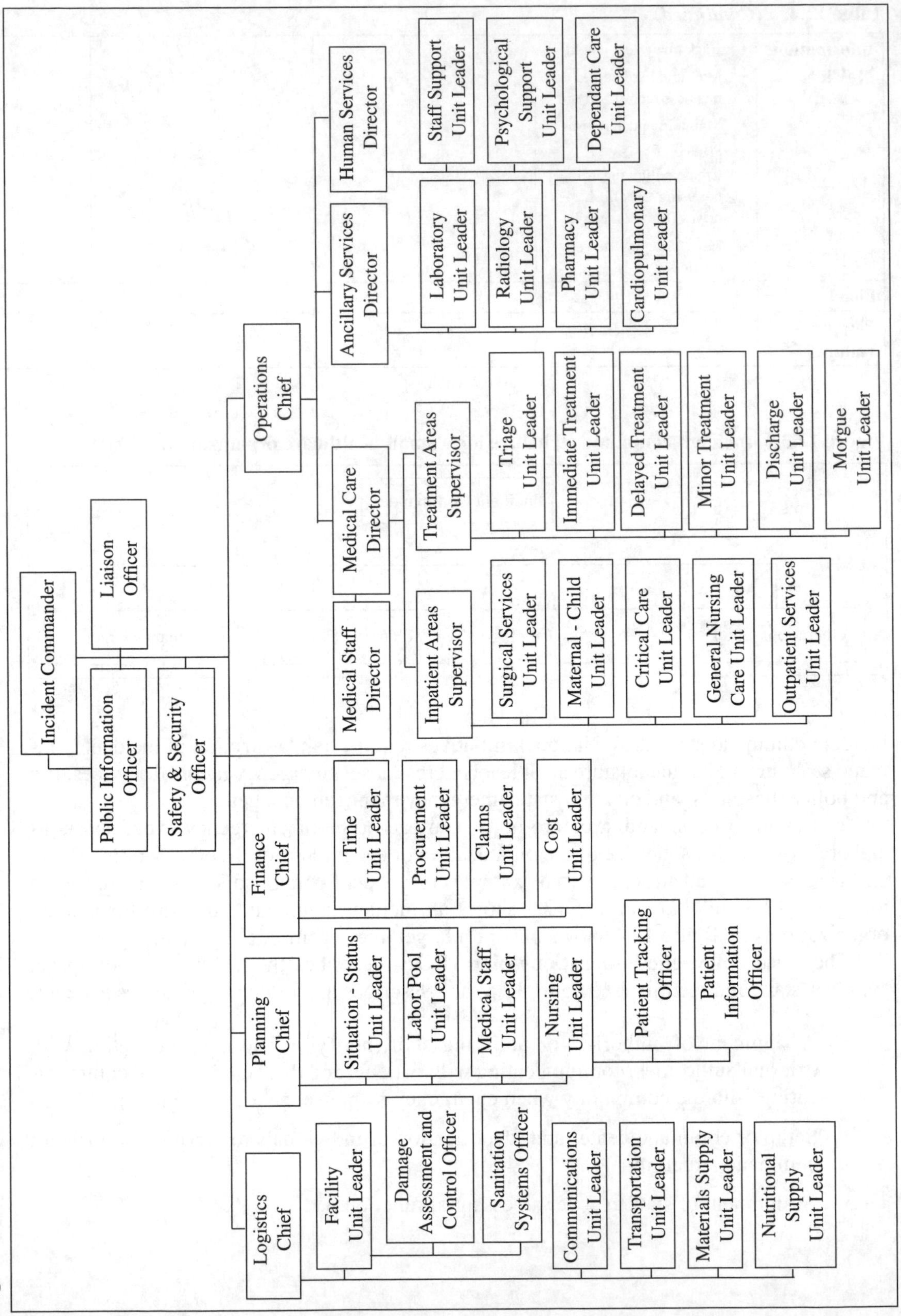

Figure 12.5.   Emergency management plan

Community Hospital of the West
EMERGENCY MANAGEMENT PLAN

MISSION STATEMENT:

Community Hospital of the West supports the Emergency Management Plan to ensure effective response to mitigate, prepare, respond, and recover from disasters or emergencies affecting the facility internally or from external events.

OBJECTIVES:

Community Hospital of the West has established, supports, and maintains an emergency preparedness program (Disaster Manual) that implements specific procedures in response to a variety of internal disasters. In the event of any type of disaster that places an unusual demand on space, supplies, security, or the facility staff, the emergency preparedness plan will be implemented.

The program integrates the center's role with the disaster plans of local, county, state, and federal emergency management authorities and facilities in proximity to Community Hospital of the West. The facility will assist external disaster victims within the capability and mission of the hospital.

SCOPE:

The emergency preparedness plan provides a mechanism to augment normal operation of the facility during an incident. The plan represents a principle-based (all hazards) response to any event, which may compromise facility operations. It may be implemented in whole or in part, or it may represent merely the first step in a more comprehensive mobilization of resources. It is intended that disaster situations be managed with as little variation from normal facility policies and procedures as possible. However, since no amount of planning can foresee every circumstance, flexibility within the guidelines of the plan is crucial.

Emergency preparedness includes the following:

1. Potential emergencies are identified from a hazard vulnerability analysis.

2. Procedures are identified for disaster readiness and management of a variety of disasters.

3. Procedures are identified for informing staff of "disaster alert" or need for disaster response.

4. Procedures are identified for individual department response to disaster.

5. Procedures are identified for evacuation.

6. Definition of the "all hazards" command structure is provided for responding to and recovery from emergencies. The command structure is referred to as the Incident Command system. The Incident Command personnel in the command center integrate the hospital's role with community-wide emergency response agencies and promote interoperability between the hospital and the community.

7. Descriptions of procedures are provided for mitigation, preparedness, response, and recovery.

8. The plan addresses four phases of emergency management: mitigation, preparedness, response, and recovery. At a minimum, the Emergency Management Plan has been developed with the involvement of facility leaders, including the Medical Director.

AUTHORITY:

The Safety Officer has the authority to intervene whenever conditions exist that pose an immediate threat to life or health or pose a threat of damage to equipment or the building.

RESPONSIBILITY:

(Continued on next page)

Figure 12.5. *(Continued)*

Community Hospital of the West
EMERGENCY MANAGEMENT PLAN

GOVERNING BOARD:

- Supports the Emergency Management Program through providing staff and resources for preparedness planning
- Receives recommendations for mitigation, preparedness, evaluation of response to disaster/drill (critiques), and recovery

SAFETY COMMITTEE ADMINISTRATION MEDICAL DIRECTOR:

- As a member of the Administration, chairs the Safety Committee
- Convenes committee twice a year (at a minimum) to implement the plan(s), train, and critique staff on their response
- With Administration and Safety Officer, assumes roles in the Incident Command Center during disasters and drills providing direction to the hospital and communicating with the community's incident command structure
- Recommends educational needs of staff, additional equipment, supplies, etc., pertaining to emergency management response
- Plans, designs, measures, assesses, and improves processes through ongoing receipt of monitoring data, written formal review of disasters/disaster drills and annual performance evaluation
- Submits reports at least quarterly to the Board, to include critiques of disasters/drills, recommendations for preparedness response, and education needs
- Updates Emergency Management Plan (Disaster Manual) as needed

SAFETY OFFICER:

- Oversees emergency management planning and reports updates and revisions to the Safety Committee
- Directs planning, implementation, and evaluation of disaster drill response
- Accepts assignment as a section chief in the incident command structure
- Attends community emergency management committees as appropriate
- Provides training to department staff in department response to disasters/drills

DEPARTMENT MANAGERS:

- Support participation of their staff in the implementation of the plan/drills
- Monitor staff compliance with the plan and participation in drills, event/incident reporting, and implementation of appropriate corrective actions

EMPLOYEES:

- Annually review disaster procedures through participation in mandatory training/education
- Take drills seriously and respond appropriately
- Take prompt action in identifying and reporting internal disasters
- Support the Emergency Management Plan by following policies and procedures, participating in drills and appropriately responding to actual events, reporting deficiencies and problems promptly, and participating in training and demonstrating competence

Figure 12.5. *(Continued)*

Community Hospital of the West
EMERGENCY MANAGEMENT PLAN

TRAINING/EDUCATION:

- New employee orientation includes information relative to the hospital response to disasters:
    - Access to the hospital
    - Employee identification
    - Situational events
    - Evacuation
- The Safety Officer will provide disaster critique feedback annually and after each disaster/drill and education for employees on disaster response and disaster-specific procedures and evacuation.

ANNUAL EVALUATION:

An evaluation of objectives, scope, performance, and effectiveness of the emergency preparedness plan and staff response is conducted annually and after each disaster/drill. This evaluation is accomplished by reviewing data sources and reports as follows:

1. Analysis of Disaster Drills; debriefing with disaster participants, involved facility staff and departments, county/state Emergency Operations staff, volunteers, etc.
2. Actual incidents within or outside the facility
3. Disaster literature/research findings
4. Information from the community, state, and/or federal agencies
5. Disaster Drill critiques
6. Department Evaluation Reports
7. Activity Log

The Safety Committee will analyze the data sources and implement appropriate actions to be taken and update the Disaster Manual.

PERFORMANCE IMPROVEMENT GOALS:

Performance goals will be established for each drill implemented, and objectives of each drill will be reviewed by the Safety Committee and submitted to the Board.

Performance Standards/Quality Improvement projects have been established for a minimum of 2 of the Safety Management programs in the Environment of Care Management.

- Management of activities related to:
    - Care and treatment of patients
    - Modifying or discontinuing services
    - Staff support (housing, incident stress, and debriefing)
    - Staff family support, child care
    - Obtaining supplies (pharmaceuticals, linens, food, and water)

- —Security

- —Communications with news media

- —Evacuation (including transportation of patients, staff, equipment, and health records)

- —Establishing alternative care sites

- —Tracking patients (disaster log)

- Credentialing of volunteers (physicians, nurses, and others not associated with the facility)

- Interhospital cooperation or transfer agreements

- Situational plans, including:

- —Radioactive, biological, and chemical isolation and decontamination

- —Communication emergencies

- —Utility failures, alternative means of meeting essential building utility needs

- —Natural disasters as identified in the HVA

- —Human-caused disasters as identified in the HVA

- —Fire response

The EOP is practiced twice a year in response to either an actual disaster or a planned drill. Exercises should stress the limits of the organization's emergency management system to assess preparedness capabilities and performance. Exercises should be plausible scenarios that are realistic and based on the organization's HVA. In organizations providing emergency services, one drill must simulate the influx of patients, and the organization must participate in one community-wide practice drill a year.

Finally, each disaster response, whether an actual emergency or a practice drill, must be critiqued. Problems identified or lessons learned during an actual event or drill should be assessed and, as appropriate, addressed in the written EOP. Administration, medical staff, and the board of trustees should approve emergency preparedness planning. In addition to drills, the organization's personnel should receive education and training as needed (at least annually).

Step 5: Monitor and Improve the Life (Fire Prevention) Safety Management Plan

Building and fire codes require facilities to be designed, constructed, maintained, and operated to minimize a fire emergency and protect patients, visitors, staff, and property from fire, smoke, and other products of combustion. The major component of the life safety management plan is a fire prevention plan that is based on appropriate design and construction of the building, fire detection, alarm and extinguishment systems, and training to provide for appropriate safety for all occupants.

The following activities are included as components of the fire prevention program (NFPA 2011):

- Inspect, test, and maintain fire detection, alarm, and protection equipment such as audible alarm systems, fire and smoke detectors, extinguishers, water flow devices, evacuation route exit signs, fire doors, and air handling and smoke management systems. This inspection, testing, and maintenance must be conducted within the time frames required by the Life Safety Code of the National Fire Protection Association (NFPA) and other codes required by state and local agencies.

- Identify, investigate, and report deficiencies and failures in the fire prevention program.

- Evaluate proposed acquisition of bedding, window coverings, furnishings, room decorations, wastebaskets, and equipment in the context of fire safety.

- Develop and implement a fire response plan through drills, education, and training of staff. Staff is trained regarding:

  —Their roles and responsibilities at the fire's point of origin and away from the point of origin

  —When and how to sound fire alarms

  —Use of fire extinguishers

  —Smoke and fire containment

  —Preparing for evacuation

- Use an easy method to train staff, such as *RACE* and *PASS*.

  —RACE stands for:

    R = Rescue patients in areas of immediate danger

    A = Activate alarms

    C = Confine fires (close doors and windows)

    E = Extinguish fires using PASS and prepare to evacuate patients

  —PASS, which is training for the use of fire extinguishers, stands for:

    P = Pull pin

    A = Aim nozzle

    S = Squeeze handle

    S = Spray base of fire

- Conduct fire drills quarterly for each shift (50 percent of the drills must be unannounced). A realistic fire scenario is prepared for each drill, and staff knowledge is evaluated. All fire drills are critiqued to identify problems and opportunities for improvement. Figure 12.6 is an example of a tracking form used to document fire

Figure 12.6.   Fire drill tracking summary

Fire Drill Summary: (Building's name) _____ With (number of) _____ smoke compartments

- Complete the table below: (A) Date of fire drill; (B) Day of week; (C) Time of day drill was held; (D) Smoke compartment from which fire drill initiated; (E) Total number of compartments observed during drill; (F) Total number of observers; (G) Was another smoke compartment monitored on the same floor and immediately adjacent to the drill site (if applicable)? (H) Was another smoke compartment monitored on the floor immediately above/below the drill site (if applicable)?
- For the fire drills, did you elect to observe all areas?   **YES   NO   N/A**   (Please circle)
- Or did you elect to randomly observe different locations using the four criteria?   **YES   NO   N/A**   (Please circle)

Fire Drill Summary		**Morning Drills**		**Afternoon Drills**		**Night Drills**
Date of fire drill	A		A		A	
Day of week	B		B		B	
Time of day	C		C		C	
Where initiated?	D		D		D	
Number of compartments observed	E		E		E	
Number of observers	F		F		F	
Adjacent compartment observed?	G	Yes No N/A	G	Yes No N/A	G	Yes No N/A
Was adjacent compartment above/below compartment observed?	H	Yes No N/A	H	Yes No N/A	H	Yes No N/A
Date of fire drill	A		A		A	
Day of week	B		B		B	
Time of day	C		C		C	
Where initiated?	D		D		D	
Number of compartments observed	E		E		E	
Number of observers	F		F		F	
Adjacent compartment observed?	G	Yes No N/A	G	Yes No N/A	G	Yes No N/A
Was adjacent compartment above/below compartment observed?	H	Yes No N/A	H	Yes No N/A	H	Yes No N/A
Date of fire drill	A		A		A	
Day of week	B		B		B	
Time of day	C		C		C	
Where initiated?	D		D		D	
Number of compartments observed?	E		E		E	
Number of observers	F		F		F	
Adjacent compartment observed?	G	Yes No N/A	G	Yes No N/A	G	Yes No N/A
Was adjacent compartment above/below compartment observed?	H	Yes No N/A	H	Yes No N/A	H	Yes No N/A

drills. A separate evaluation of staff response to each drill is documented and used in the annual evaluation of the fire safety plan.

- Oversee safety of construction and remodeling activities, including inspection for appropriate installation of fire protection systems and equipment and enforcement of safety requirements of contractors, such as hot work permits and above-ceiling permits. The facility must comply with all federal, state, and local rules; regulations; and laws.

- Conduct a life safety assessment in addition to the infection control risk assessment prior to beginning construction to determine whether the construction will interfere with life safety codes. If deficiencies or hazards are identified, appropriate activities from the Interim Life Safety Measures (ILSM) policy will be instituted. Some examples of the 11 ILSMs are:

    —Smoke-tight barriers between construction areas and the rest of the facility

    —Increased surveillance

    —Additional firefighting equipment

    —Increased number of fire drills conducted

    —Organization-wide fire safety education

- Use the Joint Commission's (2011b) Statement of Conditions (SOC) form to note when building code deficiencies affecting life safety are identified and cannot be rectified within 30 to 60 days. This documentation demonstrates the organization's intent and plan of action to rectify the life safety problem, whether it is a fire door malfunction that requires the purchase of hardware that will take longer than 30 to 60 days to arrive or other fire prevention systems failures.

Step 6: Monitor and Improve the Medical Equipment Management Program

The goals of the medical equipment management program are to provide safe and reliable equipment to patients, train care providers in the safe and effective use of the equipment, and ensure that the equipment is maintained by qualified individuals.

The written medical equipment management plan includes provisions for the following functions:

- Outlines how equipment is selected and acquired

- Establishes criteria for including equipment, regardless of ownership, on the facility inventory list. Criteria do not need to be established if the facility decides to include all equipment on the inventory. Equipment not owned by the facility may need to be examined and a safety check performed. Examples of situations in which equipment is not owned by the facility might include the following:

—Physicians may bring or purchase their own equipment to use in surgery or during other procedures.

—Patients may bring electronic devices, such as computers, TVs, and DVD players, for entertainment.

- Defines time frames for inspecting, testing, and maintaining the equipment in the inventory. The organization maintains documentation of the inspection, testing, maintenance, and repair of each piece of equipment in the inventory.

- Defines how equipment and medical device recalls will be handled.

- Provides for reporting incidents in which a medical device may have caused death, serious injury, or illness to any patient, as required by the Safe Medical Devices Act of 1990.

- Identifies processes to respond to equipment malfunction or failure

- Specifies cleaning and infection control procedures for receiving and handling equipment between patients

Previous National Patient Safety Goals now elevated to standards focus on medical equipment malfunctions: (1) the safety of using infusion pumps for pain management, and (2) the effectiveness of clinical alarm systems used in the physiological monitoring of patients (for example, cardiac monitoring and ventilators) and environmental monitoring (for example, fire alarms, door alarms, and gas pressure alarms). Facility support or clinical engineering departments should develop an inventory of clinical, life safety, and security alarms. Alarms should be evaluated for the frequency of inspecting, testing, and maintenance.

Step 7: Monitor and Improve the Utilities Management Program

The utilities management program is designed to ensure that utilities systems throughout the EOC are planned and maintained safely and comfortably; that utilities are delivered without interruption; and that mechanical systems operate safely, accurately, and reliably. A good utilities management program helps the organization minimize the risk of hospital-acquired illnesses that may be transmitted through the utility systems. Facility support personnel work closely and proactively with the infection control practitioner to control dust and to test and maintain air handlers and cooling towers. Infection control procedures also require that stained ceiling tiles, carpeting, and flooring be replaced to proactively prevent contaminates from reaching the patient.

The written utilities management program describes the following:

- The processes the organization maintains to manage the safe and reliable operation of utility systems

- The risk criteria for evaluating the operating components of the utility systems and developing an inventory. As in the medical equipment program, a facility may elect to use risk criteria but should include all utility systems in the inventory.

- The schedules for inspecting, testing, and maintaining components of the utility systems

- The emergency procedures for responding to utility disruptions or failures

- The location of schematics and facility maps that show the location of utility systems and controls for partial or complete shutdown in an emergency. The controls for shutdown in the facility should be labeled.

- Infection control and facility surveillance processes. Water-stained ceiling tiles may signify an infection control issue. Damp tiles are a medium for mold. When stained ceiling tiles are found, facility support personnel should determine, if possible, the cause of the stain and repair any problems above the ceiling before replacing tiles. One pediatric facility noted that ceiling tiles appeared to be water stained, but the cause of the problem could not be found until the infection control practitioner and the safety manager discovered that the toys to distract the children in the care environment included squirt guns.

The EOC integrates closely with the Joint Commission Patient Safety Initiatives. A safe and secure environment supports the provision of care and treatment in a healthcare organization. Important patient safety goals to be managed in the EOC program are infection control, fire safety, emergency management, medical equipment, and alarms. The infection control practitioner and the safety committee inspection team are important allies.

The EOC infection control focus is in the areas of airborne contaminants, waterborne pathogens, housekeeping procedures, and building construction issues. Figure 12.7 shows an example of an audit worksheet used to survey for issues related to the EOC plans and infection control surveillance. Physical plant changes may affect infection control for immunosuppressed or compromised patients. Preconstruction risk assessments are conducted with the infection control practitioner, safety manager, facility support staff, and construction supervisory personnel. (Additional information regarding the response to or the influx of infectious patients can be found in chapter 9 of this text.)

Facility support services should work closely with the infection control practitioner to report water system or air handling issues or concerns with drains, ice machines, carpeting, flooring, ceiling tiles and the space above the tiles, and garbage handling and storage areas.

A facility must conduct an infection control risk assessment prior to construction and have a plan in place to mitigate the effects of airborne contaminates and other infection control concerns on patients and others. The infection control professional, facility support staff, and construction personnel should routinely inspect areas affected or potentially affected by construction. The team will ensure that designated routes for construction workers are enforced and cleaned when removing garbage or bringing materials into the building and that dust barriers between construction and the rest of the facility are intact.

Figure 12.7.   Environmental tour/facility audit—clinical departments

	Location: _____ Date: _____ Survey Team: _____ Director/Manager: _____		
	Needs Correction	**Surveyor Comments**	**Management Response**
Safety			
Exit lights lit and visible			
All fire doors close and latch			
Doors found propped open			
Crash cart checked daily			
No unapproved space heaters in the area			
No items stored under sinks/no water spots or mold			
Sharps containers are no more than 2/3 full			
No tripping hazards			
No staff food/drinks in work area			
Emergency flip chart posted			
Linen cart covered; has solid bottom shelf			
No outdated supplies were found			
Hazardous Material			
Current Hazmat inventory available			
E MSDS on demand number posted and visible			
Chemicals in secondary containers are appropriately labeled			
Biohazardous trash separated from regular medical trash			
Trash labeled appropriately			
Appropriate lids on waste containers			
Spill kit available			
Fire			
Extinguishers have current inspection tag			
Hallways clear of storage, or equipment stored on one side of hall			
Fire exits, pull stations, fire doors, and extinguishers not blocked			
Waste paper disposed of properly			
Nothing stored in any stairwell			

Figure 12.7. *(Continued)*

	Needs Correction	Surveyor Comments	Management Response
All items 18" below sprinkler heads			
All items 4" off of the floor			
Furniture, Wheelchairs, Beds, Gurneys, IV Poles			
Wheels and brakes in good condition			
No broken furniture found			
Wagons clean			
Beds/cribs in good condition			
General Maintenance			
Ceiling tiles free from cracks, holes, breaks, and stains/mold • Causation? What is above the tiles? (Bathroom? Shower? etc?) Flooring free from tears, bulges, holes, etc. Random check for fire penetrations Seams on splash boards of sinks Under counter refrigerators—no dust/water Potential hazards—countertop laminate chipped or lifting Ceramic tile			
Guardrails secure			
Patient restroom grab bars secure			
Patient care equipment inspections up to date			
Electrical			
Outlet covers attached and in good condition			
All electrical cords in good condition			
Electric panels are secured and unobstructed, and no storage in closets			
Nurse call buttons functioning			
Childproof/tamper-proof outlets (GFI) in appropriate areas			
Limited use of extension cords; cords are labeled			

(Continued on next page)

Figure 12.7. *(Continued)*

	Needs Correction	Surveyor Comments	Management Response
Housekeeping			
No unlocked housekeeping closets or unattended carts in the area			
No unlabeled bottles on the cart			
Approved trash/shredding/recycling receptacles			
General cleanliness			
Refrigerator Protocol			
Refrigerator/freezer temperature checks documented appropriately			
Thermometers in place in freezer and refrigerator			
All food is covered and dated			
Food and medication are kept in separate refrigerators			
Medication			
Open multiuse bottles and vials are dated and timed			
No outdated IV solutions or medications			
Outdated formula, baby food, and supplemental feedings are disposed of			
All medication kept in locked or controlled area, including refrigerators			
All controlled substances are in double-locked cabinets			
No unattended, drawn syringes found in the area			
Medication in syringes marked with name and strength			
Oxygen and Other Medical Gases			
All medical gas cylinders secured in upright position in approved holders or chained			
All medical gas cylinders secured during transport/use			
All medical gas cylinder shut-off valves clearly marked and accessible			
Additional Comments:			

Management Signature   Date

Criteria for an Annual Evaluation

Each of the seven safety plans is to be evaluated annually, taking into consideration the objectives, scope, performance, and effectiveness of the individual program. Depending on functions performed, the policies and procedures in place, and regulatory requirements, the safety officer or the individual responsible for the plan can prepare questions that will solicit responses from evaluators on the efficacy of the program. (See table 12.5 for an example of an emergency management annual evaluation.)

Table 12.5.   Example of an emergency management annual evaluation

Criteria	Yes	No	Partial	Findings	Page 1
HOSPITAL/MEDICAL CENTER **ANNUAL EVALUATION OF THE EMERGENCY MANAGEMENT PROGRAM**					
Reviewed scope and objectives of the Emergency Management Plan.					
Reviewed current accreditation standards.					
Has the hospital conducted a Hazard Vulnerability Analysis?					
Disaster drills were conducted at least 2 times per year, 4 months apart.					
Has the hospital identified specific procedures to mitigate, prepare for, respond to, and recover from the identified procedures?					
Has the hospital defined a common command structure that links and integrates with the community?					
Does the hospital have representation in the community in regard to emergency management and preparation?					
Does the hospital have a means to notify external authorities of a possible community emergency, such as a bio-terrorist attack?					
Does the hospital have procedures to: • Notify personnel when emergency response measures are initiated? • Identify care providers during an emergency?					
Assign personnel to necessary staff positions during an emergency?					
Does the hospital have the ability to manage the following under emergency conditions: • Patient care–related activities • Staff support activities • Family support activities • Logistics in relation to critical supplies • Security					

(Continued on next page)

Table 12.5.   *(Continued)*

HOSPITAL/MEDICAL CENTER ANNUAL EVALUATION OF THE EMERGENCY MANAGEMENT PROGRAM					
Criteria	Yes	No	Partial	Findings	Page 2
Communication with the news media					
Does the hospital have a plan for evacuation if needed?					
Does the hospital have alternate care sites and agreements with other hospitals in the event of an evacuation or other emergency?					
Does the hospital have a plan to reestablish operations following an emergency?					
Does the plan identify: • Alternate means of meeting essential building needs • Backup communications • Facilities for isolation					
Alternate roles for personnel during an emergency					
Does the plan provide for orientation and education of personnel who participate in emergencies?					
Does the hospital have the ability to provide decontamination in the event of an emergency?					
Does the hospital have the appropriate facilities, equipment, and supplies for decontamination procedures?					
Does the hospital conduct emergency drills at least twice a year?					
Were problems/concerns identified during drills or actual events?					
What actions were taken to resolve them?					
Does the hospital "fit test" those who will use respirators during decontamination procedures?					
Are hospital schematics available to those who may need them during an emergency?					
Does the hospital coordinate emergency management activities with its satellite facilities?					

Objectives, as stated in each of the EOC management plans, are evaluated for current relevancy to the organization. The evaluation should state that objectives have been reviewed and considered. If a plan's objectives have not changed, it is acceptable to note "no change."

The scope of each plan is reviewed, and changes within the organization are noted, such as new security department hours, added or expanded services, or additional facilities that have been acquired, such as a new clinic that will require safety inspections, hazardous material inventory, and so forth.

Performance measurement is the foundation of the annual evaluation. Data relative to the performance improvement (PI) goals provide information for the involved staff to assess their accomplishments and compliance with regulatory standards. The data collection supports the findings of the annual evaluation. For example, if security events show an increase in lost patient belongings (as monitored under safety inspections in table 12.2), a PI goal to address the lost belongings should be included in the annual evaluation of the security plan.

The effectiveness of a plan is determined by what went well during the year, what accomplishments were achieved, whether the organization was in compliance with regulatory requirements, what procedures or policies need to be updated or implemented, and what functions need to be improved. This information, along with the data collected for performance measurement, may be the basis for determining performance goals or quality improvement projects for the following year.

Information Collection and Evaluation System

The information collection and evaluation system (ICES) shown in table 12.2 comprises many documents, facts, reports, and performance monitoring. Information collected and evaluated may include patient reports of unusual occurrence, security incident reports, employee injuries or illness reports, and the number of hazardous materials spills. The Joint Commission requires monitoring, investigation, and reporting of the following items:

- Patient or visitor injuries

- Incidents of property damage

- Occupational injuries or illnesses

- Security incidents

- Hazardous materials and waste spills and exposures

- Fire prevention problems, deficiencies, and failures

- Equipment problems, deficiencies, and failures

- Utility systems problems, deficiencies, and failures

Information collection may be the responsibility of one designated individual, such as the quality department director, the risk manager, or the safety officer. A reasonable expectation is that data collection and transmission are the responsibility of each safety plan leader. The safety committee, a multidisciplinary group, reviews the information and makes recommendations to the individual responsible for the safety plans. The safety committee ensures that the information is circulated to administration, the medical staff, and the board of trustees.

At a minimum, data should be collected on the pertinent functions or performance standards of each safety plan and submitted to the safety committee quarterly for comment and recommendations.

Real-Life Example

One Saturday morning in April, a third-party construction company was laying cable under the street about a quarter mile north of Community Hospital of the West. The workers were using an auger to drill under the roadway so that they would not need to tear up the street. Although the gas lines and electric cables in the area had been marked with blue stakes, the construction crew inadvertently damaged the main telephone cable under the street. Communications into and out of the hospital and other businesses in the area were disconnected.

The hospital did not have a cellular telephone. Because they were not able to make or receive calls, the staff at the hospital faced major problems communicating with physicians and providing care support for emergency department patients. The staff had to find a quick solution. They decided to use employees' cellular telephones and one pay phone that was still inexplicably working. Crews from the telephone company worked all day to restore service, which was reestablished at 7:30 p.m.

Because the organization had not been prepared for this type of emergency, the hospital's safety council met later to initiate the following steps:

- Purchase cellular telephones to be stored in the hospital's central communications area

- Establish and maintain an employee telephone directory, including cellular telephone numbers with departments being responsible for reporting directory updates

- Determine whether cellular telephones interfere with hospital equipment and technology, and if so, where the interferences occur

- Develop a location map with safe zones for cellular telephone use throughout the hospital

QI Toolbox Technique

Postprogram assessments are the most common method used to evaluate employee knowledge of care environment and safety area issues. The assessments are given to employees after each training session. At a minimum, every employee must attend training in each of the areas annually. Human resources systems track each employee's training attendance and record it in the employee's personnel file. (Employee training attendance may be the function of the education department, with files maintained separately. However the function is designated, training files must be available for surveyors.) Figure 12.8 shows an example of a post-training assessment tool used at Community Hospital of the West.

Some organizations have safety fairs. They set up carnival games or similar activities in which staff are asked EOC questions. Staff members who answer the questions correctly are entered into drawings or awarded small prizes. Many kinds of activities can be developed to keep safety issues in the forefront, such as participating in a community-wide mock disaster drill.

Many organizations have developed a safety response flip chart that is posted in a prominent area in each department of the facility for rapid access by personnel. Each page has emergency response information to assist employees in the first 15 to 45 minutes of an emergency.

Figure 12.8.   Post-training assessment tool used at Community Hospital of the West

INTERVIEW OF STAFF (circle questions asked)
1. What orientation did you receive on the following:
a. General safety   [ ]
b. Department safety   [ ]
c. Job-specific hazards   [ ]
2. What continuing safety education have you received?   [ ]
3. What are the emergency procedures for:
a. Bomb threat   [ ]
b. Hostage crises   [ ]
4. How are security incidents reported?   [ ]
5. Give an example of the safe use of a hazardous chemical and waste in your department.   [ ]
6. What is the procedure for reporting a hazardous materials spill?   [ ]
7. What is appropriate personal protective equipment to handle hazardous materials in your department?   [ ]
8. What is your role in the disaster plan?   [ ]
9. Describe the emergency communication system (red phones).   [ ]
10. What role and responsibilities do you have at the site of a fire?   [ ]
11. What role and responsibilities do you have away from the fire site?   [ ]
12. Describe your role in evacuation of patients and staff.   [ ]
13. Describe how to report equipment problems.   [ ]
14. Where are the MSDSs kept?   [ ]
15. Describe how to report utility failures.   [ ]

Case Study #1

During remodeling and renovation of two patient care areas at a hospital, a new nurse call system was installed. A Code Blue alarm specific to each room was a component of the new system. The other patient care areas in the hospital were to receive the new nurse call system later in the year. After installation of the new system, the nurses were instructed to begin using the Code Blue button in the patient rooms, and they were assured that the alarm and room number would automatically appear on the hospital operator's console. The new system made it unnecessary to call the operator to request a "Code Blue" and for the operator to announce the room number because it was done automatically.

Unfortunately, this was a case in which patient safety was overlooked in the excitement of receiving new technology. It was soon discovered that the room number that appeared on the console did not correspond to the room number in which the button was being pushed. The discrepancy was noted with the first Code Blue in one of the renovated areas when the room number that appeared on the console was not a recognized room number in the hospital. Use of the Code Blue button was suspended immediately. The procedure of calling the operator was reinstituted and remained in effect until all clinical areas received the new nurse call system. This gave the clinical engineering personnel time to make sure the new system was functioning appropriately, and prevented the confusion that would have resulted from maintaining two different methods of alerting the hospital operator of a Code Blue.

Case Study #2

Students should search the Internet for the MSDS information for five common household products. They should list the item description information, effects of exposure, and safe handling and disposal procedures for each of the five products. Product information may be located at http://hazard.com/msds/index.php.

Project Application

Students should identify existing environmental and safety guidelines or regulations that have implications for their projects. If the student project recommends PI training, participants should consider how they would assess the training outcomes to determine whether individuals retained important aspects of the training.

Summary

Maintaining employee knowledge and skill is a significant PI challenge in the environment of patient care and safety. Appropriate emergency response is crucial to minimizing risk to employees, patients, and medical staff. Therefore, PI activity is organized around the assessment of potential hazards and the training and retraining of personnel so that emergency procedures are initiated without question or hesitation when necessary. Employees' abilities also must be assessed consistently and frequently to ensure that their knowledge base is adequate at all times. Equipment maintenance and security management also are critical areas for continuous monitoring.

References

Joint Commission. 2011a. Emergency management and life safety chapters. *Hospital Accreditation Standards*. Oakbrook Terrace, IL: Joint Commission Resources.

Joint Commission. 2011b. Glossary. *Hospital Accreditation Standards*. Oakbrook Terrace, IL: Joint Commission Resources.

National Fire Protection Association (NFPA). 2011. *NFPA 101 Life Safety Code*. Quincy, MA: NFPA.

Safe Medical Devices Act of 1990. Public Law 101-629.

US Department of Labor, Occupational Safety and Health Administration. 1994. Hazard Communication Standard 1910.1200. http://www.osha.gov.

Resources

American National Standards Institute. http://www.ansi.org.

Centers for Disease Control and Prevention. http://www.cdc.gov.

Hinckley, C.M. 1997. Defining the best quality control system by design and inspection. *Clinical Chemistry* (435):873–879.

National Incident Management System. http://www.nims.org.

Chapter 13
Developing Staff and Human Resources

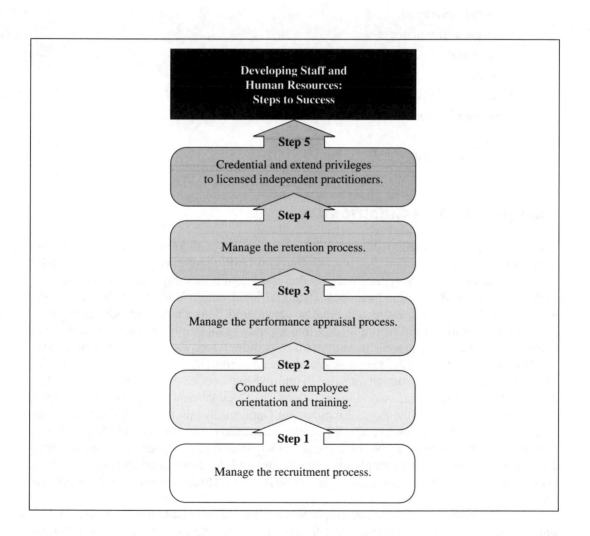

Learning Objectives

- To recognize the need to integrate performance improvement and patient safety data into the management of the human resources function in healthcare
- To identify the tools commonly used to manage the recruitment and retention of human resources
- To outline the credentialing process for independent practitioners and employed clinical staff

Key Terms

Clinical privileges

Credentialing process

Credentials

Due process

Healthcare Integrity and Protection Data Bank (HIPDB)

Licensed independent practitioner

Licenses

National Practitioner Data Bank (NPDB)

Background and Significance

The environment in which healthcare organizations manage their human resources is dictated in large part by state and federal employment laws, regulatory agencies, and market trends. Variations in the way healthcare is delivered also affect the organization's recruitment, training, and retention practices. Potential legal action undertaken by employees against healthcare organizations also must be considered. This chapter introduces information on laws, regulations, shifting market trends, and organizational policy to demonstrate some of the processes and tools used to manage people in today's healthcare environment.

During the 20th century, inequitable and unsafe employment practices were a driving force in the passage of legislation intended to improve the work environment. Legislation that addressed issues such as safe working conditions (the Occupational Safety and Health Act of 1970), wages and hours (the Equal Employment Opportunity Act of 1972), disabilities (the Americans with Disabilities Act of 1990), and medical leave (the Family and Medical Leave Act of 1993) have played a role in shaping the workplace environment and standardizing employment practices. Other employment guidelines and standards of practice in the areas of state licensure and outside accrediting agencies have evolved to direct the employer-employee relationship.

For any healthcare organization, employees are both the most important resource and the greatest potential liability. Developing effective processes related to recruitment, retention, competency, orientation, and continuing education of all staff members is a critical function of an organization's leadership, which must ensure that it employs highly skilled staff.

Effective leadership is defined as how well an organization's leaders plan, direct, integrate, and coordinate services, and how well they create a culture that focuses on continual performance improvement (PI) while at the same time maintaining a balanced budget and fiscal viability in the market. These key leadership functions are demonstrated through human resources management in the following ways:

- Defining the qualifications, competencies, and performance expectations for all staff positions

- Providing competent staff

- Ensuring orientation and other ongoing training and education

- Assessing, maintaining, and improving staff competence

- Promoting self-development and learning

Today's cutting-edge work environment encourages and empowers employees to take responsibility for improving the environment in which they work, no matter what their position in the organizational structure. PI can be a powerful concept when woven into the culture of an organization. Organizations that embrace ongoing PI do so because their leaders foster a culture of competency through staff self-development and lifelong learning. The competitive advantage for healthcare organizations today lies in their intellectual capital and organizational effectiveness. This style of motivating and developing employees is grounded in the ability of leaders to create, communicate, and model the organization's mission, vision, and values.

Steps to Success: Developing Staff and Human Resources

Historically, healthcare organizations have used a number of different criteria to determine the actual number of full-time equivalent (FTE) staff, including the patient census, the acuity of the patients being treated, licensing regulations that may outline the staff-to-patient ratio, and the qualifications of the type of staff required. In planning its budget, an organization must take into account the revenue that needs to be generated and the number of FTEs that are required to run a facility that meets licensing agreements, addresses patient safety issues, and maintains fiscal viability.

Since 2003, the Joint Commission has been developing measurable standards related to staffing effectiveness in an attempt to make maintaining prescribed staffing levels a more realistic, dynamic process. Effective staffing is complex, dynamic, and unique to each individual organization. At the core of staffing effectiveness are the competency and skill mix of the staff members currently assigned to care for a particular set of patients, as well as the associated acuity ratios (how sick the particular set of patients is) for the population in question. Staffing has a direct impact on the quality and safety of patient care. An aging workforce, which points to potential shortages of key staff, will continue to challenge and impact staffing effectiveness.

The standard approach to evaluation of effective hospital staffing includes the use of multiple hospital-specific clinical/service measures and human resources indicators as screening tools to identify potential staffing issues. There must be at least two clinical measures and two human resources indicators for each patient population, defined by internal PI activities. At a minimum, the organization identifies no fewer than two inpatient care areas for which staffing effectiveness data are collected. Identified performance measures relate to processes appropriate to the care and services provided and to problem-prone areas experienced in the past. The rationale for indicator selection is based on relevancy and sensitivity to each patient area where staffing is planned. Figure 13.1 provides a partial list of Joint Commission–approved screening indicators currently used in hospitals. The intent is that multiple indicators examined together may provide information related to staffing effectiveness. Because staffing effectiveness is considered a critical process in healthcare, the standards require that a thorough analysis be initiated whenever an organization detects or suspects significant undesirable performance or variation due to staffing issues.

Most organizations define their clinical staffing needs in two categories: direct and indirect caregivers. Examples of direct caregivers include registered nurses, licensed practical nurses, physical therapists, chaplains, and social services staff. Indirect caregivers include clinical support professionals from the pharmacy, laboratory, housekeeping, dietary, and so on. Both direct and indirect caregivers may be included in the human resources screening indicators.

Step 1: Manage the Recruitment Process

A well-defined recruitment process provides both the organization and the applicant with an opportunity to evaluate and determine their potential compatibility. The recruitment process is usually initiated to fill a vacant position, to fill a newly created position, to staff a newly instituted service, or to support increases in patient acuity or census. Organizations sometimes retain the services of an outside recruitment agency when there are shortages of qualified applicants or because of an organization's remote geographic location.

Position requisitions, position (or job) descriptions, and employment applications are the primary tools used in the recruitment process. A position requisition begins the formal communication between the human resources staff and the department or service area initiating the recruitment process. (See figure 13.2.) A detailed position requisition provides

Figure 13.1.   Partial list of hospital screening indicators used in measuring staff effectiveness

Human Resources Screens:	Clinical Service Screens:
• Agency staff use	• Adverse drug events
• Nursing care hours per patient day	• Falls with injury
• On-call or per-diem use	• Injuries to patients
• Overtime	• Length of stay
• Sick time	• Patient/family complaints
• Skill mix	• Pneumonia
• Staff injuries	• Postoperative infections
• Staff satisfaction	• Pressure ulcer prevalence
• Staff turnover rate	• Shock/cardiac arrest
• Staff vacancy rate	• Upper gastrointestinal bleeding
	• Urinary tract infection

Source: Adapted from the Joint Commission 2011 and the National Quality Forum n.d.

Figure 13.2.   Sample position requisition

PERSONNEL REQUISITION					
JOB TITLE		DATE OF REQUEST		DATE REQUIRED	
DEPARTMENT					
☐ Replacement for:					
☐ Additional Personnel:		Budgeted: ☐ Yes ☐ No			
☐ Temporary: End Date _____	☐ Full Time	☐ Part Time	☐ Exempt	☐ PRN	☐ Per Diem
Shift: Hours per week:		Suggested Pay Grade:			

Qualifications needed: education, experience, training, duties, physical fitness

	Actual:	Budgeted:	Prior Year:
YTD FTEs			
MH/STAT			
SAL $/STAT			

Reason for additional personnel or new position:

APPROVALS (must be obtained prior to offering position)	

DIRECTOR/MANAGER:
                    DATE:
	CEO:
	                    DATE:

CFO:
                    DATE:
	HUMAN RESOURCES:
	                    DATE:

NEW PERSONNEL							
To be completed by human resources					Date Required:		
Employee's Name:			Department:			Employee Number:	
Address:			Social Security Number:				
Telephone Number:			Birthdate:				
Date of Hire:			Temporary Date of Termination:				
☐ New Hire	☐ Rehire	☐ Full Time	☐ Part Time	☐ PRN	☐ Per Diem	☐ Exempt	☐ Temp.
RATE/HOUR	BIWEEKLY RATE		RACE	EEO CAT.	TAX EXEMP.	POS CODE	
COMMENTS OR SPECIAL INSTRUCTIONS:							

human resources staff with the information needed to advertise the open position, including the position title, qualifications and experience required, work schedule, and salary. Position requisitions also can be used to monitor the appropriateness of personnel requests. For example, a nonbudgeted position or a new position request may require additional documentation and administrative approval before recruitment can begin.

Position descriptions define the responsibilities of the job and the qualifications needed to fulfill those responsibilities. Qualifications may define education; licensure, certification, or registration status; and experience required. Qualifications also may include previous experience requirements, such as a pediatric nurse position requiring training and experience working with children and adolescents in particular pediatric settings.

In healthcare organizations, **credentials,** certifications, and **licenses** are qualifications of foremost importance. Clinical professionals, such as physicians, psychologists, nurses, occupational therapists, physical therapists, respiratory therapists, and social workers, as well as some ancillary services professionals, such as radiology technicians, laboratory technicians, and pharmacy technicians, are required to hold a credential or license to practice their profession.

Credentials are the recognition by healthcare organizations of previous professional practice responsibilities and experiences commonly accorded to licensed independent practitioners. Certifications are usually conferred by a national professional organization dedicated to a specific area of healthcare practice. Licenses are conferred by state regulatory agencies. Certification and licensing processes usually require an applicant to pass an examination to initially obtain the certification or license and then to maintain the certification or license through continuing education activities thereafter.

Job responsibilities describe the major tasks of the position. Responsibilities should be stated in measurable terms, which is the standard in healthcare today. A clinical position, for example, may describe a responsibility as "completing a nursing assessment on each admission within the time frame defined by policy."

In general, position descriptions provide guidance to human resources staff by defining the initial selection criteria for potential candidates. Position descriptions also provide the applicant or new employee with information about position expectations. With the support of human resources specialists, managers generally maintain position descriptions that reflect local market and current position requirements.

An employment application is provided to interested candidates who contact the organization in response to an advertised position. A review of the completed application and the applicant's resume provides human resources, and the recruiting department or service area manager, with enough information to determine whether the applicant meets the minimum position requirements. (See the example in figure 13.3.) Applicants who meet the initial position requirements and who are the most qualified are invited to interview for the position.

The interview gives the applicant and the organization an opportunity to exchange information not listed on the employment application or in the position advertisement. The organization may have additional questions specific to experience, skills, and qualifications that are not addressed in the application. The candidate, in turn, may have questions related to salary, benefits, or the organization's history. The interview provides an excellent

Figure 13.3.   **Sample employment application**

INSTRUCTIONS TO THE APPLICANT:

Please complete the application in full. You can send a resume with your completed application.

Please apply for a specific position(s) and include that position's job title(s) on the application.

APPLICANT: The federal government requires employers to collect statistical information on job applicants. Providing this information is voluntary. The information is used for statistical purposes only and will not be included in your application file. Information will be maintained and utilized in accordance with applicable laws and regulations. Refusal to provide the information below will not subject you to any adverse treatment or affect the application process in any way.

1. SEX   __ Male   __ Female

2. RACE/ETHNIC BACKGROUND (check only one):

    ___ Asian or Pacific Islander (O)
    ___ American Indian/Native American (A)
    ___ Black (not of Hispanic Origin) (B)
    ___ White (not of Hispanic Origin) (C)
    ___ Hispanic (a person whose cultural or linguistic origins are Spanish or Latin American, regardless of race, for example, Mexican, Puerto Rican, Cuban, Central or South American) (S)

3. DISABLED OR VETERAN STATUS (check all that apply):

    ___ Disabled, but not a veteran (I)
    ___ Veteran of Vietnam era (V)
    ___ Disabled veteran (D)
    ___ None of the above

___ I do not wish to provide this information.

PLEASE CONTINUE ON THE NEXT PAGE.

(Continued on next page)

Figure 13.3. *(Continued)*

_____ App#

(For office use only)

APPLICATION FOR EMPLOYMENT

All applicants selected for employment must satisfactorily pass a preemployment drug screen and criminal background check to be eligible for employment.
CHW is an Equal Opportunity and Affirmative Action Employer.
CHW hires only individuals who are authorized to work in the United States.
This application is subject to the conditions set forth in the Certification and Agreement section on the last page.

PLEASE COMPLETE APPLICATION IN FULL

DATE OF APPLICATION: _____
LAST NAME: _____ FIRST NAME: _____ MIDDLE INITIAL: _____
CURRENT ADDRESS: _____ CITY: _____ COUNTY: _____
STATE: _____ ZIP CODE: _____
SOCIAL SECURITY #: _____ HOME PHONE: (___) _____ WORK PHONE: (___) _____

SOURCE OF REFERRAL

RECRUITING METHOD: (Please check one)
__ (60) Student Work Experience   __ (05) Walk-in   __ (10) Internal Referral _____
__ (30) Newspaper   __ (80) Past Experience __ (06) Temp Employment Agency, Temp-to-hire
__ (13) Internet   __ (15) Job Line   __ (85) Community-based Organization
__ (07) Job Service   __ (20) Professional Journal __ (52) Job Elimination
__ (90) School Organization Referral

Have you ever been convicted of a felony or a misdemeanor, or have you ever plead no contest to any criminal charges?   __ Yes   __ No
Provide date, city, state, and an explanation for any "yes" responses: _____
Criminal conviction is not an absolute bar to employment but will be considered in relation to specific job requirements.

Can you perform the functions of the job for which you are applying, either with or without a reasonable accommodation?   __ Yes   __ No
Do you have any relatives employed by Community Hospital of the West?   __ Yes   __ No
If yes, where/relationship _____
Have you ever been employed by or are you currently employed by Community Hospital of the West?   __ Yes   __ No
If yes, where? _____ When? _____
Why did you leave? _____

POSITION(S) DESIRED (only two positions per application please)
TITLE: _____ Job Number:_____
TITLE: _____ Job Number:_____

WORK AVAILABILITY
MARK ALL THAT APPLY
Type of Employment   Work Schedule/Shift   Weekends __ Yes __ No   No Rotating Weekends __ Yes __ No
__ Full Time   __ Days
__ Part Time   __ Evenings
__ Temporary   __ Nights
__ On Call   Hours Available _____
Current Salary: $ _____ Minimum Salary Requirement $ _____ Date Available to Work _____

JOB SKILLS
Check all that you have experience with: PC Graphics __ Yes __ No   Word Processor __ Yes __ No
Desktop Publishing __ Yes __ No   PC __ Yes __ No   Spreadsheet __ Yes __ No
LAN __ Yes __ No   Database __ Yes __ No   Microsoft Windows® __ Yes __ No
AS/400 __ Yes __ No   Tandem __ Yes __ No   Medical Terminology __ Yes __ No
List specific software programs used: _____
Typing Speed: _____ WPM   10-Key by Touch __ Yes __ No   _____ SPM

Figure 13.3. *(Continued)*

EDUCATION

Have you graduated from high school or completed the GED equivalent? __ Yes __ No

List all degrees that you have received. List your HIGHEST DEGREE FIRST. Do NOT list degrees that you are currently working toward (see below).

MAJOR	DEGREE	SCHOOL	GRADUATION DATE

Are you currently enrolled? __ YES __ NO   Last year attended: _____   Major: _____

Check last level of school completed:

Years completed: Undergraduate: __ Freshman   __ Sophomore   __ Junior   __ Senior

Graduate: __ 1st year   __ 2nd year   __ 3rd year   __ 4th year

LICENSURE/REGISTRATION/CERTIFICATION

List all professional licenses, registrations, and certifications.

Lic/Reg/Cert Type	License #	State	Expiration Date

Do you have any pending restrictions and/or suspensions on your current professional license/registration that would restrain you from performing in this position? __ YES __ NO

Have you ever been refused professional licensure or had a license/registration suspended or revoked? __ YES __ NO

If yes, please explain: _____

List any trade or professional organizations of which you are a member, including offices held: _____

_____

List any special skills: _____

EMPLOYMENT HISTORY

Starting with your most recent employment, give a complete record of all employment and reasons for periods of unemployment.

How many years of experience do you have related to this position? _____

MAY WE CONTACT YOUR CURRENT EMPLOYER? __ YES __ NO   If no, why? _____

_____

NOTE: If your current or most recent employer is not contacted before an offer of employment is made, then any offer of employment that is made will be subject to CHW subsequently contacting such employer, and may be withdrawn based on the information received from such employer.

COMPANY NAME	ADDRESS	CITY	STATE	ZIP CODE	AREA CODE PHONE
					(____) _____

TYPE OF BUSINESS   SUPERVISOR'S NAME, TITLE & PHONE NUMBER:

_____   _____

DATE EMPLOYED: MO _____   YR _____   DATE LEFT: MO _____   YR _____

TITLE AND DUTIES: _____

REASON FOR LEAVING: _____

IF YOUR EMPLOYMENT RECORDS EXIST UNDER ANOTHER NAME, PLEASE SPECIFY: _____

FINAL SALARY: $_____

(Continued on next page)

Figure 13.3.   *(Continued)*

COMPANY NAME	ADDRESS	CITY	STATE	ZIP CODE	AREA CODE PHONE
					(_____) _____

TYPE OF BUSINESS   SUPERVISOR'S NAME, TITLE & PHONE NUMBER:
_____   _____

DATE EMPLOYED: MO _____ YR _____   DATE LEFT: MO _____ YR _____

TITLE AND DUTIES: _____

REASON FOR LEAVING: _____

IF YOUR EMPLOYMENT RECORDS EXIST UNDER ANOTHER NAME, PLEASE SPECIFY: _____

FINAL SALARY: $_____

COMPANY NAME	ADDRESS	CITY	STATE	ZIP CODE	AREA CODE PHONE
					(_____) _____

TYPE OF BUSINESS   SUPERVISOR'S NAME, TITLE & PHONE NUMBER:
_____   _____

DATE EMPLOYED: MO _____ YR _____   DATE LEFT: MO _____ YR _____

TITLE AND DUTIES: _____

REASON FOR LEAVING: _____

IF YOUR EMPLOYMENT RECORDS EXIST UNDER ANOTHER NAME, PLEASE SPECIFY: _____

FINAL SALARY: $_____

GIVE THREE ADDITIONAL WORK-RELATED REFERENCES

Name	Occupation or Title	Firm Name and Address (include city, state, and zip)	Phone
_____	_____	_____	_____
_____	_____	_____	_____
_____	_____	_____	_____

CERTIFICATION AND AGREEMENT

I certify that the information I provided in this application is complete and accurate to the best of my knowledge. I understand that any misrepresentation or omission of facts in this application disqualifies me from further consideration, or, if I am employed, is sufficient cause for dismissal. I understand that any alteration of this application in content or form may be considered cause for disqualification and/or termination.

I authorize investigation of all statements contained in this application, and understand that I may be required to provide verification (diploma, license, transcripts, type tests, etc.) of information contained in this application.

I authorize any and all persons, companies, or agencies to release to CHW any and all information they may have that is relevant to the application process. I also release all such parties from any liability that may result from furnishing information to CHW.

I understand that to be considered as a formal applicant, the position for which I am applying must be specifically identified as open, and recruitment for the position must be going on at the time this application is received by the Human Resources Department.

I understand that if I am employed with CHW, my employment will be at-will. As such, it can be terminated by me or by CHW with or without advance notice, at any time, and for any reason not prohibited by law. I agree that if I am employed by CHW, I will review the information contained in CHW's General Information Handbook.

I understand that any employment offer is contingent upon the following: (1) producing documents establishing my eligibility to work in the United States; (2) satisfactorily passing the preemployment drug screen, criminal background, and reference checks; and (3) complying with CHW's preemployment application procedures.

By either writing or typing my name and submitting this application to CHW, I acknowledge that I have read the certification and agreement and agree to abide by its terms.

NAME: _____   DATE :_____

Community Hospital of the West is an Equal Employment Opportunity/Affirmative Action Employer.

opportunity for the interviewer to evaluate the applicant's communication skills, general personality, and demeanor. During the interview process, the interviewee may be asked to sign a release for information on a background check. Most states offer this service as a risk reduction and patient safety strategy for facilities that provide physical and emotional care to vulnerable patient populations. This regulation was put into place to safeguard clients and facilities from individuals with documented histories of abuse. Potential employees in these settings must pass a criminal background check before being offered a position.

Several types of interviews can be used to screen applicants. A structured interview is conducted using a set of standard questions that are asked of all job applicants, the purpose of which is to gather comparative data. The unstructured interview uses general questions from which other questions are developed over the course of the conversation. The purpose of this type of interview is to prompt the interviewee to speak openly.

The following examples of unstructured questions may be used during an interview:

- Tell us about your previous position. In general, what kinds of duties did you perform?

- Tell us about your personal understanding of the need for maintaining the patient's rights to confidentiality.

The stress interview uses specific questions to determine how the interviewee responds under pressure. Questions in this type of interview set up specific scenarios and ask the interviewee how he or she would handle the situation. The following are examples of questions that might be asked in a stress interview:

- If a newspaper reporter came to you and wanted you to reveal information from a prominent person's health record, how would you respond?

- If an attorney came to your nursing unit and wanted to review her client's health record, what would you do?

Some types of questions should be avoided during an interview. Questions that might be interpreted as attempts to learn personal information about the applicant (such as the applicant's age, marital status, or family status) are prohibited by federal regulations. Figure 13.4 includes examples of questions that are not related to employment and would be considered discriminatory.

Some facilities add a skills-testing/competency review segment such as a coding test, medication exam, developmental age exam, or a computer literacy test to their interview process. This testing adds additional information of a concrete nature to the screening for possible candidates.

Whichever approach or combination of approaches is used, the information collected at this point in the recruitment process should be enough to determine who will advance to the next stage of the selection process. Reference checks; criminal background checks; and verifications of licensure, training, and educational requirements should be documented before any applicant is offered a position. In the past, checking past employment references sometimes yielded important new information about a candidate. Today, however,

Figure 13.4.   Appropriate and inappropriate interview questions

Examples of Appropriate Job-Related Questions	Examples of Inappropriate Questions Unrelated to the Job
• How does your education and work experience relate to the position we are discussing?	• Where were you born?
• What courses did you take in school?	• What race are you?
• What was your grade point average?	• What does your husband (or father) do for a living?
• Are you willing to work weekends?	• Are you married?
• Are you willing to work overtime?	• Do you plan to get married?
• What kind of work did you do in your previous positions?	• How old are you?
• What kind of work do you enjoy the most? The least?	• Do you have any children? How many? What are their ages?
• What areas of your work skills would you like to improve?	• Do you plan to have children?
• How do you perform under pressure?	• Is your husband likely to be transferred?
• How many people were you responsible for supervising in your previous positions?	• Who cares for your children while you are at work?
• Why did you leave your last position?	• Are you involved in any church groups?
• How do you explain the gaps in your employment history?	• Where do you live?
• Would you require any additional training to perform this position?	• Do you own or rent the place where you live?
• What are your career goals?	• What organizations do you belong to?
• What is your understanding of this area of the healthcare industry?	• Have you ever been arrested?
• What was your attendance record like in your previous positions?	
• How long have you lived in this area?	
• Are you able to work the hours required for this position?	

most organizations release only general information regarding an employee's past work performance, such as dates of employment and whether the applicant is eligible for rehire. While the information received from these contacts may be minimal in terms of a potential employee's skills, they do speak to the veracity of documentation in the resume in general and may be critical in a legal defense situation for a facility.

Some facilities utilize a point-scoring process for interviews that awards points for education, knowledge at time of interview, and experience with the specific population of patients. This system helps ensure that the top-qualified individuals will be in the running for a position.

Step 2: Conduct New Employee Orientation and Training

Orientation should be provided to every new hire, including contracted staff, agency personnel, and volunteers. New staff members are required to receive an overview of the organization as well as details about their specific job responsibilities. The organization's leaders are expected to develop a process to ensure that all new staff members are informed of performance expectations and specific responsibilities and that they are qualified to fulfill these expectations. When these issues are addressed before new staff members are allowed to perform independently, the orientation process promotes safe and effective job performance. In general, staff should be oriented to the organization's mission; vision; values; PI program; life safety procedures; infection control practices; privacy practices; policies towards patient, client, or resident abuse; specific job duties; and safety issues specific to their job assignments. Additional orientation and training may be specific to a particular type of healthcare organization, such as age-specific training for staff working with neonatal or pediatric age groups, where skills at interpreting nonverbal communication are essential.

New staff members should not work independently until they have completed orientation and demonstrated competency. Testing to assess the competency of a clinical staff member may include having the employee insert a catheter, draw blood, or use a piece of medical equipment. This type of training and orientation may include having the new employee shadow a seasoned employee for a specified period of time, complete a self-directed study course, or attend classroom instruction and then demonstrate his or her competence by performing a particular job skill a set number of times for a certified trainer.

As they are completed, orientation and demonstrated job competencies must be documented. Some organizations use a training checklist to document employee orientation. The checklist documents the names of the trainee and trainer(s), orientation dates, tasks, and demonstrated competencies. The orientation checklist should be maintained in the employee's personnel file so that it can be used in the performance appraisal process to monitor whether training and competency requirements have been met.

Aggregate data also can be compiled from training checklists to monitor organization-wide and care- or service-specific orientation and competency requirements. In hospitals, aggregate data on the levels of staff competence, relevant patterns and trends in training needs, and competence maintenance activities should be reported to the governing body at least annually. Gathering data for the competence assessment process can be accomplished through observations, demonstrations, and PI reports such as occurrence report findings, peer review findings, and staffing effectiveness and satisfaction surveys.

Policies and procedures facilitate the orientation and training of staff and form the basis for individual accountability. Policies and procedures should clearly represent and communicate the required functions and tasks the employee is expected to perform, as well as the procedures to initiate when an unacceptable incident occurs in the facility, such as a medication error. It is critical that all employees be trained in the areas of risk identification and reduction and incident reporting. Data collected from this process become the basis for much PI in healthcare facilities. (Chapter 10 discusses the application of incident reports to PI in greater detail.)

Step 3: Manage the Performance Appraisal Process

Every healthcare organization should have a process in place to periodically reassess each staff member's ability to meet the performance expectations and competencies described in his or her job description. Healthcare organizations determine how often these reassessments should occur. For example, competence can be assessed at hire; by the end of the orientation process; at regular intervals (such as once per year); when job responsibilities change; or when new or updated technologies, products, procedures, or services are introduced.

The employee performance appraisal process should be specific to the staff member's assigned responsibilities and assessed competencies. Ideally, the appraisal should include a one-on-one discussion between the employee and the supervisor or manager along with a written appraisal that provides room for employee response. The employee and the supervisor or manager should work together to develop new performance goals and to modify or enhance performance standards. The manager or supervisor should follow up with the employee to monitor his or her progress in meeting goals and performance standards through frequent, informal assessments as well as periodic formal appraisals. At a minimum, the periodic assessment should address each of the following areas of the employee's performance:

- Degree of compliance with written standards of performance as stated in the staff member's job description

- Participation in ongoing PI and patient safety activities

- Findings from competency assessment activities

Other areas, such as a staff member's strengths, weaknesses, working relationships, morale, motivation, and attendance, also may be addressed during the appraisal process.

The performance criteria used in the appraisal process should be directly linked to the employee's current position description and to the organization's mission. This process also should verify that the employee has maintained his or her credentials or licenses, as appropriate.

Organizations that have successfully implemented a PI culture have expanded the appraisal process to include team performance in tandem with individual performance. Teams may include a clinical treatment team, an administrative or leadership team, or a single department team. The appraisal process includes the team's definition of performance expectations and goals and a periodic assessment of its performance as a team rather than as individuals.

Ideally, organization-wide performance measures should be referenced and incorporated into the employee and team appraisal process. Provider- or employee-specific PI and patient safety monitoring activities may identify staff development needs. This same information reported in aggregate may identify trends in care that support the need for changes in staffing patterns, skill sets, or the care environment.

Other clinical service and human resources screening criteria used to monitor staffing effectiveness, as noted in figure 13.1, are also reviewed in preparation for the organization's annual strategic planning process.

Step 4: Manage the Retention Process

Commitment to the development and retention of human resources is of strategic importance to every healthcare organization. High retention rates communicate a strong message about the organization's values to existing and potential employees. Beyond traditional in-house orientation programs, many organizations offer tuition and professional education reimbursement as an incentive for ongoing staff development and retention. Maintaining a competitive salary and benefits package continues to be a primary leverage point in recruitment and retention programs. Organizations that go beyond traditional incentives use employee input to create reward structures to promote employee retention. Incentives such as profit sharing, job sharing, sign-on bonuses, shared leadership, and cutting-edge technological resources are a few of the trends.

Certainly, the most compelling link to employee retention is the creation of a work environment in which organizational and personal values mesh, creating a natural synergy. Teams working together with a common vision begin with a self-directed, motivated workforce. Many times, this team factor directly influences employee retention even more than salary issues do. Healthcare-related literature indicates that money is not the number one or two reason that people leave positions (Shaw et al. 1998). Employees who have been prepared for their jobs through education and who believe that they are part of a vital team that provides excellent care are willing to stay, even if their salary is not top in the field.

Another important aspect of managing employee retention in healthcare is the maintenance of employee competence. Healthcare professionals must follow many standard processes and procedures to provide quality care, while at the same time protecting patient safety. Maintaining professional knowledge and competence to perform these processes becomes of paramount importance. To accomplish this, many organizations require all employees to obtain recertification in areas specific to their clinical license, such as CPR and basic life support skills, or in areas specific to the organization's safety issues, such as fire safety, infection control, and so forth. Clinical and nonclinical staff must demonstrate their applicable competencies on an annual basis.

Managing the curriculum content, posttraining assessments, and calendar of annual updates for thousands of employees who are required to perform annual competence recertification can be a daunting task. Fortunately, there are information management tools that can assist. One such tool is a Web-based product that allows a department of education and training to:

- Define a standard curriculum for a group of employees

- Develop the curriculum in the application for distribution to the employees through a series of Microsoft® PowerPoint® slides and voice-overs

- Deliver the update training to the employee through the organization's intranet

- Administer and score assessment activities

- Track employees' current status in completing the annual update and archive records of such training for long-term reference

Step 5: Credential and Extend Privileges to Licensed Independent Practitioners

Another category of staff who works in healthcare organizations is the medical staff. Generally referred to as independent practitioners, they include individuals permitted by law and the organization to provide patient care services without direction or supervision, within the scope of their license and individually granted **clinical privileges**. Physicians, dentists, and podiatrists are the most commonly credentialed and privileged independent practitioners working in healthcare organizations. However, certified nurse-anesthetists, physician's assistants, nurse-practitioners, registered nurse-midwives, speech pathologists, dietitians, clinical psychologists, and clinical social workers also may be privileged and credentialed by the healthcare organization, as either supervised employees or contract workers.

The credentialing and privileging process for the initial appointment and reappointment of independent practitioners should be defined in the healthcare organization's medical staff bylaws and should be uniformly applied. The **credentialing process** includes obtaining, verifying, and assessing qualifications of a licensed healthcare practitioner. The primary sources of state licenses, postgraduate degrees, residency and fellowship training, specialty board status, and other healthcare affiliations should all be verified. Primary source verification involves contacting the original source of a specific credential to affirm qualifications reported by an individual healthcare practitioner. The primary source verification process is sometimes contracted out by the healthcare organization to a credentials verification organization (CVO), such as the American Medical Association Physician Master File, which verifies a physician's medical school graduation and residency completion, or the American Board of Medical Specialties, which verifies a physician's board certification. Although using such agencies may relieve the organization of the process of gathering the information, the organization is still responsible for having complete and accurate information on the applicant to substantiate privileging decisions made.

Each **licensed independent practitioner** who provides care under the auspices of a healthcare organization must do so in accordance with delineated clinical privileges based on the practitioner's training, experience, and proven clinical competence. The privilege lists sent out to applicants at initial appointment and at reappointment should be associated with the applicant's type of practice and limited to hospital-specific privileges.

The initial appointment process includes the independent practitioner requesting, completing, and submitting an application to the medical staff along with a request for delineated clinical privileges. The credentialing and privileging process is generally initiated upon completion and approval of an application for membership and request for privileges. The applicant should submit the following information:

- Education, both undergraduate and postgraduate, with names of institutions

- Training, including residencies, fellowships, and any continuing medical education or training for new skills or privileges

- Previous and current healthcare affiliations (hospitals practiced in, private office locations)

- Specialty board certifications

- Current state licenses

- Drug Enforcement Administration (DEA) registration number with expiration dates

- Professional (peer) references who have personal knowledge of the applicant's recent professional performance and experience

- Information on current health status

- Professional liability insurance coverage

- Past and present professional litigation and liability history

- Clinical privileges being requested

Letters are generally sent to at least two peer references and one healthcare organization where the applicant currently holds privileges, requesting specific information about the applicant's qualifications and competencies in relation to the privileges requested, health status, and professional working relationships as observed by the reference source.

Healthcare organizations are required by law to query for information on applicants requesting clinical privileges to the **National Practitioner Data Bank (NPDB)** and the **Healthcare Integrity and Protection Data Bank (HIPDB)**. The NPDB maintains reports on medical malpractice settlements, clinical privilege actions, and professional society membership actions against licensed healthcare providers. The HIPDB maintains reports on civil judgments, criminal convictions of licensed healthcare providers, federal and state licensing and certification actions, and exclusions from participation in federal or state healthcare programs.

Once applicant information has been source verified and references and data bank queries have been returned, the application and supporting documentation are reviewed by the organization's credentials and/or medical executive committee(s). Individual appointment and privilege delineation recommendations are then forwarded to the organization's governing body for final determination. When the application is approved, the appointment period must not exceed a period of two years. A provisional period is generally required (the medical staff bylaws should specify a time limit) for all new staff members. The performance of new staff members should be observed and monitored by an assigned proctor during the provisional period.

In 2002, the Joint Commission added a new standard that requires hospital medical staffs to initiate a process to identify and manage issues of individual physician health. This must be done separately from the disciplinary function of the medical staff. The purpose of the standard is to help facilities address the physical health of practitioners who are at risk in their industry for such job-related illnesses as addiction, stress-related physical illness, and emotional illness. Regular staff education regarding these potential illnesses is another aspect of the new standard. Facilities are required to facilitate the process for confidential diagnosis, treatment, and rehabilitation for any potentially impairing conditions such as the ones defined. These procedures must be done in compliance with any state or federal reporting regulations.

The reappraisal and reappointment process generally occurs every two years and includes a review of current licenses, DEA registration, professional liability coverage, national data bank queries, continuing medical education (as required by the state or for competency training) for new privileges, peer references, information related to claims and litigation, health, and changes in outside affiliations. Training, education, and certification, as well as the frequency with which a clinical privilege has been exercised, should show evidence of continuing proficiency for the privileges requested. An assessment of the provider's profile since the last staff appointment to verify peer review activities provides the final basis for supporting reappointment or reprivileging. Due to the nature of unannounced surveys by the Joint Commission, Centers for Medicare and Medicaid Services (CMS), and other organizations, these files should be kept up to date and monitored continuously.

An ongoing professional practice evaluation includes both administrative aspects of staff membership (for example, meeting attendance statistics, health record delinquency status, medical staff committee appointments, and practice volume statistics) and clinical performance data (for example, clinical outcome statistics, committee or department citations, peer review, and performance-monitoring reviews and actions). The evaluation allows the organization to identify professional practice trends that affect quality of care and patient safety. Such identification may require intervention by the organized medical staff. The criteria used in the ongoing professional practice evaluation may include the following (Joint Commission 2011, MS-38):

- Review of operative and other procedures performed and their outcomes

- Patterns of blood and pharmaceutical usage

- Requests for tests and procedures

- Length-of-stay patterns

- Morbidity and mortality data

- Practitioner's use of consultants

- Other relevant criteria as determined by the organized medical staff

Following review of the reappointment application information and provider profile information, the chief of staff or clinical department chairperson provides a written recommendation on reappointment and reprivileging to the credentials and/or executive committee(s) of the medical staff. These bodies then make their own recommendations and forward them to the governing body for a final decision. When a recommendation for continuing privileges is not made, or a restriction in privileges is requested, the physician must be offered due process. **Due process** provides for fair treatment through a hearing procedure that is generally outlined in the healthcare organization's medical staff bylaws. The procedure stipulates the means by which the physician's application and supporting materials will be reviewed by an impartial panel to ensure objective assessment.

Real-Life Example

Western States University Hospital recently completed a national search and recruitment effort to fill its chief clinical officer (CCO) position. The position had been vacant for six months and had experienced rapid turnover of two previous CCOs within the past two years. The members of the search team invited to participate in the recruitment effort included the chief executive medical director, the chief financial officer, the human resources director, the medical staff president, and the nurse managers from each clinical care area.

The search team followed internal policy requirements related to the recruitment process. The position description was reviewed and updated, and from it, minimum position requirements were identified and included in the advertisement posted internally and published in the local newspaper and a national nursing journal. The search team also retained the services of a national recruitment firm in an effort to fast-track the recruitment process because the organization was less than a year away from its triennial survey with the Joint Commission.

The search generated 15 applicants. The team screened the applicants and narrowed the list down to six who seemed to meet the minimum position requirements. These applicants (five of whom were out-of-state candidates) were interviewed via conference call. The selection was then narrowed to two candidates, who were invited to fly in and meet with the search team.

Of primary importance to this search team's recruitment charge was finding a CCO who had a clinical background and experience that paralleled the services provided at Western States. Experience, strong knowledge of accreditation and licensure requirements, educational background with a master's degree, past employment patterns, personal demeanor, communication style, leadership philosophy, and availability were important factors in the selection. The final candidate selected by the search team met the important criteria and minimum position requirements. Reference checks and source documents verifying the applicant's credentials confirmed the search team's decision to hire the final candidate as the CCO.

Five months into the new CCO's tenure, and six weeks before the triennial survey, Western States's director of risk and quality management resigned. Because the risk and quality position reported to the CCO, the new CCO was asked to facilitate survey preparations. Within days of this decision, the CCO requested that the leadership team recruit a local consulting group to assist in survey coordination efforts. Just two weeks before the anticipated survey, the CCO resigned.

Two main factors contributed to the CCO's resignation. First, the source documents confirming the CCO's graduate education were not in her human resources file. As personnel files were being reviewed in preparation for survey inspection, it was noted that the primary source verification of the CCO's graduate degree was incomplete. When the graduate program was contacted, it was revealed that the CCO had never completed the master's program. Second, although the CCO's curriculum vitae and references confirmed that she had 20-plus years' experience in nursing administration and Joint Commission survey work, she was unable to assume a leadership role in facilitating the nursing component of the Joint Commission survey preparation process.

Western States University Hospital has since defined what information it primary source verifies (verbal and written) when confirming education, experience, and licensure. It also has implemented a checklist for human resources to use to ensure that key action items are completed in the recruitment process. Western States University Hospital also has developed sets of interview questions that better evaluate applicants' key competencies and skill sets.

QI Toolbox Technique

Summary profiles of physician performance provide the credentials committee with significant data about specific physicians scheduled for reappointment to the medical staff. This provides the credentials committee with the information needed to make sound decisions on the performance of members of the hospital's medical staff.

The type of data captured on a physician profile summary should be unique to the healthcare organization's specific needs. The sample form in figure 13.5 is designed for a physician in the specialty area of obstetrics/gynecology (OB/GYN). It includes data about the physician's cesarean section (C-section) rate, the number of vaginal births after a cesarean section (VBACs), types of medications used, transfusion usage, record completion delinquency rates, risk management issues, and attendance at medical staff meetings. It also allows documentation of any disciplinary action against the physician that has taken place since the last credentialing process.

Case Study

The physician performance data for the Obstetric Service at Community Hospital of the West are provided in figure 13.5. Figure 13.6 gives an example of a physician profile for an individual physician, Dr. Jones. The physician index summary for Dr. Doe, an OB/GYN physician on the medical staff, is provided in figure 13.7. Using the physician index summary, students should complete as much of the information as possible on the blank physician profile (figure 13.8) for Dr. Doe. They should identify what information cannot be obtained from the physician index. Then they should determine what other sources of hospital data would have to be accessed to complete the physician profile for Dr. Doe. Finally, they should compare Dr. Doe's performance with the performance of the rest of the physicians on the Obstetric Service in the areas for which data are available. (See figure 13.5.)

Case Study Questions

1. How did Dr. Doe perform compared to the rest of the service?

2. Should Dr. Doe be reappointed to the medical staff? Why or why not?

Figure 13.5. Physician profile for OB/GYN group

COMMUNITY HOSPITAL OF THE WEST PHYSICIAN PERFORMANCE REVIEW SUMMARY FOR REAPPOINTMENT				
PHYSICIAN	*OB/GYN GROUP*		**Profile Time Frame:**	
SERVICE	*OB/GYN*		**From:**	1/1/yyyy
CATEGORY	*Active*		**To:**	12/31/yyyy
UTILIZATION:				
Admissions	*1,400*	Procedures	*598*	
Patient Days	*5,143*	VBACs	*154*	
Deliveries	*1,187*	Blood Given	*25*	
C-Sections	*137*			
OUTCOMES:				
Category	**#**	**%**	Comments:	
C-Section Rate	*137*	*11.5%*		
VBAC Rate	*154*	*11%*		
Nosocomial Inf Rate	*21*	*1.5%*		
Surgical Wound Inf Rate	*5*	*0.36%*		
Mortality Rate	*1*	*0.07%*		
PERFORMANCE REVIEW:				
Category	**# Reviewed**	**# Appropriate/%**	Comments:	
Surgical/Inv/Noninvasive Procedures	*60*	*58/96.7%*		
Medication Use	*140*	*139/99.3%*		
Blood Use	*25*	*25/100%*		
Utilization Management	*140*	*135/95.7%*		
Other Peer Review	*140*	*130/92.8%*	*Clinical Pert.*	
DATA QUALITY:				
Data Quality Monitoring			Comments:	
Delinquency (>21 days)	*15*	*7.7%*		
Suspensions	*5*	*2.6%*		
RISK/SAFETY MANAGEMENT:				
Incidents reported by other professionals/ Administration	*2*	*2/100%*	Comments:	
Litigation	*1*	*0.07%*		
MEETING ATTENDANCE:				
Medical Staff Meetings	*26*	*93%*	Comments:	
Committee Meetings	*40*	*85%*		

Figure 13.6. Physician profile for Dr. Jones

COMMUNITY HOSPITAL OF THE WEST				
PHYSICIAN PERFORMANCE REVIEW SUMMARY FOR REAPPOINTMENT				
PHYSICIAN	Bob Jones, M.D.		**Profile Time Frame:**	
SERVICE	OB/GYN		**From:**	1/1/yyyy
CATEGORY	Active		**To:**	12/31/yyyy
UTILIZATION:				
Admissions	175	Procedures	53	
Patient Days	540	VBACs	28	
Deliveries	145	Blood Given	2	
C-Sections	22			
OUTCOMES:				
Category	#	%	Comments:	
C-Section Rate	22	15.2 %		
VBAC Rate	28	80 %		
Nosocomial Inf Rate	3	1.71 %		
Surgical Wound Inf Rate	2	3.8 %		
Mortality Rate	1	0.57 %		
PERFORMANCE REVIEW:				
Category	# Reviewed	# Appropriate/%	Comments:	
Surgical/Inv/Noninvasive Procedures	6	5/83 %		
Medication Use	10	8/80 %		
Blood Use	2	2/100 %		
Utilization Management	18	18/100 %		
Other Peer Review	N/A			
DATA QUALITY:				
Data Quality Monitoring			Comments:	
Delinquency (> 21 days)	3	12.5 %		
Suspensions	1	4.2 %		
RISK/SAFETY MANAGEMENT:				
Incidents reported by other professionals/ Administration	0	0 %	Comments:	
Litigation	1	0.57 %		
MEETING ATTENDANCE:				
Medical Staff Meetings	4	100 %	Comments:	
Committee Meetings	10	80 %		

Figure 13.6. *(Continued)*

FOR COMPLETION BY SERVICE CHAIR OR CREDENTIALS COMMITTEE CHAIR			
CATEGORY	**YES**	**NO**	Comments:
Has the applicant been considered for or subject to disciplinary action since last reappointment?		✓	
Have the applicant's privileges or staff appointment been suspended, revoked, or diminished in any way, either voluntary or involuntary, since last reappointment?	✓		
Are there any currently pending challenges to any licensure or registration or the voluntary relinquishment of such?		✓	
Are there any physical or behavioral conditions or limitations?		✓	
Has the applicant exhibited satisfactory professional performance?	✓		

APPROVALS: **APPROVED?**

REVIEWER	SIGNATURE	YES	NO	DATE
Service Chair				
Credentials Chair				

Figure 13.7.   Physician index summary for Dr. Doe

Patient Age	LOS	Discharge Status	Final Dx	Diagnosis Text	Final Proc	Procedure Text
52	3	Home	6262	EXCESSIVE/FREQUENT MENSTRUATION	684	TOTAL ABDOMINAL HYSTERECTOMY
			4254	PRIMARY CARDIOMYOPATHIES	6562	REMOVAL OF REMAINING OVARY AND TUBE
			4019	ESSENTIAL HYPERTENSION, UNSPECIFIED BENIGN		
			25000	DIABETES MELLITUS WITHOUT COMPLICATION,		
			2181	INTRAMURAL LEIOMYOMA OF UTERUS		
29	4	Home	65341	FETOPELVIC DISPROPORTION, DELIVERED	741	LOW CERVICAL CESAREAN SECTION
			66111	SECONDARY UTERINE INERTIA, DELIVERED	731	SURGICAL INDUCTION OF LABOR
			65841	INFECTION OF AMNIOTIC CAVITY, DELIVERED	7309	ARTIFICIAL RUPTURE OF MEMBRANES
			64501	PROLONGED PREGNANCY, DELIVERED		
			V270	MOTHER WITH SINGLE LIVEBORN		
27	2	Home	65421	PREVIOUS CESAREAN DELIVERY, DELIVERED	736	EPISIOTOMY (with subsequent repair)
			V270	MOTHER WITH SINGLE LIVEBORN	7359	MANUALLY ASSISTED DELIVERY
					7309	ARTIFICIAL RUPTURE OF MEMBRANES
79	4	Home	6185	PROLAPSE OF VAGINAL VAULT AFTER HYSTERECTOMY	7077	VAGINAL SUSPENSION & FIXATION
			9975	URINARY COMPLICATION, NOT ELSEWHERE CLASSIFIED	5459	OTHER LYSIS OF PERITONEAL ADHESIONS
			5990	URINARY TRACT INFECTION, SITE NOT SPECIFIED		
			9973	RESPIRATORY COMPLICATION, NOT ELSEWHERE		
			5180	PULMONARY COLLAPSE (ATELECTASIS)		
			78831	URGE INCONTINENCE		
			E8788	OTHER SURGICAL OPERATION, WITH ABNORMAL		
			4019	ESSENTIAL HYPERTENSION, UNSPECIFIED BENIGN		
			5680	PERITONEAL ADHESIONS (POSTOPERATIVE)(POS		
25	4	Home	65221	BREECH PRESENTATION WITHOUT VERSION, DELIVERED	741	LOW CERVICAL CESAREAN SECTION
			64661	INFECTIONS OF GENITOURINARY TRACT IN PRE		
			6169	UNSPECIFIED INFLAMMATORY DISEASE OF CERVIX		
			66311	CORD AROUND NECK, WITH COMPRESSION, COMP		
			V270	MOTHER WITH SINGLE LIVEBORN		
39	1	Home	66331	UNSPECIFIED CORD ENTANGLEMENT, WITHOUT C	7359	MANUALLY ASSISTED DELIVERY
			64201	BENIGN ESSENTIAL HYPERTENSION COMPLICATI		
			V270	MOTHER WITH SINGLE LIVEBORN		
			4019	ESSENTIAL HYPERTENSION, UNSPECIFIED BENIGN		

Figure 13.7. *(Continued)*

Patient Age	LOS	Discharge Status	Final Dx	Diagnosis Text	Final Proc	Procedure Text
34	2	Home	64881	ABNORMAL GLUCOSE TOLERANCE IN MOTHER COM	7359	MANUALLY ASSISTED DELIVERY
			V270	MOTHER WITH SINGLE LIVEBORN	7569	REPAIR OF CURRENT OBSTETRIC LACERATION
			66401	FIRST-DEGREE PERINEAL LACERATION, DELIVERED	7309	ARTIFICIAL RUPTURE OF MEMBRANES
20	1	Home	650	NORMAL DELIVERY	7359	MANUALLY ASSISTED DELIVERY
			V270	MOTHER WITH SINGLE LIVEBORN	736	EPISIOTOMY (with subsequent repair)
36	3	Home	6398	COMPLICATION FOLLOWING ABORTION/ECTOPIC/	684	TOTAL ABDOMINAL HYSTERECTOMY
			6259	UNSPECIFIED SYMPTOM ASSOCIATED WITH FEMA		
			311	DEPRESSIVE DISORDER, NOT ELSEWHERE CLASS		
			30503	ALCOHOL ABUSE IN REMISSION		
			30593	MIXED/UNSPECIFIED DRUG ABUSE IN REMISSION		
			6262	EXCESSIVE/FREQUENT MENSTRUATION		
			2182	SUBSEROUS LEIOMYOMA OF UTERUS		
			2181	INTRAMURAL LEIOMYOMA OF UTERUS		
			78701	NAUSEA WITH VOMITING		
48	3	Home	2181	INTRAMURAL LEIOMYOMA OF UTERUS	684	TOTAL ABDOMINAL HYSTERECTOMY
			57410	CALCULUS OF GALLBLADDER WITH CHOLECYSTITIS	6561	REMOVAL OF BOTH OVARIES AND TUBES AT SAM
			6170	ENDOMETRIOSIS OF UTERUS	595	RETROPUBIC URETHRAL SUSPENSION
			2189	LEIOMYOMA OF UTERUS, UNSPECIFIED	7052	REPAIR OF RECTOCELE
			6256	STRESS INCONTINENCE, FEMALE	7092	OPERATION ON CUL-DE-SAC
			6180	PROLAPSE OF VAGINAL WALLS WITHOUT MENTION	5123	LAPAROSCOPIC CHOLECYSTECTOMY
					8753	INTRAOPERATIVE CHOLANGIOGRAM
42	2	Home	65421	PREVIOUS CESAREAN DELIVERY, DELIVERED	734	MEDICAL INDUCTION OF LABOR
			V270	MOTHER WITH SINGLE LIVEBORN	7301	INDUCTION OF LABOR BY ARTIFICIAL RUPTURE
			66331	UNSPECIFIED CORD ENTANGLEMENT, WITHOUT	7359	MANUALLY ASSISTED DELIVERY
			64881	ABNORMAL GLUCOSE TOLERANCE IN MOTHER COM	7351	MANUAL ROTATION OF FETAL HEAD
			65291	UNSPECIFIED MALPOSITION/PRESENTATION OF		
22	2	Home	66421	THIRD-DEGREE PERINEAL LACERATION, DELIVERED	7562	REPAIR OF CURRENT OBSTETRIC LACERATION O
			65681	FETAL & PLACENTAL PROBLEM, AFFECTING MAN	7359	MANUALLY ASSISTED DELIVERY
			V270	MOTHER WITH SINGLE LIVEBORN		

(Continued on next page)

Figure 13.7. *(Continued)*

Patient Age	LOS	Discharge Status	Final Dx	Diagnosis Text	Final Proc	Procedure Text
37	14	Home	65971	ABNORMALITY IN FETAL HEART RATE/RHYTHM,	741	LOW CERVICAL CESAREAN SECTION
			67131	ANTEPARTUM DEEP PHLEBOTHROMBOSIS COMPLIC	6632	BILATERAL LIGATION AND DIVISION OF FALLO
			64821	ANEMIA IN MOTHER COMPLICATING PREGNANCY,		
			65821	DELAYED DELIVERY AFTER SPONTANEOUS/UNSPEC		
			65221	BREECH PRESENTATION WITHOUT VERSION, DEL		
			64421	EARLY ONSET OF DELIVERY, DELIVERED		
			65961	ELDERLY MULTIGRAVIDA, DELIVERED		
			64891	CURRENT CONDITION IN MOTHER COMPLICATING		
			2898	DISEASE OF BLOOD/BLOOD-FORMING ORGANS		
			7821	RASH AND NONSPECIFIC SKIN ERUPTION		
			2859	ANEMIA, UNSPECIFIED		
			V270	MOTHER WITH SINGLE LIVEBORN		
			V252	STERILIZATION		
28	1	Home	66331	UNSPECIFIED CORD ENTANGLEMENT, WITHOUT	736	EPISIOTOMY (with subsequent repair)
			65921	MATERNAL PYREXIA DURING LABOR, UNSPECIFIED	734	MEDICAL INDUCTION OF LABOR
			V270	MOTHER WITH SINGLE LIVEBORN	7301	INDUCTION OF LABOR BY ARTIFICIAL RUPTURE
22	2	Home	66331	UNSPECIFIED CORD ENTANGLEMENT, WITHOUT	7309	ARTIFICIAL RUPTURE OF MEMBRANES
			65921	MATERNAL PYREXIA DURING LABOR, UNSPECIFIED	7359	MANUALLY ASSISTED DELIVERY
			V270	MOTHER WITH SINGLE LIVEBORN	7569	REPAIR OF CURRENT OBSTETRIC LACERATION
			66411	SECOND-DEGREE PERINEAL LACERATION, DELIVERED		
42	2	Home	65961	ELDERLY MULTIGRAVIDA, DELIVERED	731	SURGICAL INDUCTION OF LABOR
			V270	MOTHER WITH SINGLE LIVEBORN	7359	MANUALLY ASSISTED DELIVERY
			66551	INJURY TO PELVIC ORGANS, DELIVERED	7569	REPAIR OF CURRENT OBSTETRIC LACERATION
67	3	Home	6271	POSTMENOPAUSAL BLEEDING	684	TOTAL ABDOMINAL HYSTERECTOMY
			4465	GIANT CELL ARTERITIS	6561	REMOVAL OF BOTH OVARIES AND TUBES AT SAM
			2765	VOLUME DEPLETION DISORDER (DEHYDRATION)	5459	OTHER LYSIS OF PERITONEAL ADHESIONS
			2181	INTRAMURAL LEIOMYOMA OF UTERUS		

Figure 13.7. *(Continued)*

Patient Age	LOS	Discharge Status	Final Dx	Diagnosis Text	Final Proc	Procedure Text
			6210	POLYP OF CORPUS UTERI	684	TOTAL ABDOMINAL HYSTERECTOMY
			5680	PERITONEAL ADHESIONS (POSTOPERATIVE)(POS	6561	REMOVAL OF BOTH OVARIES AND TUBES AT SAM
			V1251	PERSONAL HISTORY OF VENOUS THROMBOSIS AN		
			49390	ASTHMA, UNSPECIFIED TYPE, WITHOUT STATUS		
51	3	Home	6270	PREMENOPAUSAL MENORRHAGIA		
			2800	IRON DEFICIENCY ANEMIA SECONDARY TO BLOOD LOSS		
			2181	INTRAMURAL LEIOMYOMA OF UTERUS		
			6208	NONINFLAMMATORY DISORDER OF OVARY/FALLOP		
			6200	FOLLICULAR CYST OF OVARY		
			6259	UNSPECIFIED SYMPTOM ASSOCIATED WITH FEMALE		
33	1	Home	66702	RETAINED PLACENTA WITHOUT HEMORRHAGE, DEL	7309	ARTIFICIAL RUPTURE OF MEMBRANES
			V270	MOTHER WITH SINGLE LIVEBORN	7351	MANUAL ROTATION OF FETAL HEAD
			65281	MALPOSITION/MALPRESENTATION OF FETUS, DELIVERED	7359	MANUALLY ASSISTED DELIVERY
			64501	PROLONGED PREGNANCY, DELIVERED	736	EPISIOTOMY (with subsequent repair)
					754	MANUAL REMOVAL OF RETAINED PLACENTA
22	2	Home	66331	UNSPECIFIED CORD ENTANGLEMENT, WITHOUT	7359	MANUALLY ASSISTED DELIVERY
			V270	MOTHER WITH SINGLE LIVEBORN	7309	ARTIFICIAL RUPTURE OF MEMBRANES
					736	EPISIOTOMY (with subsequent repair)
25	2	Home	65281	MALPOSITION/MALPRESENTATION OF FETUS, DEL	7351	MANUAL ROTATION OF FETAL HEAD
			V270	MOTHER WITH SINGLE LIVEBORN	736	EPISIOTOMY (with subsequent repair)
					7359	MANUALLY ASSISTED DELIVERY
					734	MEDICAL INDUCTION OF LABOR
					7309	ARTIFICIAL RUPTURE OF MEMBRANES
31	2	Home	66411	SECOND-DEGREE PERINEAL LACERATION, DELIV	7359	MANUALLY ASSISTED DELIVERY
			V270	MOTHER WITH SINGLE LIVEBORN	7569	REPAIR OF CURRENT OBSTETRIC LACERATION
					7301	INDUCTION OF LABOR BY ARTIFICIAL RUPTURE
40	3	Home	6172	ENDOMETRIOSIS OF FALLOPIAN TUBE	684	TOTAL ABDOMINAL HYSTERECTOMY
			2189	LEIOMYOMA OF UTERUS, UNSPECIFIED	6561	REMOVAL OF BOTH OVARIES AND TUBES AT SAM
			25000	DIABETES MELLITUS WITHOUT COMPLICATION,		
			6146	PELVIC PERITONEAL ADHESIONS, FEMALE (POS		

(Continued on next page)

Figure 13.7. *(Continued)*

Patient Age	LOS	Discharge Status	Final Dx	Diagnosis Text	Final Proc	Procedure Text
32	3	Home	65221	BREECH PRESENTATION WITHOUT VERSION, DEL	741	LOW CERVICAL CESAREAN SECTION
			66881	COMPLICATION OF ANESTHESIA/SEDATION IN L	0395	SPINAL BLOOD PATCH
			3490	REACTION TO SPINAL/LUMBAR PUNCTURE		
			64811	THYROID DYSFUNCTION IN MOTHER COMPLICATI		
			2449	UNSPECIFIED ACQUIRED HYPOTHYROIDISM		
			V270	MOTHER WITH SINGLE LIVEBORN		
81	4	Home	6185	PROLAPSE OF VAGINAL VAULT AFTER HYSTERECTOMY	7050	REPAIR OF CYSTOCELE AND RECTOCELE
			5180	PULMONARY COLLAPSE (ATELECTASIS)	595	RETROPUBIC URETHRAL SUSPENSION
			6256	STRESS INCONTINENCE, FEMALE		
			4019	ESSENTIAL HYPERTENSION, UNSPECIFIED BENIGN		
			2449	UNSPECIFIED ACQUIRED HYPOTHYROIDISM		
			71690	ARTHROPATHY, UNSPECIFIED, UNSPECIFIED SI		
			9110	TRUNK, ABRASION/FRICTION BURN, WITHOUT		
			78701	NAUSEA WITH VOMITING		
			5640	CONSTIPATION		
28	2	Home	65231	TRANSVERSE/OBLIQUE PRESENTATION OF FETUS	7309	ARTIFICIAL RUPTURE OF MEMBRANES
			66622	DELAYED & SECONDARY POSTPARTUM HEMORRHAGE	7351	MANUAL ROTATION OF FETAL HEAD
			66481	TRAUMA TO PERINEUM & VULVA, DELIVERED	7569	REPAIR OF CURRENT OBSTETRIC LACERATION
54	3	Home	V270	MOTHER WITH SINGLE LIVEBORN	7271	VACUUM EXTRACTION WITH EPISIOTOMY
			1820	MALIGNANT NEOPLASM OF CORPUS UTERI, EXCE	684	TOTAL ABDOMINAL HYSTERECTOMY
			4240	MITRAL VALVE DISORDER	7052	REPAIR OF RECTOCELE
			6182	UTEROVAGINAL PROLAPSE, INCOMPLETE	595	RETROPUBIC URETHRAL SUSPENSION
			6256	STRESS INCONTINENCE, FEMALE	6561	REMOVAL OF BOTH OVARIES AND TUBES AT SAM
			6271	POSTMENOPAUSAL BLEEDING		
			6171	ENDOMETRIOSIS OF OVARY		
			6170	ENDOMETRIOSIS OF UTERUS		
			27800	OBESITY, UNSPECIFIED		
			9095	LATE EFFECT OF ADVERSE EFFECT OF DRUG, M		
			E9470	DIETETICS CAUSING ADVERSE EFFECTS IN THE		
			E8490	INJURY OR POISONING OCCURRING AT/IN THE		

Figure 13.7. *(Continued)*

Patient Age	LOS	Discharge Status	Final Dx	Diagnosis Text	Final Proc	Procedure Text
19	1	Home	64421	EARLY ONSET OF DELIVERY, DELIVERED	7309	ARTIFICIAL RUPTURE OF MEMBRANES
			V270	MOTHER WITH SINGLE LIVEBORN	7359	MANUALLY ASSISTED DELIVERY
			65841	INFECTION OF AMNIOTIC CAVITY, DELIVERED	736	EPISIOTOMY (with subsequent repair)
37	3	Home	65221	BREECH PRESENTATION WITHOUT VERSION, DEL	741	LOW CERVICAL CESAREAN SECTION
			V270	MOTHER WITH SINGLE LIVEBORN		
			65801	OLIGOHYDRAMNIOS, DELIVERED		
24	2	Home	66421	THIRD-DEGREE PERINEAL LACERATION, DELIVE	—	—
			66331	UNSPECIFIED CORD ENTANGLEMENT, WITHOUT C		
			V270	MOTHER WITH SINGLE LIVEBORN		
21	2	Home	650	NORMAL DELIVERY	736	EPISIOTOMY (with subsequent repair)
			V270	MOTHER WITH SINGLE LIVEBORN	7359	MANUALLY ASSISTED DELIVERY
					7309	ARTIFICIAL RUPTURE OF MEMBRANES
					734	MEDICAL INDUCTION OF LABOR
39	2	Home	65941	GRAND MULTIPARITY, DELIVERED	—	—
			65961	ELDERLY MULTIGRAVIDA, DELIVERED		
			66401	FIRST-DEGREE PERINEAL LACERATION, DELIVERED		
			V270	MOTHER WITH SINGLE LIVEBORN		
			V252	STERILIZATION		
33	1	Home	650	NORMAL DELIVERY	736	EPISIOTOMY (with subsequent repair)
			V270	MOTHER WITH SINGLE LIVEBORN	7359	MANUALLY ASSISTED DELIVERY
					7309	ARTIFICIAL RUPTURE OF MEMBRANES
					734	MEDICAL INDUCTION OF LABOR
22	1	Home	66331	UNSPECIFIED CORD ENTANGLEMENT, WITHOUT C	7359	MANUALLY ASSISTED DELIVERY
			V270	MOTHER WITH SINGLE LIVEBORN	7309	ARTIFICIAL RUPTURE OF MEMBRANES
			64891	CURRENT CONDITION IN MOTHER COMPLICATING	736	EPISIOTOMY (with subsequent repair)
			V0251	CARRIER OR SUSPECTED CARRIER OF GROUP B		
20	1	Home	65811	PREMATURE RUPTURE OF MEMBRANES, DELIVERED	736	EPISIOTOMY (with subsequent repair)
			65971	ABNORMALITY IN FETAL HEART RATE/RHYTHM,	7359	MANUALLY ASSISTED DELIVERY
			64421	EARLY ONSET OF DELIVERY, DELIVERED		
			66311	CORD AROUND NECK, WITH COMPRESSION, COMP		
			64891	CURRENT CONDITION IN MOTHER COMPLICATING		
			V270	MOTHER WITH SINGLE LIVEBORN		
			V0251	CARRIER OR SUSPECTED CARRIER OF GROUP B		

(Continued on next page)

Figure 13.7. *(Continued)*

Patient Age	LOS	Discharge Status	Final Dx	Diagnosis Text	Final Proc	Procedure Text
34	3	Home	65221	BREECH PRESENTATION WITHOUT VERSION, DEL	741	LOW CERVICAL CESAREAN SECTION
			65811	PREMATURE RUPTURE OF MEMBRANES, DELIVERE	6632	BILATERAL LIGATION AND DIVISION OF FALLO
			64841	MENTAL DISORDER IN MOTHER COMPLICATING P		
			3051	TOBACCO USE DISORDER		
			V270	MOTHER WITH SINGLE LIVEBORN		
			V252	STERILIZATION		
22	1	Home	65281	MALPOSITION/MALPRESENTATION OF FETUS, DE	7351	MANUAL ROTATION OF FETAL HEAD
			65971	ABNORMALITY IN FETAL HEART RATE/RHYTHM,	7569	REPAIR OF CURRENT OBSTETRIC LACERATION
			66331	UNSPECIFIED CORD ENTANGLEMENT, WITHOUT C	7309	ARTIFICIAL RUPTURE OF MEMBRANES
			66401	FIRST-DEGREE PERINEAL LACERATION, DELIVERED	757	MANUAL EXPLORATION OF UTERINE CAVITY, PO
			V270	MOTHER WITH SINGLE LIVEBORN		
41	2	Home	64881	ABNORMAL GLUCOSE TOLERANCE IN MOTHER COM	7309	ARTIFICIAL RUPTURE OF MEMBRANES
			V270	MOTHER WITH SINGLE LIVEBORN	7351	MANUAL ROTATION OF FETAL HEAD
			64421	EARLY ONSET OF DELIVERY, DELIVERED	721	LOW FORCEPS OPERATION WITH EPISIOTOMY
			65701	POLYHYDRAMNIOS, DELIVERED		
			65951	ELDERLY PRIMIGRAVIDA, DELIVERED		
			65981	INDICATION FOR CARE/INTERVENTION RELATED		
			78703	VOMITING ALONE		
			66111	SECONDARY UTERINE INERTIA, DELIVERED		
			65671	PLACENTAL CONDITION, AFFECTING MANAGEMENT		
59	3	Home	6182	UTEROVAGINAL PROLAPSE, INCOMPLETE	6859	VAGINAL HYSTERECTOMY
			2182	SUBSEROUS LEIOMYOMA OF UTERUS	7050	REPAIR OF CYSTOCELE AND RECTOCELE
			6210	POLYP OF CORPUS UTERI	5718	SUPRAPUBIC CYSTOSTOMY
			2409	GOITER, UNSPECIFIED		
33	1	Home	66031	DEEP TRANSVERSE ARREST & PERSISTENT OCCI	7309	ARTIFICIAL RUPTURE OF MEMBRANES
			66401	FIRST-DEGREE PERINEAL LACERATION, DELIVE	7569	REPAIR OF CURRENT OBSTETRIC LACERATION
			V270	MOTHER WITH SINGLE LIVEBORN	7351	MANUAL ROTATION OF FETAL HEAD

Figure 13.7. *(Continued)*

Patient Age	LOS	Discharge Status	Final Dx	Diagnosis Text	Final Proc	Procedure Text
30	2	Home	65281	MALPOSITION/MALPRESENTATION OF FETUS, DE	721	LOW FORCEPS OPERATION WITH EPISIOTOMY
			65921	MATERNAL PYREXIA DURING LABOR, UNSPECIFIED	7359	MANUALLY ASSISTED DELIVERY
			65421	PREVIOUS CESAREAN DELIVERY, DELIVERED	757	MANUAL EXPLORATION OF UTERINE CAVITY, PO
			V270	MOTHER WITH SINGLE LIVEBORN		
67	3	Home	6180	PROLAPSE OF VAGINAL WALLS WITHOUT MENTION	7092	OPERATION ON CUL-DE-SAC
			6256	STRESS INCONTINENCE, FEMALE	7050	REPAIR OF CYSTOCELE AND RECTOCELE
			6186	VAGINAL ENTEROCELE, CONGENITAL OR ACQUIRED	595	RETROPUBIC URETHRAL SUSPENSION
81	3	Home	6181	UTERINE PROLAPSE WITHOUT MENTION OF VAGI	684	TOTAL ABDOMINAL HYSTERECTOMY
			6227	MUCOUS POLYP OF CERVIX	6561	REMOVAL OF BOTH OVARIES AND TUBES AT SAM
			6210	POLYP OF CORPUS UTERI	7092	OPERATION ON CUL-DE-SAC
			2181	INTRAMURAL LEIOMYOMA OF UTERUS		
			25000	DIABETES MELLITUS WITHOUT COMPLICATION,		
			4019	ESSENTIAL HYPERTENSION, UNSPECIFIED BENIGN		
			2724	UNSPECIFIED HYPERLIPIDEMIA		
26	1	Home	650	NORMAL DELIVERY	7359	MANUALLY ASSISTED DELIVERY
			V270	MOTHER WITH SINGLE LIVEBORN	734	MEDICAL INDUCTION OF LABOR
					736	EPISIOTOMY (with subsequent repair)
18	1	Home	66411	SECOND-DEGREE PERINEAL LACERATION, DELIVERED	7569	REPAIR OF CURRENT OBSTETRIC LACERATION
			64841	MENTAL DISORDER IN MOTHER COMPLICATING P	7359	MANUALLY ASSISTED DELIVERY
			3051	TOBACCO USE DISORDER	7309	ARTIFICIAL RUPTURE OF MEMBRANES
			V270	MOTHER WITH SINGLE LIVEBORN		
72	3	Home	1820	MALIGNANT NEOPLASM OF CORPUS UTERI, EXCE	684	TOTAL ABDOMINAL HYSTERECTOMY
			2449	UNSPECIFIED ACQUIRED HYPOTHYROIDISM	6561	REMOVAL OF BOTH OVARIES AND TUBES AT SAM
			6202	OVARIAN CYST	403	REGIONAL LYMPH NODE EXCISION
			7912	HEMOGLOBINURIA		
38	3	Home	6185	PROLAPSE OF VAGINAL VAULT AFTER HYSTEREC	7077	VAGINAL SUSPENSION & FIXATION
50	3	Home	6170	ENDOMETRIOSIS OF UTERUS	684	TOTAL ABDOMINAL HYSTERECTOMY
			2800	IRON DEFICIENCY ANEMIA SECONDARY TO BLOOD	6561	REMOVAL OF BOTH OVARIES AND TUBES AT SAM

(Continued on next page)

Figure 13.7. *(Continued)*

Patient Age	LOS	Discharge Status	Final Dx	Diagnosis Text	Final Proc	Procedure Text
			6172	ENDOMETRIOSIS OF FALLOPIAN TUBE	595	RETROPUBIC URETHRAL SUSPENSION
			6171	ENDOMETRIOSIS OF OVARY		
			6256	STRESS INCONTINENCE, FEMALE		
			6262	EXCESSIVE/FREQUENT MENSTRUATION		
			2181	INTRAMURAL LEIOMYOMA OF UTERUS		
			6160	CERVICITIS & ENDOCERVICITIS		
			6173	ENDOMETRIOSIS OF PELVIC PERITONEUM		
			6259	UNSPECIFIED SYMPTOM ASSOCIATED WITH FEMALE		
			25000	DIABETES MELLITUS WITHOUT COMPLICATION,		
			5533	DIAPHRAGMATIC HERNIA		
28	1	Home	65801	OLIGOHYDRAMNIOS, DELIVERED	721	LOW FORCEPS OPERATION WITH EPISIOTOMY
			65921	MATERNAL PYREXIA DURING LABOR, UNSPECIFI	7351	MANUAL ROTATION OF FETAL HEAD
			65281	MALPOSITION/MALPRESENTATION OF FETUS, DE	7569	REPAIR OF CURRENT OBSTETRIC LACERATION
			66951	FORCEPS/VACUUM EXTRACTOR DELIVERY WITHOUT	754	MANUAL REMOVAL OF RETAINED PLACENTA
			66411	SECOND-DEGREE PERINEAL LACERATION, DELIV	734	MEDICAL INDUCTION OF LABOR
			66331	UNSPECIFIED CORD ENTANGLEMENT, WITHOUT		
			V270	MOTHER WITH SINGLE LIVEBORN		
24	2	Home	65651	POOR FETAL GROWTH, AFFECTING MANAGEMENT	734	MEDICAL INDUCTION OF LABOR
			65921	MATERNAL PYREXIA DURING LABOR, UNSPECIFIED	7301	INDUCTION OF LABOR BY ARTIFICIAL RUPTURE
			V272	MOTHER WITH TWINS, BOTH LIVEBORN	7351	MANUAL ROTATION OF FETAL HEAD
			65281	MALPOSITION/MALPRESENTATION OF FETUS, DEL	736	EPISIOTOMY (with subsequent repair)
			V043	NEED FOR PROPHYLACTIC VACCINATION AND IN	757	MANUAL EXPLORATION OF UTERINE CAVITY, PO
					7359	MANUALLY ASSISTED DELIVERY
39	2	Home	66331	UNSPECIFIED CORD ENTANGLEMENT, WITHOUT C	736	EPISIOTOMY (with subsequent repair)
			V270	MOTHER WITH SINGLE LIVEBORN	734	MEDICAL INDUCTION OF LABOR
					7301	INDUCTION OF LABOR BY ARTIFICIAL RUPTURE
30	1	Home	66331	UNSPECIFIED CORD ENTANGLEMENT, WITHOUT C	7301	INDUCTION OF LABOR BY ARTIFICIAL RUPTURE
			V270	MOTHER WITH SINGLE LIVEBORN	734	MEDICAL INDUCTION OF LABOR
					7351	MANUAL ROTATION OF FETAL HEAD
					736	EPISIOTOMY (with subsequent repair)
					7359	MANUALLY ASSISTED DELIVERY

Figure 13.8.   Blank physician profile for case study

COMMUNITY HOSPITAL OF THE WEST PHYSICIAN PERFORMANCE REVIEW SUMMARY FOR REAPPOINTMENT				
PHYSICIAN			**Profile Time Frame:**	
SERVICE			**From:**	
CATEGORY			**To:**	
UTILIZATION:				
Admissions		Procedures		
Patient Days		VBACs		
Deliveries		Blood Given		
C-Sections				
OUTCOMES:				
Category	**#**	**%**	Comments:	
C-Section Rate				
VBAC Rate				
Nosocomial Inf Rate				
Surgical Wound Inf Rate				
Mortality Rate				
PERFORMANCE REVIEW:				
Category	**# Reviewed**	**# Appropriate/%**	Comments:	
Surgical/Inv/Noninvasive Procedures				
Medication Use				
Blood Use				
Utilization Management				
Other Peer Review				
DATA QUALITY:				
Data Quality Monitoring			Comments:	
Delinquency (>21 days)				
Suspensions				
RISK/SAFETY MANAGEMENT:				
Incidents reported by other professionals/ Administration			Comments:	
Litigation				
MEETING ATTENDANCE:				
Medical Staff Meetings			Comments:	
Committee Meetings				

(Continued on next page)

Figure 13.8.   *(Continued)*

FOR COMPLETION BY SERVICE CHAIR OR CREDENTIALS COMMITTEE CHAIR			
CATEGORY	**YES**	**NO**	Comments:
Has the applicant been considered for or subject to disciplinary action since last reappointment?			
Have the applicant's privileges or staff appointment been suspended, revoked, or diminished in any way, either voluntary or involuntary, since last reappointment?			
Are there any currently pending challenges to any licensure or registration or the voluntary relinquishment of such?			
Are there any physical or behavioral conditions or limitations?			
Has the applicant exhibited satisfactory professional performance?			

APPROVALS: **APPROVED?**

REVIEWER	**SIGNATURE**	**YES**	**NO**	**DATE**
Service Chair				
Credentials Chair				

Project Application

Students should identify any human resources issues that may have a bearing on their project. They should determine what types of issues these are and how they can obtain the data needed to evaluate them. Then they should develop recommendations for staffing.

Summary

The effective management of human resources is critically important in healthcare organizations. Quality of care depends on the processes the organization establishes and uniformly applies in its recruitment, appointment, and reappointment. Healthcare services are complex and require specialized knowledge and experience. The licenses and other credentials of the clinical professionals who provide services in healthcare organizations must be maintained and verified. The competence of licensed caregivers must be reevaluated on an annual or biennial schedule to ensure their continued ability to provide healthcare services. Healthcare organizations also must be able to demonstrate that they have contributed to the ongoing development of their employees and medical staff.

References

Americans with Disabilities Act of 1990. Public Law 101-336.

Equal Employment Opportunity Act of 1972. Public Law 92-261.

Family and Medical Leave Act of 1993. Public Law 103-3.

Joint Commission. 2011. *Hospital Accreditation Standards*. Oakbrook Terrace, IL: Joint Commission Resources.

National Quality Forum (NQF). n.d. http://www.qualityforum.org.

Occupational Safety and Health Act of 1970. (OSH Act) 29 CFR Parts 1900 to 2400.

Shaw, J.D., J.E. Delery, G.D. Jenkins, Jr., and N. Gupta. 1998. An organization-level analysis of voluntary and involuntary turnover. *Academy of Management Journal* 41(5):511–525.

Resources

Berenson, R. 1995. Profiling and performance measures: What are the legal issues? *Medical Care* 33(1):JS53–JS59 (supplement).

Delorese, A. 1995. *Leadership: The Journey Inward*. Dubuque, IA: Kendall-Hunt Publishing.

Field, R.I. 1995. Sharing clinical data for provider profiling: Protection of privacy versus the public's need to know. *Behavioral Healthcare Tomorrow* 4(3):71–73.

Hendryx, M.S., D.S. Wakefield, J.F. Murray, T. Uden-Holman, C.M. Helms, and R.L. Ludke. 1995. Using comparative clinical and economic outcome information to profile physician performance. *Health Services Management Research* 8(4):213–220.

Orsund-Gassiot, C., and S. Lindsey. 1990. *Handbook of Medical Staff Management*. Rockville, MD: Aspen Publishers.

Schachter, W. 1995. The role of provider credentialing in quality-of-care improvement and clinic risk reduction. *Behavioral Healthcare Tomorrow* 4(4):71–73.

Part III
Management of Performance Improvement Programs

Chapter 14
Organizing for Performance Improvement

Learning Objectives

- To identify both the role of an organization's leaders in performance improvement activities and the committee and reporting structures that integrate performance improvement within the organization

- To describe the various leadership configurations responsible for performance improvement activities

- To explain how healthcare organizations train and orient their governance, leaders, and employed staff in performance improvement strategies and methods

- To delineate the best ways to organize performance improvement data for effective review by a board of directors

Key Terms

Dashboard

Peer review

Strategic plan

Background and Significance

Performance improvement (PI) does not happen effortlessly. The term *continuous* is often attached to improvement efforts (as in *continuous quality improvement*) for a reason: It serves to remind healthcare workers that PI activities require organizational and individual commitment and need to be incorporated into the daily operations of the organization.

Given that PI requires commitment and continuity, which types of management environments make this happen? Many employees come from a traditional management environment, where managers direct their subordinates in exactly what to do and when to do it. The guiding principle of quality improvement in the Deming, Juran, Crosby, and Donabedian models, however, is that all members of an organization must be empowered by its leadership to contribute to the PI activities if the program is to be successful. (See the introduction to this textbook for a detailed historical discussion of the quality movement and its evolving models.)

Today, it is commonly recognized across the healthcare industry that unless the leaders are committed to maintaining PI activities in the organization and motivating employees to do the same, PI that reaps genuine benefits for the organization cannot take place. Leadership endorsement of PI is a crucial and integral contribution to an organization's continuous development.

Leading PI Activities

Healthcare organizations must put formal structures in place for meaningful PI to occur. The leaders of a healthcare organization set expectations, develop plans, and hire employees to implement procedures that assess and improve the quality of important functions. Leaders include the members of the governing body (most often termed board of "directors" or "trustees" but sometimes configured from other entities like "public commissioners"), the chief executive officer, the director of nursing, the medical director, and other senior directors or managers, as well as the leaders of the medical staff.

The board of directors has the ultimate responsibility for maintaining the quality and safety of patient care provided by its healthcare organization. The board establishes policy and directs appropriate systems to monitor and assess all services and to detect variations from acceptable standards of care or service. The board operates under a set of bylaws that provides guidance and establishes the framework for supporting quality of patient care, treatment, and services.

As in any other corporation, the board designates an executive to be its agent or managing partner. The chief executive officer (CEO), sometimes known as the administrator or executive director, is responsible for implementing board directives and for acting as board representative in managing the operations of the organization. While proper functioning of the organization remains the responsibility of the board, the CEO is a partial or full voting member of the board and is responsible for ensuring that the board is knowledgeable about its governing responsibilities. These responsibilities include understanding the structure and composition of the governing board; understanding the functioning, participation, and involvement in the oversight and operation of the organization; being aware of all federal and state laws, regulations, and standards pertinent to their roles; and understanding the organization's approach to PI.

There are three main components of a healthcare organization: the governance (board of directors and the organized medical staff), the management (leaders), and the employed staff. The key to a healthcare organization's success is the coordination and cooperation of these three groups as they work together to identify community needs and pursue organizational goals. Although responsibilities vary from group to group, all groups share common interests and must work together on planning, budgeting, capital development, expenditures, PI, and patient satisfaction. Figure 14.1 shows an example of a hospital organization chart and its organizational components.

Figure 14.1.   Example of hospital organization chart

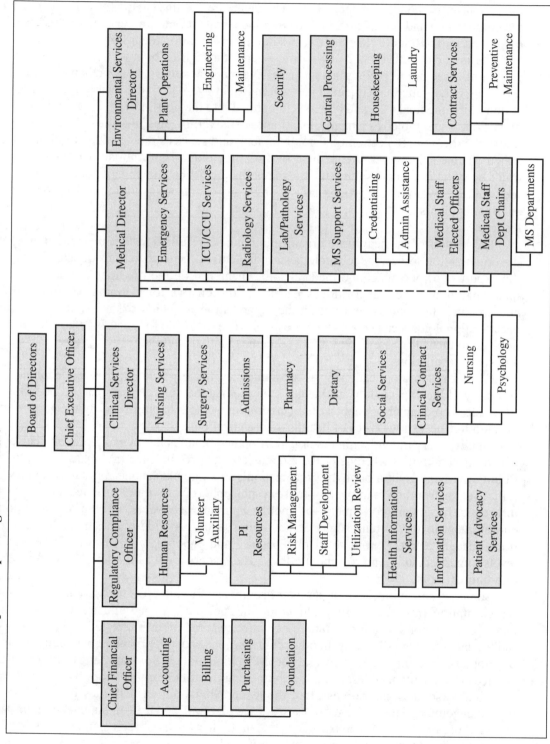

Because the board is responsible for patient care, quality, and safety, it must ensure the competence and integrity of the licensed independent practitioners (medical staff) and employed staff. (Refer to chapter 13 for additional information regarding staff competency.)

The medical staff elects its own officers and, through its bylaws, sets up an effective governing structure to accomplish its tasks. The medical staff is, in effect, an organization operating in conjunction with an organization. (Refer again to figure 14.1 to see the organization of the medical staff and how it is integrated into the hospital.) Licensed independent practitioners assembled as a medical staff are self-governing and provide clinical oversight to the healthcare organization on care, treatment, and services they provide through established channels. However, the medical staff reports to and is accountable to the organization's board of directors. Neither the board nor the medical staff can unilaterally change the medical staff bylaws; both groups must approve any changes. Planning for the provision of an organization's healthcare services, on the other hand, is a function of the organization's leaders.

The leaders of the healthcare organization must carefully consider the community that the organization serves; the technologies available to it; the expectations of customers; and the expertise of personnel and medical staff when crafting the mission, vision, and organizational goals. The organizational leaders are responsible for planning (**strategic plan**) and creating the environment within the organization in which the mission, vision, and organizational goals can be achieved. Leaders are responsible for ensuring that a process is in place to measure, assess, and improve the hospital's governance, management, clinical, and support functions.

Further reading on leadership is recommended for any student of PI in healthcare. A summary of the expectations of the leadership in healthcare organizations can be found in the leadership chapter of each set of accreditation standards published by the Joint Commission for the various types of healthcare organizations.

Ideally, every individual in the organization understands the PI principles and can contribute to PI activities when he or she recognizes the need. In some organizations, defining PI initiatives and goals around the organization's strategic plan is one approach; identifying initiatives of frontline employees—those responsible for providing products and services directly to healthcare consumers—is another approach. However, in other organizations, commitment to the PI philosophy and activities is not as widespread. In such organizations, leaders actively promote PI philosophies and encourage healthcare workers at all levels to participate in improvement efforts. The leaders are usually department managers or administrators.

Some organizations develop an interdisciplinary PI council. The council may include representation from the board of directors, the medical staff, administration, committee chairs from the organization's standing committees, and other interested and experienced individuals who lead PI efforts. In other organizations, a quality management department is developed to coordinate, oversee, and document PI activities. Some organizations retain the services of consultants to assist in developing an infrastructure that supports PI activities.

Finally, some organizations place the responsibility for PI activities in the hands of top management. This is the most conservative and traditional PI management approach. Because improvements come by mandate from higher levels of management, this is often referred to as a "top-down improvement initiative."

Whichever approach an organization follows, the community and the populations the organization serves expect that the organization will provide the highest-quality products and services possible. Accreditors and regulators want to see evidence of PI activities and the ways in which those activities have benefited the organization's customers. Ultimately, the organization's performance will be judged against that expectation.

Managing the Board of Directors' PI Activities

Most members of healthcare boards of directors are appointed from the community at large. It is unlikely that the directors will have specific knowledge of healthcare operations or organizations when they are first appointed. Even after serving for several years, most directors will not have expertise in clinical processes. Therefore, it is important that the individuals leading PI activities in healthcare organizations know how to optimally manage the board of directors' PI oversight responsibility.

The board's oversight responsibility is a difficult task. Most directors feel awkward judging the work of physicians and other clinical staff. Coordinated systems of review are imperative to assist them in making decisions about the organization's quality of care and in taking appropriate action when necessary.

According to the American Hospital Association, four key elements affect the board's ability to carry out its PI responsibilities:

- "Understanding of the quality assessment and improvement system" followed in the organization

- "Adequate reporting to the board by the staff on specific performance measures" (Figure 14.2 demonstrates one way that the results of PI monitoring can be reported.)

- "Oversight and approval of the process to ensure the continued competence of physicians and other clinical and technical staff"

- "Active questioning of the information" supplied on the quality of the care provided in the organization through performance monitoring and improvement activities (Umbdenstock 1992)

Thus, the board's ability to perform its responsibilities is of paramount importance. Carol Dye (1991) believes that education of the board should center on the following questions:

- What type of coordinated program does this facility have in place to integrate the review activities of all services for the purpose of both enhancing the quality of patient care [risk reduction] and identifying current and potential problems?

- How are the clinical and nonclinical activities of the institution monitored, and how are these two components integrated to ensure that the [PI] program is comprehensive?

- How is the [institution] organized to carry out the [PI] program? How are the services and departments organized for this function, and how are their activities coordinated?

Figure 14.2.   Defined, specific accountabilities related to PI throughout the hospital organization

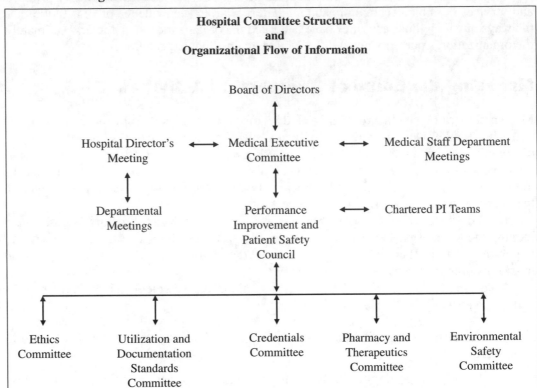

- To whom do the various committees concerned with aspects of [PI] report and how often?

- What are the institution's regular quality [monitoring] . . . activities and how often are they undertaken?

- What kinds of information [are] reported to the board, how often, and in what form? Because boards undertake much of their activities through committee structure, how [is the board] organized to receive and review information?

She goes on to say that "the board's ability to oversee [PI] functions depends on its access to timely and meaningful data. When boards are given relevant information in a form they can understand, they are in a better position to respond appropriately; that is, they are able to review, question, and set policy in an effective manner. Providing data that are concise, appropriately displayed, and organized in a comparative format will maximize the use of the board's time and assist its members in accomplishing [its oversight] activities in an efficient and effective manner" (Dye 1991, 68). Today, many PI theorists call this regular presentation of monitoring data for boards of directors a **dashboard**, much as the dashboard of your car provides minute-to-minute data on the myriad functions its various systems perform. Because many board members come from the business community, they "have become adept at reviewing financial data presented in forms such as current ratios, liquidity ratios, cash flow to total debt ratios, and so forth. Thus, for the most part, [directors] will be comfortable reviewing quality-of-care information presented in similar statistical formats. Other [directors] may benefit from having the data put into formats such as bar graphs, pie charts, and so forth that translate the statistical information into a visual image of the institution's progress. . . . When sharing data with a board of directors, it is important to remember that few [board members] are healthcare professionals. Thus, they may be unfamiliar with the data when first exposed to them. Careful attention should be paid to educating the trustees about certain concepts that govern data, such as validity, statistical confidence intervals, sample mean, and standard deviation" (Dye 1991, 68).

Dye (1991, 69) further suggests that the answers to several additional questions provide useful information for board members reviewing patient care quality and safety data:

- How were the data collected and by whom?

- How often are data collected?

- How large is the sample?

- How do these data compare to data from previous assessments?

- What do the data suggest about the quality of care? Can specific patterns be identified? Are there individual sentinel events that require action?

- Are there other reviews that need to be undertaken to provide a more complete and/or accurate picture of the [organization's] quality of care?

- What should [the organization] strive for as a final goal in a particular area? What would be an appropriate objective for improvement?

- How does [the organization] compare to other similar organizations?

The board of directors should be provided with information that answers the following questions when PI data identify adverse trends or occurrences:

- If a problem or a potential problem emerges, what actions will be taken to correct or eliminate the problem and prevent or reduce its recurrence?

- Is there an area ([service], department, procedure) that requires focused review?

- Which departments and professionals will be notified of the findings, and what roles will they have in follow-up?

- Will a report be provided to the board or an appropriate committee of the board and at what point in time?

- Have the problem, the review, and the plan of correction been documented? (Dye 1991, 69)

Ordinarily, boards of directors meet at least quarterly, while subcommittees of the board may meet more frequently. From the preceding comments, it should be obvious that performance monitoring and improvement activities should be a regular subject of inquiry and decision making at all board meetings.

Other Resources for PI Programs

In addition to the leadership and the board of directors, three other important organizational resources should be considered by healthcare organizations as they plan a PI program: standing committees of the medical staff, a new-hire and ongoing staff development program dedicated to understanding the approaches to and methods of PI, and formal quality management structures.

Standing Committees of the Medical Staff

Usually found in large healthcare organizations, standing committees of the medical staff have made significant contributions to improving quality in healthcare for many decades. Figure 14.2 provides an example of a hospital committee structure and demonstrates how important information is communicated throughout the organization.

Small organizations usually have small medical staffs and thus are not able to support standing committees dedicated solely to the quality of patient care. Consequently, a smaller organization frequently uses the executive committee of the medical staff as the "committee of the whole" to do the quality evaluation tasks traditionally executed by separate standing committees in larger organizations.

Commonly, standing committees are organized to review specific aspects of patient care services, such as ethical issues that may come up during the course of patient care; medication use—the selecting, prescribing, preparing, administering, and monitoring; and the rate of healthcare-associated (nosocomial) infections. Standing committees are usually chaired by a physician who specializes in an area related to the purview of the committee. Committee members are usually drawn from the medical staff, nursing units, and administrative areas related to that specialty.

Routine review of care is usually undertaken by standing committees according to a preestablished protocol (peer review plan) stipulating criteria by which cases are selected for review. Special review of particular cases also is undertaken when negative outcomes have been identified through administrative channels or through referral from other organizational care review processes. The intent of the review is to identify case-specific patterns of care that could have achieved better outcomes had the care processes involved been better designed or implemented. Review also seeks to identify the need for education or the use of clinical practice guidelines among the clinicians or others involved in the particular area of care.

For example, one common area of care review currently focuses on cesarean section delivery of newborns. Contemporary obstetrical clinical practice guidelines define situations in which cesarean section delivery is appropriate because of the risk involved to infant and mother. When cesarean section is utilized in questionable circumstances, it is the responsibility of the obstetrical staff to determine appropriateness and make recommendations to the clinicians involved regarding better practice decisions. In healthcare settings, this type of review by colleagues is referred to as **peer review.** (See the discussion of peer review in chapter 21.) Findings from peer reviews are aggregated and reported to the executive committee of the medical staff as well as to clinicians' professional files for consideration in the recredentialing process. (See the discussion of credentialing in chapter 13.) Nursing and operations administrators also consider these findings when issues uncover opportunities for improving nursing or other patient care functions. Because standing committee reviews and findings are clear evidence that medical staff is involved in PI activities, it is important that the reviews and findings be documented in committee meeting minutes and reflected in the PI program documentation.

PI Education

In addition to ensuring that the mission, vision, and organizational goals are communicated throughout the organization, the leaders should provide staff training in basic approaches to PI. Most healthcare organizations have a two-part training program that employees follow as part of the organization's new-hire orientation process, which is then repeated or supplemented annually for all staff. Generally, this training is a required competency. Frequently, organizations link the PI competency to the annual performance appraisal process, where employees are rated on their participation on PI teams and completion of training.

The organization's leaders also need to meet established PI competencies. Training for leaders is frequently conducted with the expectation that the leaders understand and can conduct training themselves on the organization's established PI framework. Leaders also are expected to provide support and resources for staff involvement in PI activities.

Formal Quality Management Structures

Consideration of a formal quality management structure usually revolves around the question of whether an organization should develop a PI department. The answer to this question, in turn, depends on a number of factors.

First, PI activities are data and information intensive. (See the discussion of information management in chapter 16.) A PI department can help an organization manage PI-related information and activities. It can become the centralized repository of information from PI activities, and its staff can coordinate the preparation of reports that turn data collection into information for committee and board analysis and decision making. Staff of this department also can facilitate the PI committee's responsibilities and can be the organization's experts in facilitating PI team activities and using QI toolbox techniques. They can educate leaders and staff on the principles of PI, data collection, data analysis, and any regulatory changes as they occur. Finally, they can take the lead in the development of functional and cross-functional PI teams, and organization-wide reporting of PI activities to quality councils and boards of directors. When used effectively within an existing PI culture, these resource departments support a healthcare organization's PI initiatives.

However, it is important to consider whether an organization is developing a PI department to deflect and perhaps hide its unwillingness to commit to a more authentic

PI culture. Some organizations develop PI departments to keep from having to develop organization-wide, multidisciplinary, integrated PI processes and to avoid having to deal with issues inherent in developing a more empowered nonmanagement staff.

Creating an authentic PI culture is a daunting task for many organizations even when the leaders are committed to the process. Commitment begins with establishing an educational process for the entire organization in the application of PI techniques. Creating a PI department allows the organization to centralize its quality efforts.

In an organization with a healthy, evolving PI culture, the PI department oversees PI efforts, ensures that individual departments complete their PI activities and meet reporting deadlines, and monitors the organizational culture to make sure that a healthy PI philosophy develops.

Case Study

When a large regional medical center became part of an integrated delivery system that had a central board of directors, the medical center's board began to struggle with its revised role. The new organizational environment included several outpatient clinics, multispecialty physician practices, and an insurance entity. Many of the current board members had served the organization since the medical center was built, and board activities always had been performed in a certain way. The administration rigidly controlled board meetings. Board members did not ask questions and routinely approved committee reports. The reports covered topics such as the organization's financial status and future financial plans, physician credentialing, care quality monitoring, new policies, and plans for a new hospital.

A new board member with a healthcare background was appointed after extensive screening and a personal interview with the executive committee. She was not part of the local business power structure, and the administration was concerned that her appointment might not be a wise move. During her first board meeting, two very interesting reports were given. One report detailed some reengineering projects. One of these involved redesigning nursing staffing patterns, decreasing the number of registered nurses (RNs) and replacing them with licensed practical nurses (LPNs) and certified nursing assistants (CNAs). The current quality report documented a very high quality of care and positive patient satisfaction surveys. Data excerpted from this report can be seen in the "1st Quarter" column of table 14.1. Given that this was her first board meeting, the new board member remained silent and did not ask questions.

Within four months, the new nursing staffing pattern had been launched. Data excerpted from the quality indicators report presented to the board can be seen in the "2nd Quarter" column of table 14.1. The new board member was very concerned and decided to ask the nurse administrator presenting the quality report the values, which show a negative trend, were for the nursing units with the new nursing staffing patterns. The administrator reported that there was a direct correlation. This answer initiated discussion among other board members who were accustomed to using quality indicators in their businesses. This was the first substantive board-level discussion that the new board member had seen. One board member wanted to know whether any data had been gathered from patient focus groups. Another board member asked whether the average length-of-stay data had increased, and

Table 14.1.   Case study data

Quality Performance Measure	1st Quarter	2nd Quarter
Medication errors	3.20%	10.42%
Patient falls	4.21%	8.56%
Cesarean sections	14.21%	17.87%
Rate of vaginal births after c-section	18.27%	15.72%
Nosocomial infections	1.78%	4.85%
X-ray discrepancies	0.15%	0.21%
Patient Satisfaction Measure	**1st Quarter**	**2nd Quarter**
Overall service	40.52%	20.74%
Overall clinical	86.72%	70.82%
Overall quality of service	45.40%	22.34%
Food	30.56%	32.54%
Overall cleanliness	85.89%	83.26%

someone else asked about a cost–benefit analysis of the new staffing patterns. Following the usual process, the chair called for approval of the report and presentation of the next item on the agenda.

Case Study Questions

1. What changes or patterns do you see in the data? What remedies might be suggested for any problems?

2. Has the CEO carried out his or her responsibility for educating the board? Why or why not?

3. Depending on the answer to question 2, what strategies would you recommend at this point?

4. What quality data should be reported and utilized by this board of directors?

5. Given this administration's style and leadership approach, do you think the minutes of the board meeting reflect actual board meeting discussions?

Summary

Several important aspects of PI programs should be reflected in the organizational structure. First and foremost, it is important for a healthcare organization to determine the roles of its leadership group and governing board within the PI program. A significant amount of board development is needed with respect to understanding healthcare processes and issues and analyzing PI data and information. Some organizations use their standing medical staff committees as important adjuncts to team-based PI activities. Some develop formal PI departments in support of PI activities.

References

Dye, C. 1991. Quality assurance data management: The trustees' role. Chapter 7 in *Quantitative Methods in Quality Management*. Edited by Longo, D.R., and D. Bohr. Chicago: American Hospital Publishing.

Umbdenstock, R.J. 1992. *So You're on the Hospital Board!* Chicago: American Hospital Publishing.

Resources

Arrington, B., K. Gautam, and W.M. McCabe. 1995. Continually improving governance. *Hospital and Health Services Administration* 40(1):95–110.

Crosby, P.B. 1980. *Quality Is Free*. New York: Mentor Books.

Crosby, P.B. 1984. *Quality without Tears*. New York: Plume Books.

Deming, W.E. 1986. *Out of the Crisis*. Cambridge, MA: MIT Press. First published in 1982 as *Quality, Productivity, and Competitive Position*.

Donabedian, A. 1966. Evaluating the quality of medical care. *Milbank Quarterly* 44:166–203.

Donabedian, A. 1980. *The Definition of Quality and Approaches to Its Management. Volume 1: Explorations in Quality Assessment and Monitoring*. Ann Arbor, MI: Health Administration Press.

Gardner, K., ed. 2003. *The Excellent Board: Practical Solutions for Healthcare Trustees and CEOs*. Chicago: American Hospital Publishing.

Holland, T.P., R.A. Ritvo, and A.R. Kovner. 1997. *Improving Board Effectiveness: Practical Lessons for Nonprofit Health Care Organizations*. Chicago: American Hospital Publishing.

Joint Commission. 2008. *2009 Comprehensive Accreditation Manual for Hospitals (CAMU): The Official Handbook*. Oakbrook Terrace, IL: Joint Commission Resources.

Juran, J.M. 1945. *Management of Inspection and Quality Control*. New York: Harper & Brothers.

Juran, J.M. 1951. *Quality Control Handbook*. New York: McGraw-Hill.

Juran, J.M. 1964. *Managerial Breakthrough*. New York: McGraw-Hill.

Juran, J.M. 1967. *Management of Quality Control*. New York: Joseph M. Juran.

Juran, J.M. 1970. *Quality Planning and Analysis*. New York: McGraw-Hill.

Juran, J.M. 1980. *Upper Management and Quality*. New York: Joseph M. Juran.

Juran, J.M. 1988. *Juran on Planning for Quality*. New York: Free Press.

Pointer, D.D., and J.E. Orlikoff. 1999. *Board Work: Governing Health Care Organizations*. San Francisco: Jossey-Bass.

Pointer, D.D., and J.E. Orlikoff. 2002. *Getting to Great: Principles of Health Care Organization Governance*. San Francisco: Jossey-Bass.

Chapter 15
Navigating the Accreditation, Certification, or Licensure Process

Learning Objectives

- To differentiate between compulsory and voluntary reviews

- To explain the performance improvement perspectives of accreditation, certification, and licensure organizations

- To describe the various approaches of accreditation, certification, and licensure agencies to the site visit and survey

- To identify approaches that lead to success in the survey process

Key Terms

Accreditation

Accreditation standards

Certification

Compliance

Compulsory reviews

Conditions of Participation

Deemed status

Document review

Exit conference

Licensure

Opening conference

Quality improvement organizations (QIOs)

Site visit

Survey team
Tracer methodology
Voluntary reviews

Background and Significance

The complexities of accreditation, certification, and licensure requirements can have a significant impact on healthcare organizations. Few healthcare professionals work in the industry for long without taking part in one of these three processes. This chapter provides a basic introduction to the concepts and processes involved.

Accreditation is the act of granting approval to a healthcare organization. The approval is based on whether the organization has met a set of voluntary standards developed by the accreditation agency. The Joint Commission is an example of an accreditation agency. Accreditation confirms the quality of the services that healthcare organizations provide. For example, hospitals accredited by the Joint Commission have a competitive advantage over nonaccredited hospitals in their geographical area because the Joint Commission "stamp of approval" lets the consumer know he or she is getting care from an organization meeting higher standards.

Licensure is a state's act of granting a healthcare organization or an individual healthcare practitioner permission to provide services of a defined scope in a limited geographical area. State governments issue licenses based on regulations specific to healthcare practices. For example, states issue licenses to individual hospitals, physicians, and nurses. It is illegal for organizations and professionals to provide healthcare services without a license.

Certification grants approval for a healthcare organization to provide services to a specific group of beneficiaries. For example, healthcare organizations must meet the federal *Conditions of Participation* to receive funding through the Medicare and Medicaid programs. These programs are administered by the Centers for Medicare and Medicaid Services (CMS), which is an agency of the Department of Health and Human Services.

Healthcare Accreditation, Certification, and Licensure Standards

In healthcare today, many different agencies develop and monitor standards on the quality of healthcare services. These agencies accomplish their missions through a comprehensive review process. Some of the review processes are compulsory, and others are voluntary. **Compulsory reviews** are performed to fulfill legal or licensure requirements. **Voluntary reviews** are conducted at the request of the healthcare facility seeking accreditation or certification.

Every accreditation, certification, and licensure agency develops written standards or regulations that serve as the basis of the review process. It is imperative that healthcare facilities monitor any changes and updates to the various standards and regulations and keep current sets of them on hand at all times to help maintain compliance status. **Compliance** is the process of meeting a prescribed set of standards or regulations to maintain active accreditation, licensure, or certification status. The materials may be provided in manuals, such as the Joint Commission's (2011a) *Hospital Accreditation Standards*, or in state and federal regulations, such as the CMS (2006) *Conditions of Participation*.

The Joint Commission and Its Accreditation Activities

The Joint Commission has been the most visible organization responsible for accrediting healthcare organizations since the mid-1950s. The Joint Commission (2011a, 2) describes its mission as follows:

> To continuously improve health care for the public, in collaboration with other stakeholders, by evaluating health care organizations and inspiring them to excel in providing safe and effective care of the highest quality and value.

The primary focus of the Joint Commission at this time is to determine whether organizations seeking accreditation are continually monitoring and improving the quality of care they provide. The Joint Commission requires that this continual improvement process be in place throughout the entire organization, from the governing body down, as well as across all department lines.

The structure of a typical Joint Commission (2011a, 3) **accreditation standards** manual contains the following major chapter topics:

- Organizational leadership
- Provision of care, treatment, and services
- Medication management
- Infection prevention and control
- Information management
- Medical staff
- Nursing
- Performance improvement
- National Patient Safety Goals
- Environment of care
- Emergency management
- Life safety
- Record of care, treatment, and services
- Rights and responsibilities of the individual
- Human Resources
- Transplant safety
- Waived testing

Within each chapter, the standards associated with each topic are cited and then elaborated upon with "elements of performance" (EP) that directly communicate the intent of the Joint Commission with respect to each standard. In addition, a scoring guideline is provided that allows the organization to score itself on each EP and thus get a sum total on each standard.

Commission on Accreditation of Rehabilitation Facilities

In 1966, the Commission on Accreditation of Rehabilitation Facilities (CARF) was established. CARF is a private, not-for-profit organization committed to developing and maintaining practical customer-focused standards to help organizations measure and improve the quality, value, and outcomes of behavioral health and medical rehabilitation programs. CARF accreditation is based on an organization's commitment to continually enhance the quality of its services and programs and to focus on customer satisfaction.

American Osteopathic Association

The American Osteopathic Association (AOA) implemented the accreditation of healthcare organizations in 1945. Initially, the primary initiative of the AOA was to ensure that osteopathic students received their training through rotating internships and residencies in facilities that provided high-quality patient care. The AOA has since developed accreditation standards for hospitals, ambulatory care facilities, ambulatory surgery centers, behavioral health facilities, substance abuse treatment facilities, and physical rehabilitation facilities.

National Committee for Quality Assurance

The National Committee for Quality Assurance (NCQA) began accrediting managed care organizations in 1991. Since then, the NCQA's activities have broadened to include accreditation of managed behavioral health organizations and credentials verification for physician organizations. As a private, not-for-profit organization, the NCQA is dedicated to improving the quality of healthcare by assessing and reporting on the nation's managed care plans. Its efforts are focused on the development of performance measurements in key areas such as member satisfaction, quality of care, access, and service. The NCQA uses the Health Plan Employer Data and Information Set (HEDIS) to accomplish these assessments of managed healthcare plans. The performance measures in HEDIS are related to significant public health issues and are a basis for purchasers and consumers to compare the performance of healthcare plans. For example, Western States University Hospital has a contractual relationship with a municipal managed care health plan in its region. Each year, health plan quality management officials come to University Hospital to review cases against selected HEDIS screens for health maintenance. Commonly, it reviews screens for adolescent well care, comprehensive diabetes mellitus care, well child <15 months care, prenatal and postpartum care, cervical cancer screening, well child 3 to 6 years care, and childhood immunizations administration. This information is used in the negotiations for contract renewal, and Western States University Hospital receives information from the health plan on how well it is meeting the required screens. In turn, HEDIS data, along with NCQA accreditation, provide organizations such as this municipal government a method for selecting healthcare plans or providers based on demonstrated value rather than simply on cost.

Accreditation Association for Ambulatory Health Care

The Accreditation Association for Ambulatory Health Care (AAAHC) surveys and accredits ambulatory medical facilities and managed care organizations. These include multispecialty and single-specialty group practices, health maintenance organizations, dental groups, occupational health services, community and student health services, independent practice associations, diagnostic imaging centers, and radiation oncology centers. However, its primary focus for accreditation is ambulatory surgery centers.

CMS *Conditions of Participation*

Every healthcare organization that provides services to Medicare and Medicaid beneficiaries must demonstrate compliance with the CMS *Conditions of Participation* (2006). The compliance process is known as certification, and it is usually carried out by state departments of health. The *Conditions of Participation* for healthcare facilities cover issues related to medical necessity, level of care, and quality of care. CMS also contracts with nongovernmental agencies across the country to monitor the care provided by independent healthcare practitioners. These agencies, called **quality improvement organizations (QIOs),** retrospectively review patient records to ensure that the care provided by practitioners meets the federal standards for medical necessity, level of care, and quality of care.

State Licensure

Every healthcare facility must have a license to operate within the state in which it is located. This license grants the facility the legal authority to provide healthcare services within its scope of services. To maintain its licensed status, the organization must adhere to the state regulations that govern issues related to staffing, physical facilities, services provided, documentation requirements, and quality of care. The regulations are usually monitored and evaluated on an annual basis by the licensing agencies of state departments of health. Many state health departments today publish "report cards" on the performance of the organizations that they license on Web sites maintained by these agencies.

Development of Policies and Procedures to Meet Multiple Standards and Regulations

At a minimum, healthcare organizations must consider state licensure regulations when they develop policies and procedures that relate to the documentation and quality of their healthcare services. When a facility provides care to Medicare and Medicaid patients, it also must determine which of the *Conditions of Participation* (CMS 2006) apply. When a facility is accredited by the Joint Commission, CARF, AOA, or some other accreditation organization, those standards also must be taken into consideration.

To ensure compliance, the healthcare organization must continually review its operating policies and procedures to make sure they reflect ongoing changes to accreditation standards and federal and state regulations that may affect the scope of care and services provided. The organization should identify the most stringent standard or regulation on each aspect of care and base its organizational policies and procedures on that standard or regulation. For example, when a healthcare facility is setting its policy on charting by exception, it must review the state licensure regulations for its requirements. Then the organization must review the *Conditions of Participation* regulations for its requirements. Finally, it must review all relevant accreditation standards. The strictest of all standards should be written into the policy and procedure for chart documentation by exception.

Surviving the Survey Process

Ongoing foresight and planning are the keys to successful completion of accreditation and licensure reviews. The leaders of the healthcare organization must stay focused on the organization's accreditation, certification, and licensure status to ensure that these issues are not overlooked in the flurry of day-to-day operations. Preparation for accreditation and licensure processes cannot be accomplished a few weeks before the organization is due for review. A solid accreditation and licensure infrastructure must be built and maintained so that the organization is ready for an inspection at any time.

Some accreditation processes are scheduled and others are unannounced. The Joint Commission's progression over the years from scheduled triennial surveys to periodic self-assessments and unannounced surveys by 2009 represents a gradual paradigm shift in its attitude toward survey readiness, which has become increasingly stringent. State agencies representing state licensing or federal Medicare and Medicaid certification programs also may conduct unannounced surveys. State licensing agencies make unannounced visits to healthcare organizations in response to complaints and reports of sentinel or never events.

CMS accepts accreditation by AAAHC, AOA, CARF, and the Joint Commission in granting what it calls **deemed status.** When granting deemed status, CMS assumes that the organization meets the *Conditions of Participation* if it is currently accredited by one of these organizations. Regional offices of CMS, however, frequently review psychiatric facilities accredited by CARF for compliance with the *Conditions of Participation.* Additionally, CMS will conduct a validation survey with roughly 10 percent of organizations that obtain deemed status through Joint Commission accreditation for *Conditions of Participation* compliance. Many state licensing agencies routinely survey organizations in order to qualify them for deemed status.

A review process with any of these agencies is more than just an issue of appearances. The reviewing agency becomes part of, and observes, the normal day-to-day operations of the healthcare organization. Surveyors from the Joint Commission, for example, want to be assured that the facility's leadership and staff can successfully execute organizational policies and procedures. They want to be assured that the leadership and staff are continuously monitoring and improving organizational performance and that those improvements are tied to the organization's strategic plan. Therefore, surveyors will want to validate these aspects as operative in the organization when they arrive for a review.

Although state licensure surveys may be more focused on a facility's ability to meet department of health regulations, the emphasis is still on high-quality care. It is important to remember that the goal of reviewers is to help healthcare organizations consider their own performance. Members of the organization are often too close to everyday activities and events to recognize important trends or consequences of the organization's inaction.

There is no standard review process for accrediting and licensing agencies. Processes may change from year to year as philosophies change within the agencies. In general, voluntary accreditation processes, such as those of the Joint Commission and CARF, are more flexible and tailored to the type of organization being reviewed. Governmental processes tend to be more bureaucratic.

Following is an overview of the more prominent accreditation and licensure processes.

Accreditation of Acute Care and Other Facilities: The Joint Commission

Currently, the Joint Commission's accreditation survey process is an unscheduled one. This approach shifts the organization's focus from survey preparation to continuous survey readiness since Joint Commission surveyors may show up at any time during a predefined window of opportunity to perform the accreditation survey. An organization interested in becoming accredited by the Joint Commission must file an application that provides information on the type of organization it is, the services it provides, certain statistical characteristics, and the names of its executive officers.

Most organizations undergo a **site visit** every three years; however, with the Joint Commission's move to unannounced surveys in 2006, the survey cycle includes a midpoint self-assessment. This self-assessment facilitates a more continuous, efficient accreditation process. The organization evaluates itself against applicable standards and submits a written progress report to the Joint Commission. As part of this assessment, the organization also must submit a corrective action plan. The organization's chief executive officer must attest to the accuracy of the self-assessment and corrective action plan. At the time of the triennial survey, surveyors will devote their time to validating the resolution of action plans submitted.

Hospitals must notify the state licensure organization of the occurrence of a Joint Commission site visit and must announce it to the public through a newspaper advertisement and postings throughout the facility. This announcement allows the public the opportunity to schedule and meet with the **survey team** to discuss any issues of concern. Failure to post these notifications may impact the final accreditation decision. The Joint Commission may also preschedule the state licensing organization to accompany its survey for CMS *Conditions of Participation* validation.

The composition of the Joint Commission survey team will vary depending on the size of the organization. It may include a physician, an administrator, a registered nurse, and other master's-level clinicians. Representatives from state licensing agencies who have arranged to join the survey for their own examination of the organization for licensing and CMS validation purposes may bring physician, nurse, pharmacist, nutritionist, or life safety surveyors. Beginning in 2005, most survey teams included an expert in environment of care and life safety issues. The Joint Commission surveyors have many years of experience practicing in the healthcare industry. Every surveyor undergoes considerable training in Joint Commission accreditation processes prior to being assigned to a survey team. In 2002, the Joint Commission began requiring surveyors to successfully complete a surveyor certification examination to participate in healthcare organization surveys.

Surveyors tailor review activities to the characteristics and services of the organization under review. These activities are based on information, data, and the corrective action plans provided in the midpoint self-assessment. It is important to remember that Joint Commission processes are not static from year to year, because the Joint Commission institutes regular improvements in its own survey processes. Any healthcare professional preparing for a Joint Commission accreditation survey must be aware of the current requirements, constraints, and expectations of surveyors.

The survey process lasts three to five days, depending on the size and complexity of the organization. For a large and highly complex organization, such as a university medical center, the accreditation survey activities most likely will last five days.

The site visit begins with an opening preliminary planning session at which the surveyors review current documentation from the organization. Depending on the type of organization to be surveyed, they would expect to review lists of sites eligible for survey and the services provided at each site, performance improvement (PI) data from the last 12 months, infection-related data, environment of care data, patient and resident rosters, and data specifically developed for the organization's compliance with Joint Commission standards ("measure of success" data). Following the preliminary planning session, the organization's leaders are expected to provide an overview of the organization's mission and vision, strategic goals and objectives, current experiences and outcomes, and performance monitoring and improvement activities. If the organization is experiencing significant new challenges in any areas, it is expected to identify those areas for the surveyors. Information about the organization's recent achievements is very important as well, because the surveyors want an accurate picture of the status of the organization.

Surveyors are interested in seeing how all members of the organization collaborate to provide healthcare services and products, how they measure the quality of those services and products, and how they identify and develop opportunities for improvement. Therefore, the **opening conference** is an important opportunity for the organization to set the tone for the survey process.

Surveyors come with knowledge of the organization from its midpoint self-assessment action plan, any consumer complaints reported to the Joint Commission, previous accreditation data, core measure data, and other information related to the organization's performance. Having this knowledge allows surveyors to tailor the on-site survey process to critical areas of focus (priority focus areas, or PFAs), including processes, systems, and structures within the healthcare organization known to significantly impact patient safety and quality of care. The on-site survey utilizes a **tracer methodology** that permits assessment of operational systems and processes in relation to the actual experiences of selected patients currently under the organization's care. Patients are selected on the basis of the current census of patients that the organization identifies as typical of its case mix. As cases are examined in relation to the actual care processes, the surveyor may identify performance issues or trends in one or more steps of the process or in the interfaces between processes. Patients on subsequent days may be selected on the basis of issues raised.

The Joint Commission's accreditation process emphasizes a systems approach to evaluate continuous improvement in key safety and quality areas. The performance reports of accredited organizations emphasize information that demonstrates an organization's commitment to quality and safety, such as achieving the National Patient Safety Goals (NPSGs), performing well in mandated core measures, or obtaining disease-specific care certification.

Surveyors visit patient care settings and conduct interviews with selected patients, department and program staff, and the organization's leaders. During the patient-specific tracer interviews on nursing units and in clinics, the surveyors gain firsthand knowledge about how well staff understands current objectives of treatment for the patient and how well that treatment is coordinated across all of the care modalities available in a modern healthcare organization. During interviews of various staff members and organization leaders, surveyors gain insight into the organization's recent successes and current challenges. They expect to gain insight into the management philosophy of the organization and the means by which the organization implements change as a result of PI. As surveyors "trace" caregiving to specific patients in patient care settings, their mission is to verify at the first-line level of employees the status of the organization as conveyed in presurvey documents and in the opening conference. They want to see that staff members who are in direct contact with patients know and carry out policies and procedures that managers and leadership have developed for the important issues that healthcare organizations encounter. Taking the patient's care in its specific context, surveyors want staff to be able to explain how the patient came to be in the hospital, what the current diagnoses and therapies are (particularly medications), and the rationales for their use. If the patient came through the emergency department, they may want to visit the area where the patient was treated and examine its processes. If the patient required surgery in the operating suite, they may want to visit that care site and examine its processes. If the patient had a procedure in interventional radiology, they may want to visit the radiologic suite and examine its processes as they relate to the tracer patient's specific care. They will expect to see all areas adhering to policy regarding staff communication, patient's rights, and patient safety in addition to the everyday processes of providing patient care.

As the tracer activities progress, general themes may begin to emerge, showing that staff may not be as well prepared or as conversant as is necessary. Table 15.1 shows aspects of the nursing process that emerged at Western States University Hospital during the first day's tracer activities. These themes were communicated to nurse managers so that on subsequent days, staff could be better prepared to discuss these aspects with surveyors.

Table 15.2 notes themes regarding all staff that emerged on the first day of tracer activities at Western States.

Trigger issues encountered during visits to care settings and tracer activities are reviewed with staff and leadership during special issues-resolution sessions at the end

Table 15.1. Nursing themes and actions

Accreditation and Licensing Survey—Nursing	
Common Theme	**Action**
Date/time of progress notes and orders	Review all orders and notes.
Do not use abbreviations	Review all orders.
Legibility of notes	
Pain assessments	Know your policy practice on when an assessment/reassessment is done and where it is documented in your area.
Admission/discharge criteria	Know your area's criteria; refer to your Statement of Conditions.
Restraints	We start with least restrictive. All four-side rails up is considered a restraint!
Hand hygiene	Artificial nails are not allowed in ICU, OR, NICU, and ED units.
High-alert medications	Focus on insulin administration (especially drips).
Infant security	Articulate your role in Code Pink, 6C, and 6H; know your policy regarding ID badges, family, lists, exits, etc.
Moderate sedation	Know the policy in your area. Concentrate on preprocedure assessments (especially airway).
Thinning charts	Review charts and ensure that what is required to be in a chart after it is thinned remains in chart. Refer to Nursing Policy 11.5, Thinning of Patient Charts on Unit.
Staffing	Managers and charge nurses should be able to speak to your practice.
Fire extinguishers	Ensure staff know the location of the fire extinguishers. All Behavioral Health staff should have keys to the fire extinguishers.
Communication between levels of care	Know your organization's practice of communicating pertinent clinical data to the next level of care, to the primary care provider, and to referral findings.
Assessment for falls	Ensure that patients have risk assessments for falls, and communicate information on high-risk patients to the next level of care or to their diagnostic care areas.
Infection control	Know the surveillance in your area. Specific risk assessment and monitoring for long-term care.
Medication storage	Ensure that used inhalers are covered/capped.
Loose needles	All needles need to be in a locked area so that staff and/or patients do not have access to them.
Infant security; rescue drills	Look into "apron" that will hold four infants for one staff to evacuate.
Assessment and reassessment	Ensure that all data required to be collected for an assessment are completed. Reassess in appropriate time frame and document your findings.
Documentation	Ensure that all care is documented, for example, dressing change.

Table 15.2.   Multidisciplinary themes and actions

Accreditation and Licensing Survey—Multidisciplinary	
Common Theme	**Action**
Range orders	Articulate the process when writing and administrating a range order.
Post anesthesia notes by an attending	Notes required in chart within 48 hours.
Emergency Department length of stay	
Medication lists	Remember that we have a hybrid charting system (paper and electronic). Outpatient is to focus the surveyors on the LCR medication list.
Problem list (outpatient)	Remember that we have a hybrid charting system (paper and electronic). Outpatient is to focus the surveyors on the LCR problem list.
Dietary consults	Ensure consults are done in the time frame required by policy.
Lab results	Know your lab results, why you are treating, and when you will need to repeat a test, especially microbiology (know the organism) and the antibiotic.
Nutrition assessment	Know your practice as to when a nutrition assessment is completed and when a referral is needed.
Provider privileges	Remember to always look up a provider's privileges on the Medical Staff Web site prior to the procedure.
Do Not Resuscitate orders	Document patient or family involvement in decision making.
Staffing effectiveness	Articulate our two HR indicators (hours per patient day [HPPD] and per diem staff) and two Clinical Indicators (patient falls and patient complaints). Initially, we looked at entire hospital—no correlation. Narrowed it down to areas where falls and patient complaints were common—no correlation. Now we're looking at time of day and whether overtime is a factor.
Performance improvement	Direct surveyor to PI storyboards and articulate the process: data before—process/intervention—data after.
Sample medications	Know your practice and the policy.
Forms	Identify short history forms in procedure areas that could/should be consistent across the organization.
Clean/dirty utility areas	If in the same room, ensure proper designation.
Oxygen containers on wheels	If possible, keep all portable O_2 in the O_2 (yellow) storage areas.
Patient charts/white boards	Locating patient charts outside patient rooms is a potential breach of patient confidentiality. White boards have too many patient identifiers.
Respiration therapy assessments/reassessments	Articulate your practice for a full assessment, especially if level of care changes.
"Time Out"	Ensure that this is documented for all required invasive procedures.
Preventive maintenance of biomedical equipment	Ensure that equipment is up to date. Biomed to maintain records

(Continued on next page)

Table 15.2. *(Continued)*

Common Theme	Action
Functional assessment—referrals for OT/PT/speech	Know your process for how to make referrals and document referrals.
Fire extinguishers	Ensure staff know the locations of the fire extinguishers. All Behavioral Health staff should have keys to the fire extinguishers.
Communication among levels of care	Know your practice of communicating pertinent clinical data to the next level of care, to the primary care provider, and referral findings.
Infection control	Know the surveillance in your area. Specific risk assessment and monitoring for long-term care

of each day. These day-end discussion sessions among surveyors and leadership may resolve issues to the surveyors' satisfaction. If issues appear significant or systemic, surveyors may request to review closed patient records retrospectively to get a picture of how the organization has handled the same issues in the same kinds of patients over time. Alternatively, they may request reports of organizational sampling around the trigger issue from the past or concurrent to the survey. Some of the trigger issues on which Joint Commission surveyors focus include patient rights, communication, medication use, information management, and general safety in the care environment. Whatever the trigger issues are, the organization's leaders must be aware of them and must implement a corrective action plan.

In addition to individual patient tracer activities, surveyors also conduct leadership interviews and "system tracers." Leadership interviews typically involve talking to top administration and medical staff officials about overall systems issues. For example, the medical staff leadership interview reviews in detail the credentialing activities and processes and medical staff oversight of teaching programs. The environment of care leadership interview reviews all aspects of the organization's environment of care and disaster management processes. (See chapter 12.) Results of ongoing monitoring are reviewed, and PI activities are discussed.

System tracers convene responsible individuals from across the organization to examine the following organizational issues relevant to patient care:

- The medication management system tracer reviews all aspects of the appropriate and safe preparation, distribution, and administration of medications in the organization. (See chapter 11.)

- The data management system tracer examines how the organization uses data and information for quality and PI activities as well as for ongoing monitoring of important functions. (See chapter 16.)

- The infection control system tracer examines the infection control program, processes, interventions, and outcomes. (See chapter 9.)

After completion of the tracers, system tracers, interviews, and visits to patient care areas, the survey team sequesters itself to consider its findings. It develops a preliminary report of the on-site survey and identifies any deficiencies that it perceives are evident in the organization.

After the team develops the preliminary report, surveyors, members of the organization's leadership team, and a representative from the state's licensing agency, if applicable, reconvene for an **exit conference.** During the exit conference, Joint Commission surveyors summarize their findings and explain any deficiencies identified during the site visit. Leaders have a short opportunity to discuss the surveyors' perspectives or to provide additional information related to any deficiencies. Deficiencies are reported to the organization as Requirements for Improvement (RFIs). Finally, the surveyors report the probable accreditation decision of the Joint Commission on the basis of the survey findings.

The Joint Commission (2011a) uses the following five categories to report its decisions on accreditation:

- *Accredited*: The organization has complied with Joint Commission performance standards, and its RFIs are at a level not sufficient to cause provisional accreditation status.

    Within 45 days of the final report of accreditation status, the organization must prepare a written plan of correction for each cited RFI and must show an appropriate measure of success to demonstrate that the RFI has been corrected. The organization then must monitor the measure for an additional four months after submitting the correction plan to the Commission, and the results of this monitoring must be reported to the Joint Commission. Upon submitting successful monitoring data as evidence of correction, the organization may have its accreditation status revised by the Commission, depending on the nature of the remaining deficiencies and the accreditation status initially granted.

- *Accreditation with follow-up survey*: The organization is not in compliance with specific standards and requires a follow-up survey within 30 days to 6 months. The organization must address the identified problem areas in an evidence of compliance report that details what the organization has changed to bring itself into compliance with the standards.

- *Contingent accreditation*: The organization did not meet all of the Joint Commission's standards at the time of the on-site survey and had a level of standards noncompliance and RFIs in excess of the published levels for that year. Although organizations that receive conditional accreditation may appeal, they must also remedy the noncompliance to the satisfaction of the Commission and, in most cases, are subject to a follow-up survey in 30 days.

- *Preliminary denial of accreditation*: The organization is in significant noncompliance with Joint Commission standards in multiple performance areas, with RFIs in excess of the published levels for that year. This accreditation decision is subject to appeal, and the organization has the opportunity to present additional information or evidence of compliance prior to accreditation denial. The accreditation decision on appeal also may result in decisions other than accreditation denied.

- *Denial of accreditation*: All available appeal procedures have been exhausted, and the organization has been denied accreditation.

All other Joint Commission–sponsored accreditations follow the same basic survey process as outlined for acute care. Site visits begin with an opening conference, proceed to care unit visits using tracer methodology (which can include a client's home in home health accreditation), and close with an exit conference.

Public Disclosure

All organizations currently accredited by the Joint Commission have quality reports published by the Commission on its public Web site, http://www.qualitycheck.org. Here, consumers can see how the organization has performed on implementing NPSGs and meeting core measures, and they can see the organization's accreditation history (Joint Commission 2011b).

Certification and Licensure of Long-Term Care Facilities: State Departments of Health

Long-term care facilities are subject to government-directed certification and licensure programs. Licensure regulations are published by each state, and long-term care facilities are expected to comply with the regulations. In addition to state regulations, the federal government developed its own set of regulations in 1974 in an attempt to improve the care provided in long-term care facilities that receive federal Medicare and Medicaid funds.

State departments of health usually conduct unscheduled reviews of long-term care facilities. All long-term care facilities must have a license to provide services in the states in which they operate, and usually licenses are renewed annually. Facility administrators understand that the state department of health will return for the next annual review within 15 months of the previous on-site review.

Long-term care facilities that receive Medicare and Medicaid funding must achieve certification of compliance with the *Conditions of Participation* as well. State departments of health also conduct Medicare and Medicaid certification reviews, which may or may not be performed concurrent with licensure review. Scheduling of certification reviews depends on the organizational structure of the state department of health. When there have been complaints from residents, families, or employees against a long-term care facility, department of health surveyors may visit at any time to perform a special investigation. Department of health survey teams commonly consist of two surveyors who have nursing, pharmacy, nutritionist, or clinical laboratory backgrounds. If the review is not conducted in response to a complaint, the survey process encompasses all aspects of facility operations. The surveyors determine at the time of the site visit which of those operations will be investigated.

CMS is currently moving all state survey agencies to a more data-driven process using the Quality Indicator Survey (QIS) (see chapter 8). The QIS is a two-staged survey process designed to produce a standardized resident-centered, outcome-oriented quality review. Automated steps guide surveyors through the survey process, identifying focused areas for further review (CMS 2007). In California, the annual site visit begins with the posting of survey notification on facility doors and at every nursing station. The notification requests that anyone—whether resident, staff member, or visitor—who has issues or perspectives to communicate to the surveyors make himself or herself known. An opening conference is held with the facility's administrators and the director of nursing to explain the purpose of the survey and outline the sequence of the survey activities.

Long-term care site surveyors always look for evidence of three trigger issues: very high percentages of patients suffering from dehydration, decubitus ulcers in low-risk residents, and fecal impaction. Current federal regulations mandate the primary importance of these issues in the long-term care setting. Whether the facility has very high percentages is determined on the basis of the Facility Quality Indicator Survey. The report is compiled from information provided to state departments of health via the Minimum Data Set (MDS) for Long-Term Care. An MDS must be maintained for every resident of a long-term care facility. (See the earlier discussion of this subject in chapter 8.) Focused review of the health records of residents with these conditions is carried out when excessive numbers are identified.

After delineating survey objectives, the surveyors begin examining facility operations. The president of the facility's residents' council is interviewed to determine whether any issues have been raised by residents since the last site review. If there is not a residents' council, then individual residents may be interviewed. Surveyors visit ancillary departments, such as nutrition services, and review operations for continuing adherence to public health standards. Surveyors visit nursing units and review resident records as deemed necessary. Records are reviewed for compliance with state regulations regarding such issues as annual care plan review by physicians, authentication of physicians' orders, proper administration of medication by nurses, and appropriate charting of care by nursing assistants.

When their review activities are complete, the surveyors reconvene with the facility's administrators and director of nursing to summarize their findings. Any deficiencies that require citations also are discussed at this time.

Accreditation of Psychiatric and Rehabilitative Care Facilities: CARF

Accreditation reviews by CARF (2008) are usually scheduled in advance. Organizations interested in CARF accreditation must file an application that provides its organizational type, the services it provides, statistical and textual descriptions of its characteristics, and the names of individuals who make up its leadership. Most CARF-accredited organizations undergo a site visit every three years.

The CARF survey team commonly includes three members, although additional members may be added for special purposes unique to the applying organization. Typically, the team is made up of professionals from other CARF-accredited organizations. Their areas of expertise are similar to those in which the organization undergoing accreditation specializes. For example, when the organization under review is an inpatient psychiatric institution, the surveyors have psychiatric inpatient experience and have practiced as administrators or clinicians in that setting. Surveyors undergo considerable training in CARF accreditation processes before they are assigned to a survey team.

In contrast to the Joint Commission process, the CARF accreditation process is much more flexible and is highly tailored to the patient care services and communities of interest of the organization. Although a template review schedule is followed, within each segment of the schedule the activities pursued depend on the characteristics of the organization applying for accreditation.

The CARF accreditation site visit begins with an opening conference. CARF requires that the opening conference be accessible to all communities of interest in the organization. Interested participants may include payers, staff members, referring agencies, members of the community, and patients. The surveyors expect that these constituencies will be allowed to voice concerns and issues during the opening conference. The survey team then outlines the activities it wants to pursue over the ensuing two or three days of the site survey.

The second part of the CARF accreditation is the **document review.** The document review examines policies and procedures, administrative rules and regulations, administrative records, human resources records, and the case records of patients.

The third part of the survey involves interviews with program staff and patients. The surveyors seek to validate the information gathered from the document review and to determine whether staff or patients have any important issues regarding patient care services.

Finally, the CARF process ends with an exit interview with the organization's leaders. Surveyors identify any deficiencies that have been uncovered and present an overall summary of their findings.

Certification: Compliance with the CMS
Conditions of Participation

Some healthcare organizations in the United States do not undergo an accreditation process. Others have undergone accreditation with an accrediting agency but have been identified by federal Medicare officials as requiring specific review for compliance with the CMS *Conditions of Participation*.

Surveys to determine a facility's compliance with the *Conditions of Participation* are carried out by state healthcare certification and licensure agencies. As with the state certification and licensure processes discussed earlier, state department of health reviews are typically unannounced. The survey team visits the healthcare facility as necessary either on an annual basis or in response to complaints from patients or employees. In addition to the surveyors commonly used by the department of health in a given state, regional Medicare agencies may provide one or two Medicare officials.

During the opening conference, the Medicare officials make it known that the review is for the purpose of determining compliance with the *Conditions of Participation*. They then generally leave and do not participate in the on-site survey activities. Judgments about compliance are left to the state certification surveyors.

Real-Life Example

Table 15.3 provides an example of how applicable standards can be reviewed as a basis for developing an organization's policies and procedures to meet multiple standards. The hospital for which this analysis was developed treats patients at many levels of care (inpatient hospitalization, partial hospitalization, outpatient group-home environment, and so on). Hospital administrators wanted to develop a policy for charting by exception that would meet all applicable regulations and standards. Each regulatory and accrediting agency's standards

Table 15.3. Regulations pertaining to charting by exception

Regulatory Body	Regulation	Comments
Medicare *Conditions of Participation*	"All records must document the following as appropriate. . . . All practitioners' orders, nursing notes, reports of treatment, medication records, radiology and laboratory reports, and vital signs and other information necessary to monitor the patient's condition."	Regulations do not require specific documentation for progress notes and other information. The documentation must, however, be sufficient to follow the care process.
	Special medical record requirements for psychiatric hospitals: "The special medical record requirement applicable to psychiatric hospitals was designed so that 'active psychiatric treatment' could be identified. The clinical records, therefore, should provide evidence of individualized treatment or a diagnostic plan that could reasonably be expected to improve the patient's condition."	These standards are more specific to your treatment setting but still do not appear to prohibit charting by exception.
	"The treatment received by the patient must be documented in such a way to assure that all active therapeutic efforts are included." Surveyors are to verify that all treatment profiled is recorded by the team member(s) providing services. The treatment provided should be clearly documented as well as the patient's response to the treatment.	The standard does not prohibit charting by exception. It does define what charting must be able to accomplish; that is, it must describe the treatment (what was done) and how the patient reacted. This can be done in charting by exception if carefully defined and consistently formatted.
	Surveyors are instructed to verify that progress notes indicate how the patient is responding to the treatment being carried out. Specifically, the progress notes recorded by the professional staff responsible for the patient's treatment must give a chronology.	See comments above.

(Continued on next page)

Table 15.3. *(Continued)*

Regulatory Body	Regulation	Comments
Medicare *Conditions of Participation* (continued)	"The records of the persons served should communicate appropriate information in a form that is clear, complete, and current. The record of each person served should include: . . . Reports of initial and ongoing assessments, . . . signed and dated reports from each care giver."	The standard does not prohibit charting by exception. It does define what charting must be able to accomplish; that is, charting must communicate appropriate information in a form that is clear, complete, and current. This can be done in charting by exception if carefully defined and monitored.
The Joint Commission	"(RC.01.01.01) The clinical record contains enough information to identify the individual, support the diagnosis, justify the treatment, document the course and results, and facilitate continuity of care among health care providers."	
	"(RC.01.02.01) . . . Progress notes made by the clinical staff and other authorized individuals and used as the basis for treatment and habilitation plan development and review. . . . (RC.02.01.01) All reassessments, when necessary. . . . Any observations relevant to care. . . ."	
State Regulations	"Information contained in the medical record shall be complete and sufficiently detailed relative to the patient's history, examination, laboratory and other diagnostic tests, diagnosis and treatment to facilitate continuity of care."	
	Medical records service or department: "Progress notes: Shall give a chronological picture of patient's progress and shall delineate the course and results of treatment. Patient's condition shall determine frequency."	
	Special requirements for inpatient psychiatric services	Standards address assessments, written individualized treatment plans, and written aftercare plans when appropriate. They do not address progress notes and other documentation specifically.
SUMMARY: None of the regulations reviewed above have specifically defined time frames for documentation of care or how progress notes need to be completed. Charting by exception, if well planned and implemented, can be used while maintaining compliance.		

were reviewed and then organized in a tabular format that allows easy viewing to determine which standard sets the strictest requirements. None of the standards consulted prohibit the use of charting-by-exception methodologies.

Case Study

Henry McConnell has been an administrator surveyor with the Joint Commission for five years. He currently serves on a survey team reviewing a large midwestern tertiary care facility. The survey is going well, and he and the nurse member of the team are visiting the patient care areas of the facility. The chief operating officer (COO) and the director of nursing (DON) accompany the two surveyors to various nursing units. They decide to visit the inpatient psychiatric unit.

This particular inpatient psychiatric unit cares for people with psychotic and other severe emotional disturbances. Many of the patients on the unit frequently suffer hallucinations. Others have had prehospital episodes of violence toward others. The unit is known in psychiatric medicine as a "locked facility," meaning that special keys are necessary to enter or exit the unit.

As McConnell and his fellow nurse surveyor approach the unit with the COO and the DON, the COO comments on the level of acute psychiatric patients that the institution commonly houses in the unit. She points out that the double doors are made of metal with wired glass windows and that the doors are locked from both sides. She makes a production of getting out her set of keys to the unit so that they can enter, making sure that the two surveyors see that the doorknobs will not open the doors and that one can enter only with a key. After they all pass through the doors, she turns around to show them that the doors have closed securely behind them.

They then turn to go onto the unit to do the review. The COO and the DON walk carefully out in front of the surveyors toward the nursing station, the surveyors following a little ways behind. One of the first things McConnell observes is a 3-foot-long red-handled fireman's axe located about 5 feet inside the doorway and up near the ceiling.

Case Study Questions

1. How did the axe get there?

2. What common characteristic of healthcare organizations discussed in the "Background and Significance" section of this chapter is exhibited in this case?

3. How could a potentially dangerous situation such as this be avoided?

Project Application

Community Hospital of the West is evaluating its medical staff rules and regulations in the area of physician documentation, specifically, dictated reports. This hospital has an accredited rehabilitation unit, so CARF regulations apply. Students should review the state licensure rules, the CMS *Conditions of Participation*, Joint Commission standards, and the CARF standards for these documentation requirements. Then they should prepare a comparative report of the standards and make a recommendation as to what the new policy should be.

Summary

Accreditation, licensure, and certification activities are a significant component of contemporary quality management programs in healthcare organizations. A variety of accreditation and licensing agencies exist, including the Joint Commission, CARF, the AOA, the NCQA, the AAAHC, and state departments of health. All of these agencies publish standards that organizations must meet in order to be awarded or maintain accreditation or licensure. Compliance with these accreditation standards and licensure regulations should be built into the healthcare organization's operating policies and procedures and PI activities.

References

Centers for Medicare and Medicaid Services. 2006. *Conditions of Participation*. http://www.cms.hhs.gov/CFCsANDCOPs/06_Hospitals.asp#TopOfPage.

Centers for Medicare and Medicaid Services. 2007. Evaluation of the Quality Indicator Survey (QIS) contract #500-00-0032, TO#7, final report (December). https://www.cms.gov/CertificationandComplianc/Downloads/QISExecSummary.pdf.

Commission on Accreditation of Rehabilitation Facilities. 2008. *CARF Accreditation Sourcebook, 2008*. Tucson, AZ: CARF.

Joint Commission. 2011a. *Hospital Accreditation Standards*. Oakbrook Terrace, IL: Joint Commission Resources.

Joint Commission. 2011b. Facts about the Joint Commission on Accreditation of Healthcare Organizations. http://www.jointcommission.org.

Resources

Accreditation Association for Ambulatory Health Care. 2011. http://www.aaahc.org.

American Osteopathic Association. 2011. http://www.osteopathic.org/Pages/default.aspx.

Brennan, T.A. 1998. The role of regulation in quality improvement. *Milbank Quarterly* 76(4):709–731.

Commission on Accreditation of Rehabilitation Facilities. 2011. http://www.carf.org/home/.

Grant, P.N., and W.R. Hirsch. 2002. *Medicare Provider-Sponsored Organizations: A Practical Guide to Development and Certification*. San Francisco: Jossey-Bass.

Jencks, S.F. 1994. The government's role in hospital accountability for quality of care. *Joint Commission Journal of Quality Improvement* 20(7):364–369.

Kelly, M.A. 1993. Thorough preparation key to successful surveys. *Health Facility Management* 6(2):38–44.

National Committee for Quality Assurance. 2011. http://www.ncqa.org.

Chapter 16
Implementing Effective Information Management Tools for Performance Improvement

Learning Objectives

- To identify the reasons that contemporary information technologies are important to quality improvement in healthcare

- To describe the information management tools commonly used in the performance improvement process

- To describe current developments in healthcare information technologies that will enhance performance improvement activities in the future

- To enumerate how information resources management professionals can help performance improvement teams pursue their improvement activities

Key Terms

Data collection

Information management standards

Background and Significance

Performance improvement (PI) in healthcare is an information-intensive activity. Because PI models are based on the continuous monitoring and assessment of performance measures, the effective management of the data and information collected is crucial to the success of the PI program. Developing effective data and information management systems requires a clear picture of the ramifications of data and information management for PI activities.

Healthcare organizations collect all kinds of data in routine, day-to-day patient care, operations, and administrative activities. According to Elliott (1999, 210) and Johns (1997, 53):

> The basic unit of recording in healthcare is an *event*. An event is the observation of an occurrence, subjective characteristic, or objective measurement relevant to an individual's health status that can be described by numeric values, words, character strings, images, or sounds. The observation may be made by a healthcare worker, healthcare professional, diagnostic/therapeutic instrument, or a patient/client and family/associates. Commonly, events are further described by type, date and time, observer, and individual observed. It is the web of these recorded events regarding patient after patient that forms the basic data of the healthcare information system.
>
> Data, however, are facts, simple facts. They are singular units of *knowledge* that never provide a reliable and valid knowledge-picture of an entity—in this case patients and their various health aspects—in its entirety. They rarely provide a competent knowledge-picture of even one aspect of an entity. In addition, data often must be put in the context of their observation before their real meaning is understood. Understanding of the meaning of data in context transforms the data into information. Johns notes that this transformation comes by means of formatting, filtering, and manipulation: changing the configuration in context, selecting pertinent aspects, or recombining aspects of the data to more clearly delineate its meaning. Johns also notes that after the data-to-information transformation, the result is "useful to a particular task"; that is, it helps individuals to make decisions. What then, is knowledge? In information sciences, it is commonly held that knowledge consists of the collection of information about an entity, the abstract concepts of which have been validated by the consensus of multiple interpreters. Here, Johns refers to "a combination of rules, relationships, ideas, and experiences" that, again, facilitate decision making.

Management of information resources for PI purposes must facilitate the transformation from data to information and from information to knowledge. **Data collection** in healthcare organizations falls into one of three categories:

- *Patient-specific*: Pertains to the care services provided to each patient

- *Aggregated*: Summarizes the experiences of many patients regarding a set of aspects of their care

- *Comparative*: Uses aggregate data to describe the experiences of unique types of patients with one or more aspects of their care

But these data are only meaningful in context; they must be formatted, filtered, and manipulated to be transformed into information and knowledge that can be used in PI programs.

Transformation of Data into Knowledge

How do the formatting, filtering, and manipulating occur? Fortunately, today's information management technologies enhance that transformation when they are deployed appropriately for that purpose by a healthcare organization. Careful consideration must be given to the support that information technologies can provide.

First, the QI toolbox techniques discussed in part II of this text can help with the tasks of manipulating and interpreting data. The QI toolbox techniques showcase excellent tools that make it possible for PI teams to see what the data are really showing. Looking at a mass of numbers and picking out the salient points and trends is usually difficult. The QI toolbox techniques make it easier to organize data, work through them to uncover meaningful information, and present them in a way that other people can understand.

Aggregating and performing basic statistical analysis can be facilitated by computer-based spreadsheet applications. PI teams can download data from computer-based healthcare information systems and perform ratio and correlation analysis or other statistical analyses on the data or compare the outcomes of different groups.

Standardized reporting formats can be developed to track important measures that the organization has selected for periodic review. Figure 16.1 is an example of a PI report used by a hospital to track its important measures on a quarterly basis. With spreadsheet applications, potential scenarios also can be developed to examine possible outcomes of changes in healthcare processes. Presentation development and word-processing applications make it easy for PI teams to communicate effectively with others in the organization and to document progress on a project as it occurs.

Internet access and various indexing search engines provide information to PI teams on the resources contained in journals and in professional healthcare literature. With Internet access, benchmarking against other organizations' PI accomplishments is a simple process.

Ideally, the healthcare information resources supporting PI activities are based in an environment that has enhanced communications and information management technologies already implemented. Most healthcare performance measures are used to assess everyday healthcare service activities, so the easiest and most effective places to find data about those measures is in the already-deployed information systems that support those service activities. For example, if a PI team wanted to assess the effectiveness of blood transfusion services, probably the best place to find data about those services would be in the blood bank component of clinical laboratory systems. If a PI team wanted to assess the effectiveness of wound care, the most likely place to find data about that service would be in the nursing component of clinical information systems.

However, healthcare organizations have found over the past few years that stand-alone information systems are difficult to use for PI activities. The examination and improvement of a process often involve the analysis of data and information from a variety of organizational information resources. Thus, the objective has become to provide integrated configuration and access to information resources from a variety of systems across the organization. Important developments that can assist an organization in this objective are discussed in the following sections of this chapter.

Data Repositories

In the late 1990s, some healthcare organizations began to develop data repositories to facilitate PI activities and long-range strategic planning. Organizations that have deployed this technology are copying every instantiation of every datum collected in the course of

Figure 16.1.   Example of a routine PI report for a community hospital

General Statistics

Statistics	Jan–March 2011	April–June 2011	July–Sept 2011	Oct–Dec 2011	2011 Average	2010 Average
Admissions	625	711	802	775	728.25	747.25
Discharges	789	690	766	759	751.00	789.25
Patient days	1,657	1,671	1,623	1,611	1,640.50	1,910.00
Lost work hours	0*	33*	22*	17*	18*	17*
Observation patients	146	125	137	144	138.00	153.25
Inpatient mortality rate	1.32%	1.35%	1.03%	0.81%	1.13%	1.11%
Deliveries	234	221	232	245	233.00	268.25
Emergency department visits	5,523	5,683	5,890	5,789	5,721.25	6,232.50
Inpatient/outpatient operative encounters	687	664	665	676	673.00	728.75
Outpatient operative encounters	546	524	530	568	542.00	585.25

Patient Care

Measure	Benchmark	Jan–March 2011	April–June 2011	July–Sept 2011	Oct–Dec 2011	2011 Average	2010 Average
Discrepancies: Preop/postop/pathological (op report indicates specimen removed)	100% (I)	37%	47%	86%	85%	64%	40%
Procedure appropriateness: Criteria met	100% (I)	100%	100%	100%	100%	100%	100%
Patient preparation for procedure: Adequate	100% (I)	86%	79%	87%	89%	85%	83%
Procedure performance and patient monitoring: Intraoperative incidents	0% (I)	0.13%	0.0%	0.38%	0.29%	0.20%	0.21%
Procedure performance and patient monitoring: Unplanned returns to OR (M)	0% (M)	0.13%	0.13%	0.38%	1.1%	0.44%	0.27%
Postprocedure care: Complications of postprocedure care	0% (I)	0.26%	0.40%	0.25%	0.43%	0.34%	0.03%
Postprocedure patient education completed	100% (I)	51%	67%	75%	74%	67%	67%

Figure 16.1. *(Continued)*

Patient Care *(continued)*

Medication Use							
Prescribing or ordering: Orders changed as result of MD clarification	NI	NI	89%	95.4%	93.8%	92.7%	89%
Preparing and dispensing: Dispensing errors	0% (I)	0%	≤1%	0%	0%	≤0.25%	≤1%
Preparing and dispensing: Medication delivery time—preop antibiotics within 2 hours of surgery (hips, knees, appendectomies, hysterectomies)	≤2 hours (N)	89%	93%	93%	91%	92%	87%
Administering: DUE—appropriateness of dosage	90% (I)	73%	67%	73.8%	81.0%	73.7%	89.0%
Monitoring the effects on patients: Adverse reactions	0.1% (I)	0.04%	0.09%	1.0%	0.22%	0.34%	0.36%
Monitoring the effects on patients: Drug–drug interactions	NI	23	2	4	1	7.5	16.0
Monitoring the effects on patients: Drug–food interactions	NI	7	23	44	62	34.0	20.0
Adverse effects during anesthesia	NI	NI	NI	NI	NI	NI	NI
Use of Restraints							
Documented evidence of less restrictive measures used	NI	3	3	11	6	6	NI
Use of Blood and Blood Components							
Ordering: Blood usage appropriate	100% (I)	100%	100%	100%	100%	100%	100%
Distributing, handling, and dispensing	NI	NI	NI	NI	NI	NI	NI
Administering: Blood slips completed and on chart	100% (I)	88.2%	81%	82.6%	86.4%	84.6%	85.7%
Administration: Cross-match:transfusion ratio	≤2:1 (I)	1.8:1	1.6:1	2.2:1	1.8:1	1.9:1	2.0:1
Monitoring blood and blood component effects on patients: Potential transfusion reactions	NI	0.0%	0.0%	0.0%	0.0%	0.0%	0.0%
Monitoring blood and blood component effects on patients: Confirmed transfusion reactions	0% (I)	0.0%	0.0%	0.0%	0.0%	0.0%	0.0%

(Continued on next page)

Figure 16.1. (*Continued*)

Continuum of Care

Measure	Benchmark	Jan–March 2011	April–June 2011	July–Sept 2011	Oct–Dec 2011	2011 Average	2010 Average
Utilization management: Patients admitted as inpatients not meeting appropriateness criteria on initial review	100% (I)	NI	NI	NI	NI	NI	NI
Utilization management: Continuing stay criteria met	100% (I)	NI	NI	NI	NI	NI	NI
Utilization management: Patients remaining inpatients after discharge criteria met	100% (I)	NI	NI	NI	NI	NI	NI

Important Processes and Outcomes

Measure	Benchmark	Jan–March 2011	April–June 2011	July–Sept 2011	Oct–Dec 2011	2011 Average	2010 Average
Autopsy results: Number performed/number met criteria	100% (I)	NI	NI	NI	NI	NI	NI
Critical occurrences	—	0	1	0	0	0.25	0
C-section rate (O)	12% (M); 17% (N)	15.3%	12.8%	11.8%	12.4%	13.1%	12.1%
VBAC rate (O)	50% (M); 36% (N)	37.5%	38%	38%	34%	37%	50%
Primary C-section rate (O)	6.5% (O)	9.7%	7.8%	5.7%	6.1%	7.3%	7.9%
Percentage of total C-section (O)	50% (O)	56.9%	55.8%	42.5%	43.6%	49.7%	59.2%
Repeat C-section rate (O)	65% (O)	62.5%	62.1%	62.2%	65.9%	63.2%	50.0%
X-ray discrepancies resulting in change of care (O)	1.0% (O)	0.7%	0.42%	0.36%	0.4%	0.5%	NI
Unplanned return to emergency department within 72 hours (M)	0.6% (O)	0.53%	0.5%	0.7%	0.7%	0.6%	0.6%
Patients in emergency department more than 6 hours (M)	12% (I)	14.7%	10%	13.1%	8.8%	11.7%	12.0%
Unplanned return to special care unit (M)	0.0% (I)	1.9%	2.3%	1.8%	2.5%	2.1%	NI
Unplanned admits from outpatient surgery (M)	2.0% (I)	2.3%	1.9%	2.4%	6.9%	3.4%	1.8%
Cancelled surgeries (M)	1.4% (I)	1.0%	1.0%	1.9%	1.6%	1.4%	1.3%
Cancelled endoscopies (M)	1.1% (I)	1.2%	1.9%	1%	1.4%	1.4%	1.1%

Figure 16.1. *(Continued)*

Quality Control Activities

Measure	Benchmark	Jan–March 2011	April–June 2011	July–Sept 2011	Oct–Dec 2011	2011 Average	2010 Average
Clinical lab: Number of QC functions completed/number required	100% (I)	0.0%	1.54%	0.78%	2.0%	1.1%	1.2%
Diagnostic radiology: Number of QC functions completed/number required	100% (I)	NI	NI	NI	NI	NI	NI
Dietary: Number of QC functions completed/number required	100% (I)	NI	NI	NI	NI	NI	NI
Equipment used to administer medication: Number of QC functions completed/number required	100% (I)	NI	NI	NI	NI	NI	NI
Pharmacy equipment used to prepare medication: Number of QC functions completed/number required	100% (I)	NI	NI	NI	NI	NI	NI
Equipment malfunctions	0% (I)	NI	1	0	6	2	3

Patient Rights

Measure	Benchmark	Jan–March 2011	April–June 2011	July–Sept 2011	Oct–Dec 2011	2011 Average	2010 Average
Overall patient satisfaction	68% (I)	67.2%	63.8%	68.3%	73.8%	68.3%	63.0%
Advance directives: Patients asked whether they have an advance directive	100% (I)	67.7%	68.6%	66.7%	82.6%	71.4%	NI
Advance directives: Patients provided information about advance directives	100% (I)	100%	100%	100%	100%	100%	NI

Human Resources

Measure	Benchmark	Jan–March 2011	April–June 2011	July–Sept 2011	Oct–Dec 2011	2011 Average	2010 Average
Employee satisfaction: Overall annual employee satisfaction rate	NI	NI	NI	NI	NI	NI	NI
Annual turnover rate	NI	8.6%	9.7%	5.6%	8.6%	8.1%	41.0%
Complete new hire orientation	100% (I)	100%	100%	100%	100%	100%	100%

(Continued on next page)

Figure 16.1. *(Continued)*

Information Management

Measure	Benchmark	Jan–March 2011	April–June 2011	July–Sept 2011	Oct–Dec 2011	2011 Average	2010 Average
Data quality monitoring: Documentation appropriateness	90% (I)	95.3%	97.1%	95.4%	97.8%	96.4%	NI
Medical record delinquency: Overall	50% (J)	8.7%	8.4%	8.8%	11.1%	9.3%	11.1%
Medical record delinquency: History and physicals	≤2% (I)	1.0%	0.3%	0.3%	0.12%	0.43%	0.6%
Medical record delinquency: Operative reports	≤2% (I)	3.0%	4.1%	3.6%	4.8%	3.9%	2.9%
Verbal orders countersigned	100% (I)	68.0%	NI	81.3%	95.6%	81.6%	NI
Medical records dated (all entries)	90% (I)	48%	NI	53%	NI	51%	NI

Surveillance, Prevention, and Infection Control

Measure	Benchmark	Jan–March 2011	April–June 2011	July–Sept 2011	Oct–Dec 2011	2011 Average	2010 Average
Nosocomial surgical site infection rate	2.5% (I)	0.8%	1.2%	0.6%	2.2%	1.2%	1.2%
Postop nosocomial pneumonia rate	1.0% (I)	0.0%	0.3%	0.3%	0.6%	0.3%	0.13%

New Programs

Measure	Benchmark	Jan–March 2011	April–June 2011	July–Sept 2011	Oct–Dec 2011	2011 Average	2010 Average
Measures of new program effectiveness	NI	NI	NI	NI	NI	NI	NI

Benchmarking Key: N = national; J = Joint Commission; I = internal; O = ORYX; M = Maryland Quality Indicator Project; NI = no information

*Number of incidents per 200,000 hours worked

providing healthcare services to customers. In addition, they are collecting the secondary data acquired in the course of using the technologies to support care, such as those collected to provide audit trails and to support other administrative aspects of running information systems. Which users entered data, which access terminal was used, and the date and time of entry are key examples of this type of administrative data. As these repositories become more common in healthcare information systems implementations, they will provide healthcare professionals involved in PI activities with timely data and information that can be used continuously to monitor the quality of many different aspects of the care they provide.

Many healthcare organizations, however, have not yet implemented such information technology resources. In their absence, organizations must design information collection and transmission systems that can effectively support PI initiatives. Many routine reports produced in healthcare organizations should be made available across departments and across PI teams. The health records of specific patients contain immense stores of data about all aspects of patient care. These paper-based records are repositories as well, but they cannot be accessed as easily as a computer-based repository. Systems must be developed to make these data available in spite of the fact that the organization does not have computer-based patient records.

Intranet-Based Communication Technologies

Everyone in the organization who is concerned with quality issues must be kept apprised of the current status of PI activities. A PI team working on one issue in a specific work unit of the organization may discover important information that could be used by another PI team working on a different issue in a different work unit. Without good communication of PI activities throughout the organization, the second team might capture information that has already been captured or analyze collected data that have already been analyzed, thereby wasting time and money.

Deploying intranet-based communication technologies can help keep everyone in the organization apprised of the current status of PI projects. Intranets are wide-area or local-area network-based resources that allow members of a healthcare organization access to information resources from a variety of contexts within the organization. Only valid users from within the organization should have access to intranet-based materials. Commonly, the presentation of materials uses the standard interface of the Internet and Web browsers, but other presentations may be supported by the intranet.

Using the Internet configuration can facilitate communication about PI activities. Each PI project can be accorded Web pages (URLs) on the intranet where PI team members can upload project documentation or presentations as various milestones are achieved. Team members also can share data that they have collected for their project with other teams who can use the data for their projects. At any time, the organization's members can look up the status of PI projects within the organization and review which projects have been completed.

Standardization and Support of Information Management Tools

Another important aspect of utilizing information systems in PI activities is standardization. Frequently, the leader of each PI team will want to use his or her personal favorite information management technology. This is understandable, given that each leader may have developed expertise in using particular products. However, statistical analysis applications are available from several vendors.

This situation points to the need for organizations to standardize data collection and analysis technologies across all PI activities. Standardization facilitates the use of data by multiple individuals and multiple teams. Sharing can decrease the time and cost of PI activities for the organization. To accomplish sharing ability, organizations should carefully consider the most appropriate kind of information technology support.

Today, of course, most organizations use office software that includes both word-processing and spreadsheet applications. Software should be standardized across all departments. Statistical analysis and graphing applications also should be acquired to facilitate analysis of data sets collected during PI team activities. All staff involved in PI activities should have Internet access so they can search periodicals and scientific journals. The National Library of Medicine provides online access to its clinical and scientific journal index through its PubMed search engine. Other indices for social, biological, and physical science as well as healthcare profession publications are available through the Web sites of university or public libraries.

User support must be provided for all information technology resources. Expert users should be identified and made available to PI teams to optimize the use of these technologies. Training sessions should be held periodically to acquaint staff across the organization with techniques for data analysis and statistical packages.

Information Warehouses

A recent development related to the issues of standardization and duplication in health information resources management is the deployment of information warehouses. Information warehouses allow organizations to store reports, presentations, profiles, and graphics interpreted and developed from stores of data for reuse in subsequent organizational activities. For example, a report developed by a PI team on the occurrence of methicillin-resistant *Staphylococcus aureus* infection in a neonatal intensive care unit subsequently could be used by the perinatal morbidity and mortality committee in a monthly review of infant morbidity. A marketing report on the need for services pertinent to women and children in an organization's locale could be used by a PI team that wants to delineate the important aspects of customer satisfaction with women's and children's services.

Providing online access to information warehouses via intranets and Web browsers facilitates information resource distribution. Browser search engines allow users within the organization to search for previously compiled and interpreted information on any subject contained in the warehouses. Any materials available in a warehouse can be printed and redistributed to PI team members. Materials in electronic formats can be downloaded and reused in word processors, spreadsheets, graphics presentations, or statistical applications.

Comparative Performance Data

As discussed in part I of this textbook, benchmarking can make an important contribution to the improvement of performance in healthcare organizations. Benchmarking is so important that the Joint Commission and the Centers for Medicare and Medicaid Services (CMS) have placed renewed emphasis on it by requiring that accredited and participating organizations, respectively, participate in national benchmarking activities through the core measures projects and patient satisfaction surveying. In turn, the organizations have access to data from these measures databases. The organization then can compare its performance with the performance of similar organizations. The comparison can assure the organization that it is performing up to industry standards or help the organization identify opportunities for improvement.

The Joint Commission and CMS have identified several sets of core measures—sets of patient care characteristics that reflect the quality of care an organization can provide for important diagnoses. Pneumonia, congestive heart failure, and myocardial infarction are examples of current core measure sets about which accredited organizations are required to collect data. Organizations can either transmit the data directly to the Joint Commission and CMS or use a vendor recognized by the Joint Commission and CMS. Some vendors have developed their data entry applications on the Internet. In this case, the organization would identify in its computer-based or paper health records the value of the given measure and enter the values for each measure on the Web page for that diagnosis on the vendor's Web site. After the organization enters the necessary number of cases, the vendor analyzes the data, develops summary reporting, and forwards the data and analysis back to the organization and to the Joint Commission. The summary reporting details how well the organization performed with respect to the measure in terms of percentage of compliance with the measure and shows how well the organization performed with respect to other similar organizations. (See figures 16.2 and 16.3.)

"Recently, The Joint Commission has categorized its performance measures into *accountability* and *non-accountability* measures. This approach places more emphasis on an organization's performance on accountability measures—quality measures that meet four criteria designed to identify measures that produce the greatest positive impact on patient outcomes when hospitals demonstrate improvement:

- **Research:** Strong scientific evidence exists demonstrating that compliance with a given process of care improves health outcomes (either directly or by reducing risk of adverse outcomes).

- **Proximity:** The process being measured is closely connected to the outcome it impacts; there are relatively few clinical processes that occur after the one that is measured and before the improved outcome occurs.

Figure 16.2.   Pneumonia core measure set

Performance Measure Name	Description
Pneumococcal/Vaccination	Pneumonia patients, age 65 and older, who were screened for pneumococcal vaccine status and were administered the vaccine prior to discharge, if indicated
Blood cultures performed within 24 hours prior to or 24 hours after hospital arrival for patients who were transferred or admitted to the ICU within 24 hours of hospital arrival	Pneumonia patients transferred or admitted to the ICU within 24 hours of hospital arrival, who had blood cultures performed within 24 hours prior to or 24 hours after hospital arrival
Blood cultures performed in the Emergency Department prior to initial antibiotic received in hospital	Pneumonia patients whose initial emergency room blood culture specimen was collected prior to first hospital dose of antibiotics. This measure focuses on the treatment provided to Emergency Department patients prior to admission orders.
Adult smoking cessation advice/ Counseling	Pneumonia patients with a history of smoking cigarettes who are given smoking cessation advice or counseling during hospital stay. For the purposes of this measure, a smoker is defined as someone who has smoked cigarettes anytime during the year prior to hospital arrival.
Antibiotic timing (median)	Median time from arrival at the hospital to the administration of the first dose of antibiotic at the hospital
Initial antibiotic received within 6 hours of hospital arrival	Pneumonia patients who receive their first dose of antibiotics within 6 hours after arrival at the hospital
Initial antibiotic selection for immunocompetent patient–ICU/ non-ICU	Immunocompetent patients with community-acquired pneumonia who receive an initial antibiotic regimen during the first 24 hours that is consistent with current guidelines
Influenza vaccination	Patients, age 50 or older, discharged during Oct, Nov, Dec, Jan, Feb, or Mar who were screened for flu vaccine status and vaccinated if indicated

Source: Joint Commission 2011a.

- **Accuracy:** The measure accurately assesses whether the evidence-based process has actually been provided. That is, the measure should be capable of judging whether the process has been delivered with sufficient effectiveness to make improved outcomes likely. . . .

- **Adverse effects:** The measure construct is designed to minimize or eliminate unintended adverse effects.

Non-accountability measures (for example, providing smoking cessation advice) are more suitable for secondary uses, such as exploration or learning within individual health care organizations and are good advice in terms of appropriate patient care." Going forward, only accountability measures will be evaluated statistically and reported on the Quality Check Web site for use in rating an organization against national experience or against other similar organizations (Joint Commission 2011b).

In addition to the activities of the Joint Commission and CMS, many other agencies and organizations contribute benchmark frameworks for use in PI activities. Please see figure 16.4 for a discussion of many of these organizations.

Figure 16.3.   Acute myocardial infarction (AMI) core measure set

Performance Measure Name	Description
Aspirin at arrival	Acute myocardial infarction (AMI) patients without aspirin contraindications who received aspirin within 24 hours before or after hospital arrival
Aspirin prescribed at discharge	AMI patients without aspirin contraindications who were prescribed aspirin at hospital discharge
ACEI or ARB for LVSD	AMI patients with left ventricular systolic dysfunction (LVSD) who are prescribed an angiotensin converting enzyme inhibitor (ACEI) or angiotensin receptor blocker (ARB) at hospital discharge. For purposes of this measure, LVSD is defined as chart documentation of a left ventricular ejection fraction (LVEF) less than 40% or a narrative description of left ventricular systolic (LVS) function consistent with moderate or severe systolic dysfunction.
Adult smoking cessation advice/ Counseling	AMI patients with a history of smoking cigarettes, who were given smoking cessation advice or counseling during hospital stay
Beta blocker prescribed at discharge	AMI patients without beta blocker contraindications who were prescribed a beta blocker at hospital discharge
Median time to fibrinolysis	Median time from arrival to administration of fibrinolytic agent in patients with ST-segment elevation or left bundle branch block (LBBB) on the electrocardiogram (ECG) performed closest to hospital arrival time
Fibrinolytic therapy received within 30 minutes of hospital arrival	AMI patients receiving fibrinolytic therapy during the hospital stay and having a time from hospital arrival to fibrinolysis of 30 minutes or less
Median time to primary PCI	Median time from arrival to primary percutaneous coronary intervention (PCI) in patients with ST-segment elevation or LBBB on the ECG performed closest to hospital arrival time
Primary PCI received within 90 minutes of hospital arrival	AMI patients receiving PCI during the hospital stay with a time from hospital arrival to PCI of 90 minutes or less
Inpatient mortality	AMI patients who expired during hospital stay
Statin prescribed at discharge	AMI patients who are prescribed a statin at hospital discharge
LDL cholesterol assessment	AMI patients with documentation of low-density lipoprotein cholesterol (LDL-c) level in the hospital record or documentation that LDL-c testing was done during the hospital stay or is planned for after discharge
Lipid-lowering therapy at discharge	AMI patients with elevated low-density lipoprotein cholesterol (LDL-c $\geq$100 mg/dL or narrative equivalent) who are prescribed a lipid-lowering medication at hospital discharge

Source: Joint Commission 2011a.

Figure 16.4.   A guide to US quality measurement organizations

With the federal government ramping up efforts to further tie healthcare reimbursement to quality of care through initiatives like value-based purchasing and accountable care organizations, quality measurement organizations are gaining more national prominence. Many organizations develop, endorse, implement, and promote performance measures. Trying to decipher and understand the interplay of organizations involved with quality measures can be challenging. The following list serves as a current guide to the country's quality improvement and measurement efforts.

Healthcare Quality Organizations

Agency for Healthcare Research and Quality (AHRQ)

http://www.ahrq.gov

AHRQ develops strategies for quality measurement and improvement by:

- Supporting more than 90 projects in a multiyear effort to improve patient safety.

- Overseeing the Patient Safety Task Force, a federal effort to integrate research, data collection, and analysis of medical errors and promote interagency collaboration in reducing the number of injuries resulting from these errors.

- Facilitating patient safety organizations (PSOs), which share the goal of improving the quality and safety of healthcare delivery. Organizations eligible to become PSOs include public or private entities, profit or not-for-profit entities, provider entities such as hospital chains, and other entities that establish special components to serve as PSOs.

By providing both privilege and confidentiality, PSOs create a secure environment where clinicians and healthcare organizations can collect, aggregate, and analyze data, thereby improving quality by identifying and reducing the risks and hazards associated with patient care.

PSOs provide hospitals, health data organizations, and states with enhanced quality assessment tools that they can use with their own hospital administrative data to highlight potential quality concerns and track changes over time in three areas: ambulatory care sensitive conditions, inpatient quality (volume, mortality, and resource use), and patient safety.

Ambulatory Care Quality Alliance (AQA)

http://www.aqaalliance.org

AQA improves healthcare quality and patient safety through a collaborative process in which key stakeholders agree on a strategy for measuring performance at the physician or group level; collecting and aggregating data in the least burdensome way; and reporting meaningful information to consumers, physicians, and other stakeholders to inform choices and improve outcomes.

Centers for Medicare and Medicaid Services (CMS)

http://www.cms.gov/QualityInitiativesGenInfo

CMS conducts a variety of quality initiatives targeting hospitals, physician offices, nursing homes, home health agencies, and end-stage renal disease facilities. Physicians and other eligible professionals can participate in the Physician Quality Reporting Initiative (PQRI), the Hospital Inpatient Quality Reporting program, and the electronic health record (EHR) meaningful use incentive program.

CMS quality measures address both Medicare and Medicaid populations. Medicaid quality and care management programs are run by state organizations, though not all states have such programs. AHRQ helps states develop quality measurement programs.

While CMS typically uses quality measures endorsed by the National Quality Forum, if a certain measure doesn't exist, CMS will develop it.

Health IT (HIT) Standards Committee Clinical Quality Workgroup

http://healthit.hhs.gov

The HIT Standards Committee serves as an advisory body to the Office of the National Coordinator for Health IT. Its Clinical Quality Workgroup makes recommendations to the committee on the quality measures that should be included in the meaningful use program and EHR certification requirements.

Figure 16.4. *(Continued)*

Hospital Quality Alliance (HQA)
http://www.hospitalqualityalliance.org
HQA improves the quality of care provided by the nation's hospitals by measuring and publicly reporting on that care. Quality performance information collected from the more than 4,000 participating hospitals is reported on Hospital Compare, a Web site tool developed by CMS.
Institute for Healthcare Improvement (IHI)
http://www.ihi.org
IHI focuses on identifying and testing new models of care to reduce waste, address healthcare disparities, and save lives. The nonprofit organization achieves these goals by promoting measureable healthcare progress. An example of its work is the IHI Improvement Map, an initiative to "help hospitals make sense of countless requirements and focus on high-leverage changes to transform care."
Institute of Medicine (IOM)
http://www.iom.edu
IOM advises the nation's public and healthcare decision makers on ways to improve health. The independent, nonprofit organization has written foundational reports focusing on quality issues that have changed healthcare, including "Crossing the Quality Chasm: A New Health System for the 21st Century," "For the Public's Health: The Role of Measurement in Action and Accountability," and "Health Professions Education: A Bridge to Quality."
Joint Commission
http://www.jointcommission.org
The Joint Commission identifies, tests, and specifies standardized performance measures. It engages in performance measurement research and development activities.
The Commission presides over a growing national comparative performance measurement database that can inform internal healthcare organization quality improvement activities, external accountability, and pay-for-performance programs and advance research.
Leapfrog Group
http://www.leapfroggroup.org
Leapfrog mobilizes employer purchasing power to promote healthcare safety, quality, and customer value and recognize improvements with rewards. Leapfrog is a voluntary program that works with employer members to encourage transparency and easy access to healthcare information as well as rewards for hospitals that have a proven record of high-quality care.
Participating hospitals can take part in Leapfrog's public reporting initiatives, which provide quality benchmarks for both healthcare providers and employer purchasers.
National Committee for Quality Assurance (NCQA)
http://web.ncqa.org
NCQA provides programs and services that reflect a straightforward formula for improvement: Measure. Analyze. Improve. Repeat. NCQA develops quality standards and performance measures for a broad range of healthcare entities. These measures and standards are the tools that organizations and individuals can use to identify opportunities for improvement.
NCQA is also the developer of the Healthcare Effectiveness Data and Information Set (HEDIS), a tool used by more than 90 percent of America's health plans to measure performance on important dimensions of care and service.

(Continued on next page)

Figure 16.4. *(Continued)*

National Committee on Vital and Health Statistics (NCVHS) Subcommittee on Quality http://www.ncvhs.hhs.gov/wg-qual.htm NCVHS assists and advises the secretary of Health and Human Services on health data, statistics, privacy, national health information policy, and the Department of Health and Human Services' strategy to address these issues. The subcommittee addresses information needs related to assessing and improving the quality of care and services and improving public access to those services and outcomes of care.
National Priorities Partnership (NPP) http://www.nationalprioritiespartnership.org NPP developed a core set of national priorities and goals that center on improving healthcare in areas of payment, public reporting, quality improvement, and consumer engagement. Its work has successfully influenced many aspects of healthcare reform in areas of patient and family engagement in healthcare and population health reporting.
National Quality Forum (NQF) http://www.qualityforum.org NQF improves the quality of American healthcare by setting national priorities and goals for performance improvement, endorsing national consensus standards for measuring and publicly reporting on performance, and promoting the attainment of national goals through education and outreach programs. NQF does not develop measures but endorses measures using a consensus standards process.
Physician Consortium for Performance Improvement (PCPI) http://www.ama-assn.org PCPI enhances quality of care and patient safety by developing, testing, and maintaining evidence-based clinical performance measures and providing measurement resources for physicians. PCPI was convened by the American Medical Association. PCPI measure development processes are viewed as a gold standard in the industry. Its 266 measures are available for 43 clinical topics and conditions, from asthma to radiology to stroke.
Premier http://www.premierinc.com An alliance of healthcare providers, Premier collects clinical and financial data from participating hospitals to establish a quality performance baseline. Web-based tools allow hospitals to use Premier's database to compare their performance in specific areas with peers and best performers, find opportunities for improvement, and track the results of their efforts. The Food and Drug Administration uses this data warehouse for drug surveillance, and CMS uses it to evaluate next-generation payment models. The Premier QUEST program uses quality measures, such as frequency of readmissions, to measure 200 participating hospitals' performance.
Quality Alliance Steering Committee (QASC) http://www.healthqualityalliance.org QASC implements measures that improve the quality and efficiency of healthcare in the United States. Made up of quality alliances and healthcare stakeholders, it developed the High-Value Health Care Project, which works to make consistent and useful information about the quality and cost of healthcare widely available to patients, physicians, hospitals, health insurers, and others who need information about healthcare delivery.

Figure 16.4. *(Continued)*

Quality Improvement Organizations (QIOs)
http://www.cms.gov/QualityImprovementOrgs
QIOs help implement CMS Medicare quality programs, support providers, and improve the quality of healthcare for Medicare consumers.
CMS contracts with one organization in each state to serve as a private, mostly not-for-profit organization. The organization is staffed by healthcare professionals trained to review medical care and help beneficiaries with complaints about the quality of care in various organizations. In part, QIOs use quality measures to help implement improvements in healthcare organizations.

Regional Extension Centers
http://healthit.hhs.gov/portal/server.pt/community/healthit_hhs_gov__rec_program/1495
Working under federal contracts, regional extension centers provide outreach and support services to eligible hospitals and eligible professionals to support adoption and meaningful use of health IT. Their work includes the use of technology to improve healthcare quality and to enable organizations to submit quality measure data to the federal government for the payment of EHR implementation incentives.

AHIMA Resources on Quality Measurement
http://www.ahima.org/advocacy/dataquality.aspx
AHIMA's Advocacy and Public Policy Web site tracks a variety of data quality management and data content issues, including quality measurement initiatives. The site offers an overview of standards and activities, resource links, and analysis.

Source: Viola and Kallem 2011.

Information Resources Management Professionals

Regardless of the configuration of a healthcare organization's technical infrastructure, the staff involved in PI activities should recognize important resources already developed within the organization, such as health information services managers, information systems managers, knowledge-based librarians, and privacy officers. These information management professionals are usually already working in the organization and possess a wealth of professional expertise that can be extremely useful in PI activities.

Information resources management professionals can assist quality improvement programs in a variety of ways. First, they can help train PI teams to utilize appropriate sources for finding data or other information regarding an improvement opportunity. They can assist the team in evaluating the quality of the data extracted from internal sources and the reliability of information retrieved from external sources. When software applications are acquired to support specific PI activities, these professionals can assist in the development of system requirements and requests for proposal. When new information technology applications are developed to track PI measures, information resources management professionals can be called on to oversee development with an organization-appropriate cost–benefit analysis.

Although much of the data and information collected, analyzed, and discussed in PI processes is "protected," as noted in chapter 21 ("Understanding the Legal Implications of Performance Improvement"), it is important to note the privacy responsibilities that the Health Insurance Portability and Accountability Act (HIPAA) places on this type of information when collateral disclosures are allowed to occur outside of formal PI structures in an organization. There may also be data-gathering situations in which protected health information (PHI) from patient, resident, or client health records is specifically matched with other data from marketing or satisfaction surveys that would require the special protection of HIPAA to be exercised. Organizational privacy officers may need to be consulted by PI teams to be sure PHI is used, stored, and disclosed appropriately to meet the requirements of federal and state laws and regulations. The privacy officers may also be of assistance in treating PI data as appropriate to their status as research versus quality improvement information, also discussed in chapter 21.

Joint Commission Information Management Standards

Effective information management for PI entails an understanding of the Joint Commission's (2011b) **information management standards.** The information management chapter of the accreditation standards was developed during the mid-1990s to focus healthcare organizations on the importance of information systems issues in the provision of high-quality patient care. Any healthcare organization that uses accreditation as a component of its PI program must ensure that it meets these standards. Even healthcare organizations that do not seek Joint Commission accreditation as a component of their PI programs would be wise to consider the standards in developing PI systems and procedures.

The Joint Commission information management standards focus on information systems issues, not on information systems. The systems implemented may be computer based or paper based. Either way, solutions to these issues must be developed and consciously implemented in healthcare organizations so that information systems can contribute properly to high-quality patient care.

Information management standards address areas in which information resources management contributes to high-quality and improved patient care. Each first-level standard is cited and followed by relevant elaboration of its intent as summarized by the Joint Commission (2011b):

IM.01.01.01 The [healthcare organization] plans for managing information.

Intent: Healthcare organizations vary in size, complexity, governance, structure, decision-making processes, and resources. Information management systems and processes vary accordingly. The [organization] bases its information management processes on a thorough analysis of internal and external information needs. The analysis considers what data and information are needed within and among departments, the medical staff, the administration, and the governing body, as well as what information is needed to support relationships with outside services, companies, and agencies. Leaders seek input from staff in a variety of areas and services.

Appropriate individuals ensure that required data and information are provided efficiently for patient care, research, education, and management at every level.

IM.01.01.03 The [healthcare organization] plans for continuity of its information management processes.

Intent: The organization has a written plan for managing interruption to its information processes whether paper-based, electronic, or a hybrid of each [that] include[s] downtime and backup procedures.

IM.02.01.01 The [healthcare organization] protects the privacy of health information.

IM.02.01.03 The [healthcare organization] maintains the security and integrity of health information.

Intent: The healthcare organization maintains the security and confidentiality of data and information and is especially careful about preserving the confidentiality of sensitive data and information. The balance between data sharing and data confidentiality is addressed. The [healthcare organization] determines the level of security and confidentiality maintained for different categories of information. Access to each category of information is based on need and defined by job title and function. Policy and procedure are developed regarding the retention and destruction of the various types of information developed and maintained by the organization.

IM.02.02.01 The [healthcare organization] effectively manages the collection of health information and retrieves, disseminates, and transmits health information in usable formats.

Intent: Standardizing terminology, definitions, vocabulary, and nomenclature facilitates comparison of data and information within and among organizations. Abbreviations and symbols are also standardized. Uniformly applied and accepted definitions, codes, classifications, and terminology support data aggregation and analysis and provide criteria for decision analysis.

IM.02.02.03 The [healthcare organization] retrieves, disseminates, and transmits health information in useful formats.

Intent: Quality control systems are used to monitor data content and collection activities and to ensure timely and economical data collection. Standardization is consistent with recognized state and federal standards. The [healthcare organization] minimizes bias in data and regularly assesses the data's reliability, validity, and accuracy. To maximize the benefits of data capture and report generation, information management processes exhibit the following characteristics: unique identification, accuracy, completeness, timeliness, interoperability, retrievability, authentication, accountability, auditability, confidentiality, and security.

IM.03.01.01 Knowledge-based information resources are available, current, and authoritative.

Intent: Knowledge-based information, often referred to as "literature," includes journal literature, reference information, and research data. . . . Knowledge-based information is authoritative and up to date. It supports clinical and management decision making, performance improvement activities, patient and family education, continuing education of staff, and research. . . . Appropriate knowledge-based information is acquired, assembled, and transmitted to users . . . [is accessible and in appropriate formats].

IM.04.01.01 The organization maintains accurate health information.

The organization has processes in place to check the accuracy of health information.

In the 2011 Joint Commission Accreditation Standards, all of the standards and elements of performance regarding documentation of patient care, treatment, and services were moved to a new chapter, "Record of Care, Treatment, and Services":

RC.01.01.01 The [healthcare organization] maintains complete and accurate medical records for each individual patient.

Intent: Information management processes provide for the use of patient-specific data and information to facilitate patient care, serve as a financial and legal record, aid in clinical research, support decision analysis, and guide professional and organizational performance improvement. Components of the complete medical record are defined. All components are specifically identified as belonging to the patient from and about whom they were collected. The information supports the patient's diagnoses, care, treatment, and services. The information supports continuity of care. If the record is composed of multiple formats, assembly of the information in all those formats is facilitated and location of all components is documented.

RC.01.02.01 Entries in the medical record are authenticated.

Intent: Only authorized individuals make entries in the medical record. Authors of each entry are identified and each authenticates his or her entry by written signature, electronic signature, rubber-stamp signature, or computer key.

RC.01.03.01 Documentation in the medical record is entered in a timely manner, including time frames for completion of all components.

RC.01.04.01 The [healthcare organization] audits its medical records.

Intent: Ongoing review of medical records is performed regularly at the point of care. Medical record delinquency is measured at regular intervals.

RC.01.05.01 The [healthcare organization] retains its medical records.

RC.02.01.01   The medical record contains information that reflects the patient's care, treatment, and services.

Intent: The medical record contains demographic information, clinical information, advance directives, consents, and record of communications with the patient. Operative or other high-risk procedures and the use of moderate or deep sedation or anesthesia are documented. Use of restraint and/or seclusion is specifically documented including orders for use, results of monitoring, and unanticipated changes in condition. There is a summary list for each patient who receives continuing ambulatory care services.

RC.02.01.03   The patient's medical record documents operative or other high-risk procedures and the use of moderate or deep sedation or anesthesia.

RC.02.01.03   For hospitals that do not use accreditation for deemed status purposes: The medical record contains documentation of the use of restraint and/or seclusion.

RC.02.01.07   The medical record contains a summary list for each patient who receives continuing ambulatory care services.

RC.02.03.07   Qualified staff receive and record verbal orders.

RC.02.04.01   The hospital documents the patient's discharge information.

Intent: In order to provide information for subsequent caregivers and facilitate continuity of care, the medical record contains a concise discharge summary, list of procedures performed, summary of care, treatment, and services provided, and information regarding home-going instructions, medications, and follow-up appointments and testing.

In addition to the information management standards and the record of care, treatment, and services standards, there are also standards regarding the use of data and information in the PI function. The 2011 edition of the Joint Commission accreditation manual cites the following standards:

PI.01.01.01   The [healthcare organization] collects data to monitor its performance.

PI.02.01.01   The [healthcare organization] compiles and analyzes data.

PI.03.01.01   The [healthcare organization] improves performance on an ongoing basis.

PI.04.01.01   The [healthcare organization] uses data from clinical/service screening indicators and human resource screening indicators to assess and continuously improve staffing effectiveness.

Each of the principal standards previously cited has multiple subdivisions that discuss and provide examples of the issues involved with the standard. PI healthcare students should remember these standards and should refer to current and future Joint Commission accreditation manuals for a more detailed discussion.

Case Study

The following excerpt is from a consultant's report on the status of information technologies at Community Hospital of the West:

Infrastructure: As is true with many organizations trying to keep up with the rapid developments in information technology, Community Hospital of the West has a variety of hardware and software that is used in its departments. Computer workstations are widely used across the organization, but in many departments the computer workstations are too old to provide an adequate platform for the later versions of software that would most effectively support departmental reporting responsibilities. There is no organization-wide local-area network in place. Software applications and versions are not standardized across the organization, and so members of different departments cannot share data and information in electronic formats. This forces members of the organization to duplicate report-generation efforts when reports contain the same or similar data. An office suite application available to users on a local-area network could help solve this problem.

The absence of a local-area network and an administrative database accessible to department managers means that reports must be prepared in the generating department, output on paper, and then input again in administrative departments to be utilized in administrative applications. An administrative database served by a network to all departments would require data to be gathered only once and then would be made available for subsequent users and purposes without redefinition or reprocessing. All of the logs that the organization currently generates, many of which are on an hourly or daily basis, could be more effectively administered and accessed if they were in electronic formats.

Organizational Knowledge of Computing Applications: Although there is broad distribution of hardware and software across the organization, organizational knowledge regarding the use of available software has not been optimized. Many of the respondents in the interviews stated that they had access to a computer workstation but had not had adequate training on using the applications. Consequently, most reporting is done without the use of software applications (some is even done on a typewriter) where the use of software could accomplish the process more effectively and efficiently. This situation is intensified because there are so many different versions of the same software being used across the organization. There is no health information management (HIM) expert to assist personnel in solving their information processing problems. Maintaining all the different versions of all the different applications is essentially impossible for information systems personnel.

Interfacing and Use of Existing Databases: Several respondents felt that access to existing databases would improve the performance of their administrative reporting activities. This issue is one that many organizations face as they try to make database information available and accessible, yet maintain data integrity and security. In particular, four of the respondents noted that they felt their productivity reporting could be more effectively accomplished if it was pulled from the payroll database. Some felt that information should be made available from financial and patient care systems and shared directly with an administrative database.

Archival of Administrative Reporting: The organization does not appear to have an archiving policy. Departmental staff decides for themselves how long they should keep reports that they generate or receive. The archival period varies widely from no archival at all to decades. Many departments receive and archive reports for which they have no use, do not know the author, and do not know the purpose. Most administrative reporting is paper based. If the organization had an administrative database, archiving many, if not all, reports could be accomplished electronically, increasing the availability, reliability, and security of administrative information for long-term use. There is no formal distinction made at this time between information that is valuable in the long term and that for short-term monitoring purposes only.

Case Study Questions

1. What issues does the consultant's report raise that may have an impact on PI activities in this facility?

2. Compare the case study situation with the Joint Commission information management standards. What issues does this analysis raise?

Summary

Because PI activities are information intensive, healthcare organizations must pay special attention to managing information resources to support improvements. Ideally, the organization would make available common business-oriented applications, such as spreadsheets and word-processing software, as well as statistical analysis and presentation packages. Many organizations make information available across the organization via intranets and archive clinical information system data permanently in data repositories, making them available for PI activities. Information resources also must allow access to national comparative data collections for organizations accredited by the Joint Commission or participating in federal Medicare or Medicaid programs. Organizations must ensure that they meet the other Joint Commission information management standards as well. Information resources management personnel, such as directors of health information services and information systems and institutional librarians with expertise in healthcare literature, also should work to support PI activities.

References

Elliott, C. 1999. Introducing the electronic health record user community. Chapter 11 in *Electronic Health Records: Changing the Vision*. Edited by Murphy, G.F., M.A. Hanken, and K. Waters. New York: W.B. Saunders.

Johns, M. 1997. *Information Management for Health Professions*. Albany, NY: Delmar.

Joint Commission. 2011a. *Specifications Manual for National Hospital Inpatient Quality Measures*. http://www.jointcommission.org/specifications_manual_for_national_hospital_inpatient_quality_measures/.

Joint Commission. 2011b. *Hospital Accreditation Standards*. Oakbrook Terrace, IL: Joint Commission Resources.

Viola, A., and C. Kallem. 2011. A guide to US quality measurement organizations. *Journal of AHIMA* 82(4):40–42.

Resources

Armoni, A., ed. 2000. *Healthcare Information Systems: Challenges of the New Millennium.* Hershey, PA: Idea Group.

Johns, M. 2001. *Information Management for Health Professions,* 2nd ed. Albany, NY: Delmar.

National Library of Medicine. http://www.ncbi.nlm.nih.gov/sites/entrez.

Shapiro, J. 2000. *Guide to Effective Healthcare Information and Management Systems and the Role of the Chief Information Officer.* Chicago: Healthcare Information Management Systems Society.

Stegwee, R., and T. Spil. 2001. *Strategies for Healthcare Information Systems.* Hershey, PA: Idea Group.

Chapter 17
Managing Healthcare Performance Improvement Projects

Learning Objectives

- To describe the function of project management in performance improvement programs

- To identify specific knowledge and skills required for team leadership

- To describe project life cycles and the group dynamics of team life cycles

- To identify the steps a team leader should follow to successfully implement and complete a project

- To describe the importance of closure with regard to reporting back to organizational leadership

Background and Significance

Initiating a performance improvement (PI) program requires a project team that will be responsible for formulating and implementing the program. Thus, to perform effectively, PI team members need to develop project management skills.

Project management is defined in a number of ways—from a narrowly focused approach with a small, task-oriented team to a much broader, organization-wide philosophy that is reflected in organizational culture, behavior, and structure. Project management as a discipline is rooted in engineering and is oriented toward quantitative application methods. Over time, project management has embraced organizational behavior as a critical element of the knowledge and skills necessary for successful implementation of a project.

PI projects in modern healthcare organizations range from small efforts involving only a few departments to larger ones that affect the organization in very significant ways. Healthcare professionals are likely to be assigned to project teams and, in some cases, may lead them.

When a PI team is formed (as discussed in chapters 1 and 3), the life cycle of the team and the project begins. Generally, the organization leadership first determines the composition of the team. Then team roles are established. The mission of the team should be developed in alignment with the organization's overall mission and vision.

Project Management and Organizational Structure

Organizational culture and structure are critical to the success of project management. Bureaucratic organizations with highly structured hierarchies are less accepting of the project management concept than is a more dynamic and flexible organization. Organizations in which employees regularly interact across organizational boundaries are more likely to be open to project management, and their employees will likely perform better on project teams.

Project Life Cycle

The length of time a project will take over its entire life cycle varies depending on the scope and size of the project. Large building projects may take months or years, but most projects will last from a few weeks to a few months. The life cycle of a project is composed of several phases; the number of phases and their definitions vary depending on who is outlining the phases and the industry involved. Most projects have between four and six phases.

A Guide to the Project Management Body of Knowledge (PMBOK® Guide), updated in 2008 by the Project Management Institute (PMI) Standards Committee, compares several life-cycle phases representative of different industries. Some experts in the field of project management have chosen to focus on a series of processes from the *PMBOK Guide* that organize project management into four life-cycle phases: initiation, planning, execution (implementation), and closure (Globerson and Zweifael 2002; Keeling 2002). These four phases are appropriate for projects in service industries such as healthcare delivery. For the sake of simplicity, these four phases are used in this chapter.

Initiation

The initiation phase begins with the determination that a gap exists between organization performance and expected outcomes. The leadership then identifies an opportunity for improvement and assesses the feasibility of the project.

Sponsorship
One or more individuals in an organization normally sponsor a project. The personal commitment a sponsor brings to a project coincides with the degree of empowerment a project manager will have. Sponsorship by top leadership, therefore, must be characterized by commitment and clear articulation of expectations.

Team Member Selection
Leadership will select members for the project team and identify any other resources needed to complete the project. Team members should be selected by identifying individuals who possess a variety of skills and expertise. If all project team members are selected

from the same department and have similar experience and skills, the team runs the risk of overlooking viable alternative solutions that might be raised by a team with more diverse experience and skills. Organizational leadership usually completes much of the initiation phase, during which preliminary definitions of the project objectives, activities, and expectations are prepared. Once formed, the team refines these processes.

Mission Statement

If a mission statement has not been articulated by leadership, the project team's first priority is to establish one at the beginning of the team's life cycle. A clear mission and vision statement will serve as a guide in the development of objectives and goals.

Project Phases and Processes

Once a project team has been formed, project management steps similar to the cycle of a team-based PI process are followed. There are seven steps in the cycle of PI team processes:

1. Identify an improvement opportunity.

2. Research and define performance expectations.

3. Design and redesign process/education.

4. Implement process/education.

5. Measure performance.

6. Document and communicate findings.

7. Analyze and compare internal and external data.

These steps parallel the phases of a project. As a project progresses through the series of steps, it moves from one phase to the next. Figure 17.1 lists the processes that occur with each of the four phases of a project.

Team Group Dynamics

Just as a project is often defined by its phases, the project team will experience a series of stages and adjustments at various times throughout the life of the project. The project team leader and members will be better prepared to complete the project if they understand the group dynamics of team development. A newly formed team will normally go through all stages of team development, regardless of how well the members know one another.

Models of team development uniformly define four stages of progression (Montebello and Buzzotta 1993):

1. *Cautious affiliation*: This is the forming stage, in which team members tend to be very polite as they get to know one another. This also is a time in which the team members assess one another's strengths and weaknesses.

2. *Competitiveness*: This is the storming stage, in which conflicts emerge. Without effective leadership and the ability to resolve conflicts, it is difficult for teams to get past this stage. They will either stay in conflict or revert to a phony politeness. Regardless of how they react, the productivity of the team is limited during this stage.

Figure 17.1. The PI process cycle

Phase	Processes (Steps)
Initiation	1. Identify a PI opportunity 2. Determine feasibility of the project 3. Define project objectives and scope 4. Select team members 5. Create vision and mission statement
Planning	6. Identify activities (tasks) the team will perform, and estimate the duration of activities 7. Develop final system requirements and criteria for standards of success 8. Develop a schedule and cost estimates 9. Perform tasks and track progress 10. Develop training plan and implementation plan
Execution (Implementation)	11. Present recommendations to leadership 12. Execute implementation plan 13. Begin training 14. Track and monitor progress 15. Revise project as needed
Closure	16. Communicate results (final report) 17. Celebrate successes 18. Continue evaluation and control and identify new opportunities for improvement

3. *Harmonious cohesiveness*: This is the norming stage, in which team members learn to communicate and collaborate. They become more focused on the task at hand. Members begin to feel as though they are a contributing part of the team. They also begin to establish rules of engagement with one another.

4. *Collaborative teamwork*: This is the performing stage, where a group of individuals begins to collaborate as a team. Team members come to understand group norms, and communication becomes more efficient and effective. In highly effective teams there is less conversation and more action. Individuals take pride in the results produced by the team.

The team leader needs to be prepared for the natural shift in dynamics of a group as it matures, and he or she must be able to facilitate team development. Team leaders should allocate time for forming, storming, norming, and performing every time the team meets (Glacel 1997). This progression of stages is not necessarily linear. Even though a team may mature to norming or performing, events may occur that cause the team to revert to storming.

Allotting a few minutes at the beginning of each meeting to "check in" can help move the team along toward greater maturity. Checking in can be as simple as asking each team member to tell the team what he or she is prepared to bring to the meeting that day. If there is a change of even one team member, the team returns to the forming stage and the progression through the four stages begins again.

Some authors add a fifth stage, called *adjourning*, to this process. Adjourning marks the dissolution of a group. If handled appropriately, it provides positive closure for the team members. This is a time to celebrate successes and recognize team member contributions and accomplishments.

Leadership

A successful team leader must possess job task competencies and behavioral competencies (Cheng et al. 2005). A technically competent individual may not necessarily be a good project team leader unless he or she also possesses behavioral competencies that enable him or her to understand team dynamics and positively influence team members. Situational leadership is a useful model for understanding and leading project teams (Hersey et al. 2000). A team leader who understands which level of maturity his or her team has reached can select an appropriate, effective leadership style. The team leader should be more task oriented and directive with newly formed groups, and more relationship oriented and supportive of team members as they mature.

The project team leader is usually an employee from a functional area of the organization who is assigned responsibility for leading the team to completion of a project. This may put the leader in a position that divides attention and loyalty between the project team and the parent organization if the vision, goals, and objectives of the two do not align. A key role for the team leader is to bring these three elements into harmony.

Planning

Organization leadership should make clear to the project team members the importance of the project and the expected impact on the organization. However, once objectives for the project are established, the team should feel free to proceed without interference from leadership. Periodic feedback through reports and briefings can be scheduled to keep leadership informed about the progress of the project. (Chapter 5 discusses meeting minutes and reports that can be effective in keeping leadership informed regarding the team's progress.)

A critical element of the planning phase is the identification of final system requirements or criteria that set standards for measuring success. Without these standards in place, determining whether a project has succeeded becomes difficult.

Design

The most important contribution that team members can make during the design phase is the development of alternative solutions. If the organizational culture truly embraces PI and problem solving, a team will be able to develop alternative solutions and work through a step-by-step process to decide which alternative provides the optimal solution.

As alternatives are developed and discussed, the cost of implementing a recommended solution should be considered. Costs should be divided into two categories: fixed and operating. Fixed costs are one-time expenses associated with buying new equipment and getting started. Operating costs are incurred to sustain the project on an ongoing basis.

Once the team decides to recommend an optimal solution, it needs to develop a schedule for implementation. This is a critical element of the planning function in project management. Planning must identify tasks, their duration, and who will be responsible for them.

Gantt Charts

An effective tool for planning and tracking the implementation of a project is the Gantt chart (discussed in chapter 7). A recent development in healthcare project management is the use of the project management methodology for planning and tracking inpatient care.

Dr. Darren Kaufman points out that each hospital admission is a one-time event and is a project that can be managed in four stages: clinical assessment, planning, scheduling, and tracking. This is particularly useful when tracking patients with multiple diagnoses. Dr. Kaufman (2005) has incorporated the use of Gantt charts similar to the chart in figure 17.3 of this text to track patients during their hospitalization.

PERT Charts

If a more quantitative approach is required, the Program Evaluation and Review Technique (PERT) may be used. This is also called Critical Path Method (CPM). The PERT technique provides a structure that requires the project team to identify the order and projected duration of activities needed to complete a project. The most helpful element of PERT is that it identifies those critical activities that must be completed on time in order for the entire project to meet its final deadline.

PERT charts depict a network of activities, represented by arrows, as shown in figure 17.2. The numbers above the arrows represent the time required to complete the activities. Duration time is usually measured in hours or days. To construct a PERT chart, the PI team must identify all activities required and determine which activities precede one another. The letters below the arrows represent the activity. The circles, ovals, or bubbles, called events, represent the beginning of an activity.

Some activities may be concurrent. These are called parallel activities. By following any path of arrows through the network from start to finish and adding the duration times of each activity, you can determine the total amount of time that series of activities will require. The path with the greatest total duration time is called the critical path and represents the longest amount of time required to complete the total project. The critical path in figure 17.2 is the sequence "a ⟶ d ⟶ g ⟶ h ⟶ i," which will require 23 days. Both PERT and Gantt charts require the planner to identify critical tasks, the duration of each task, and the expected completion dates. This scheduling process must consider those tasks that must be performed in order to complete the project at the proposed time, as well as the duration of each critical task. The costs associated with the tasks and the resources needed to complete them must also be considered. Within the critical path, noncritical tasks may be scheduled as resources to accomplish them become available and as their prerequisite tasks are completed.

Figure 17.2. PERT chart

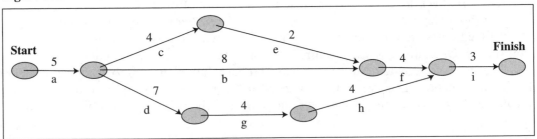

Execution

Once project planning is completed, execution (or implementation) begins. This is where installation of equipment or construction begins, and any policy or procedure manuals should be prepared for distribution. Specifications developed in the design (planning) phase should be finalized. Any new systems or processes should be tested for performance.

Individuals involved in implementation and continued operation of a new or reorganized system need training. Thus, the implementation plan should include training and identify who will be trained. The training portion of the implementation plan should identify the content of the training, training objectives, and expected outcomes. If any QI toolbox techniques are to be implemented, they should be part of the training plan.

Execution of "a project has milestones, and to achieve these milestones we must commit resources to certain tasks to achieve certain predefined goals (scope); many of these tasks will be related (dependencies) and to complete tasks we will often need to overcome obstacles (risks) in a timely manner" (Gunasekaran 2008). There are, however, some techniques that can help make the execution of the project plan go as smoothly as possible.

First, define the critical success criteria for each phase. This means identifying and defining the processes, products, and outcomes of each phase of the project plan that need to be accomplished in order to actually know that a phase is complete and operational. Processes are those actions that people take to make the project actually run. Products are those tangible or intangible outputs that the project produces from the work of its processes and personnel, and are defined by the nature of the project undertaken. Outcomes are those elements of change in an organization and its constituent parts that result from undertaking the project.

Second, organize the work on a weekly and monthly basis. "Organizations as a whole can manage change efforts at a monthly level. The project plan should be developed with a monthly milestone discipline that can be communicated and managed with [organizational] leadership. Once the . . . leadership is engaged with the key monthly milestones, they can assist in work prioritization and ensure key deliverables are completed. The project team, however, must have weekly milestones to complete project tasks so that work can be adjusted on a weekly basis to ensure monthly milestones are met" (Gunasekaran 2008). Often, one will see project managers distribute two- and three-year Gantt charts representing the milestones that the project must allegedly meet in order to be successful in the allotted organizational time frame. However, few individuals in an organization are truly able to relate to this kind of presentation on a day-to-day basis. They need to know what they need to accomplish each week and each month in order to keep the project moving, particularly when the project is large enough to last several years. Project managers who want to keep their teams focused and motivated need to chunk the project objectives into smaller windows of time in order for the team members involved to understand what is expected and then really make it happen. Remember that old adage "How do you eat an elephant? . . . One bite at a time!"

Third, make the project calendar public. "It is crucial that all levels of . . . leadership have access to the project timeline with monthly milestone details. This will allow the leadership to better understand the implementation and allow them to better plan their other operational decisions and activities. On the project team, make the project plan and weekly work assignments of all team members available to the entire team. This will promote greater visibility and critical thinking by the project team about the work" (Gunasekaran 2008). It also allows everyone on the team to see how their contributions dovetail with everyone else's assignments and how crucial their responsible participation really is.

Fourth, standardize status reporting for the entire organization. "A well-designed status report can help move a project forward more rapidly than any other project activity. When [organizational and project] leadership are empowered with specific, practical knowledge of what needs to be done, significant organizational obstacles can be overcome. The key to the status report is to tailor it [to] the appropriate audience with the appropriate level of detail to help the reader become informed and take action. For [organizational] leadership, this should be tied to the monthly milestones and should follow a twice-a-month frequency. . . . Within the [project leadership], status reports should be weekly" (Gunasekaran 2008).

Fifth, manage resource conflicts. Critical path PERT charts can assist in determining what development or phase of a project needs to be completed before another development or phase. But that is just the first step because, sometimes, different phases require the same resources in order to reach completion. Resources may be such things as the attendance of highly specialized personnel like electricians or programmers, whose expertise is rare and exclusive, or they may be physical equipment that takes a long process or time period to acquire. Alternately, they may be physical spaces or buildings that have to be remodeled before they can be used for the project. Remember, when an organization modifies physical resources, it also must leave time and money to meet local and state regulatory requirements and acquire permits, adding more time to the entire process. In any of these cases, management of project timelines is crucial to a project's success. Managing the project calendar and schedule ensures that criteria are successfully accomplished on a weekly as well as a project-wide basis.

Measurement Techniques

A number of the QI toolbox techniques discussed throughout part II of this text can be used to measure performance continuously and to evaluate the success or failure of newly implemented processes or systems. The charts and graphs discussed in chapter 4 are useful for organizing collected data into a meaningful presentation when providing feedback to organizational leadership.

Measurement should also be undertaken on a weekly and monthly basis against the project calendar discussed in the preceding section. It may be as simple as checking off the success criteria as they are accomplished on a weekly or monthly basis, or it may turn to more sophisticated techniques such as run charts as the project actually gears up and begins functioning as it was (or was not) designed to function.

Closure

In closure, stage four of project management, the new system or process is used by the customer. This is the phase in which the project shifts to become an integrated part of organizational operations. During the operational phase, management must continually monitor performance and determine whether the new system or process meets established performance criteria.

Evaluation and Control

As a project shifts from planning to execution to closure, testing performance results against finalized standards must not be ignored. Too often this is where the organization becomes distracted with other issues or new events and does not follow up on the success or failure of the project. This is one reason a project fails.

The project becomes the standard way of doing things in the closure phase. Team members return to their functional roles or move on to newly assigned roles if the project is one that changes their old functional roles. This is the phase in which the lessons learned are cataloged and documented. As the established project continues, it must be evaluated continually to determine whether performance is meeting established criteria and standards. During the process of evaluating results and outcomes, the organization looks for new improvement and innovation opportunities. When a new PI opportunity is identified, a new project is initiated.

Real-Life Example

In the aftermath of September 11, 2001, the Joint Commission broadened accreditation requirements to include specific plans for response to bioterrorism. The Centers for Disease Control and Prevention, Health Resources and Services Administration, and the Department of Homeland Security have been working together to ensure that state and local health departments, hospitals, and other health agencies are able to mount a collective response to bioterrorism events.

A 150-bed community hospital, located approximately 35 miles from a large medical center in another county, has been approached by the county health officer to develop a bioterrorism response plan. Although the hospital has conducted annual disaster drills in compliance with previous Joint Commission standards, the drills were mass casualty exercises based on the scenario of a major fire in an industrial setting, natural disasters, or a transportation accident involving large numbers of injured patients. Previous exercises did not address exposure of large numbers of patients to biological or chemical agents due to a terrorist act.

The hospital administrator and the county health officer agree that there is a need to enhance and broaden the scope of disaster planning to include issues that would require significant decontamination of patients or strict quarantine of patients exposed to biological or chemical agents. The hospital administrator has agreed to appoint a project team that will work with the county health officer to expand the existing disaster plan to include bioterrorism threats.

The county health officer has authorization to spend funds from the Department of Homeland Security to purchase supplies and equipment that the hospital would need in the event of an attack. This includes items such as decontamination equipment and personal protective equipment for hospital personnel assigned to bioterrorist response teams. To qualify for the funds, the hospital must coordinate with county health officer and develop a plan for responding to a bioterrorist attack using the framework developed by Homeland Security, called the National Incident Management System (NIMS), adoption of which is a condition for federal preparedness assistance and funding. For years, the hospital had been using the Incident Command System to orchestrate a response to local disaster situations, but now, the response plan needs to be broadened to work with multiple agencies in the region to manage the possibly dispersed nature of a biochemical terrorist event.

Because federal funding is involved, the plan must be complete and in place within 12 weeks or the funds will be withdrawn and reallocated to other regions of the country. The hospital is scheduled for a Joint Commission survey in about 9 months, an additional incentive to complete the project in a timely manner.

During the initiation phase of the project, the hospital administrator and the county health officer agree upon the mission to develop an implementation plan for policies and procedures that prepare the hospital to effectively respond to an external bioterrorist attack involving biological or chemical agents. The combination of individuals selected for the hospital project team is based on ensuring that all of the required components of the Incident Command System under unified command are represented. The hospital administrator has decided to appoint the director of emergency services as the hospital project team leader. The team leader will be expected to work closely with the county health officer along with the leadership of fire, police, EMS, and public works agencies in directing the team's activities. The county health officer will be the overall coordinator of the regional multidisciplinary project team. Under a unified command, agencies will work together through the designated members to analyze intelligence information and establish a common set of objectives and strategies for a single Incident Action Plan. In the case of a real bioterrorism event, it would be likely that the director of emergency services would fill the roll of operations section chief for hospital incident activities.

The director of health information services is selected to represent the functions of the public information officer (PIO). The PIO is responsible for interfacing with the public and the media and with other agencies and organizations with incident-related information requirements. The PIO develops accurate and complete information on the incident's cause, size, current situation, and other matters of general interest for both internal and external consumption.

The infection control nurse's activities become even more important in a bioterrorist attack in collecting data and training staff on procedures that will control further spread of disease and illness from a patient infected by a biological agent. The infection control nurse is selected for the project team to support the operations section chief with technical information and processes for handling the bioterrorism event.

The director of physical facilities, in support of the operations section chief, is responsible for ensuring that portable decontamination tents and other equipment can be unstored and deployed efficiently in the case of a real event. He or she also must be able to effectively control heating, ventilation, and air conditioning systems that can be shut down and secured in the event of a bioterrorist threat to the hospital's internal environment from contaminants floating in the external air.

Finally, the director of materials management is selected for the team to represent the Logistics Section, responsible for all support requirements, including communications support, medical support to incident personnel, food for incident personnel, and supplies and ground support.

As part of the initiation phase, the hospital administrator brings the selected members of the project team together for orientation. At this point, the planning phase begins. The team will meet to brainstorm and identify problems. Figure 17.3 is a Gantt chart that

Figure 17.3. Gantt chart depicting four phases of a project

Phase / Tasks	Responsible Parties	1	2	3	4	5	6	7	8	9	10	11	12
Initiation		◀━━━━▶											
First meeting of team leaders	Hospital administrator and county health officer	▼											
Mission statement	Hospital administrator	━━											
Team member selection and appointment of team leader	Hospital administrator		━━										
Team orientation meeting	County health officer			▼									
Planning				◀━━━━━━▶									
Planning meeting to brainstorm and identify problem(s)	Emergency services		▼										
Assign individual tasks	Emergency services		▼										
FEMA coordination planning	County health officer				━━━━━━━━								
Admission and medical information management	Health information				━━━━								
Equipment storage and access	Physical facilities				━━━━								
Infection management	Infection control				━━━━								
Identify locations suitable for patients	Physical facilities and nursing				━━━━								
HVAC issues	Physical facilities				━━━━								
Media management	Public affairs				━━━━								
Develop training plan	Emergency services					━━━━━━							
Execution									◀━━━━━━▶				
Collect team input and write the final plan	All team members								━━━				
Training	All team members								━━━━━━				
Closure												◀━━▶	
Submit plan for federal funding												▼	
Rehearsal exercise	All team members and hospital staff											▼	
Prepare and submit final report	Emergency services												━━▼
Begin ongoing evaluation													▼

depicts the four phases of the project and the tasks to be accomplished in each phase. In the planning phase, the subtasks are assigned to individual team members based on their areas of expertise and responsibility.

As team members bring information and expertise back to the team, the plan begins to take shape and the team prepares to move into the execution phase. The predominant tasks of the execution phase are writing the final draft of the plan and training staff in preparation for future exercises and the possibility of an actual terrorist attack.

During the last phase, closure, the team and hospital leadership evaluate the results of the project. The rehearsal exercise will be documented so that the lessons learned can be applied to opportunities for continued improvement and demonstrate to the Joint Commission surveyors that an annual exercise meeting the new standards has been conducted.

Why Projects Fail

The Center for Project Management (n.d.) has published the seven deadly sins of project failure on its Web site:

1. Mistaking half-baked ideas for viable projects
2. Dictating unrealistic project deadlines
3. Assigning underskilled project managers to highly complex projects
4. Not ensuring solid business sponsorship
5. Not monitoring project vital signs
6. Failing to develop a robust project process architecture
7. Not establishing a comprehensive project portfolio

Some of the sins are self-explanatory. Failing to secure solid business sponsorship places responsibility squarely on an organization's senior leadership. As mentioned earlier, executive-level commitment and support of a project are critical to its success. Without the backing of leadership, implementing a new project will be difficult, if not impossible, because of the natural resistance to change that occurs in most organizations.

Developing a viable project process shows that the organization has developed guidelines for standardized and repeatable processes of beginning and completing projects. Project team leaders should not have to start from scratch with each new project. A comprehensive project portfolio consists of a set of files organized into at least six areas that leadership and project team leaders are able to reference. The portfolio should include a file of ideas, charters (or proposed projects), projects in execution, completed projects, suspended projects, and canceled projects. With this collection of information, a project manager can compare his or her project with past successes and failures and other activities going on throughout the organization.

It is just as important to plan and organize a team for success as it is to avoid those things that lead to failure. Following is a list of six key steps that can lead to a winning strategy:

1. Organize for success.

   Again, the problem must be defined specifically before any project planning occurs. This should be addressed as part of the project planning.

2. Create a project plan.

3.   Develop a means to track performance against the plan.

4.   Implement the plan.

5.   Train and retrain, if necessary.

6.   Anticipate and prepare for the culture shock associated with change (Zimmer 1999).

Getting organized and having a well-conceived plan in place are essential. To find out whether the project is progressing satisfactorily, the team needs to implement a monitoring system that measures success criteria against outcomes.

The last step cannot be ignored. It is a natural force in humans and organizations to initially resist change. Leadership must be prepared to effectively counter resistance and continue the process of implementation and improvement.

As mentioned earlier in this chapter, some organizations are more receptive to change than others. The organization's leadership, project sponsors, and team members must champion the project and be persistent in seeing it through to full implementation.

Case Study

A community health clinic located in a city of 250,000 provides the bulk of Medicaid and homeless care to the community. The clinic maintains approximately 27,000 active health records and has a staff of 90 employees. The professional clinical staff includes five family practice physicians, seven physician's assistants, and four clinical nurse-practitioners.

The clinic management was recently notified that it is eligible to receive funding to convert its existing computer systems to a new integrated system that includes electronic health records. Until this point, all records have been paper, and records' tracking throughout the clinic has been manual. Billing and financial management processes have been maintained on separate systems. Clinic appointments were maintained on another system. The office applications consisted of outdated word-processing and spreadsheet software. The database software was not integrated with other software.

The proposal for the new integrated system includes office management applications such as word processing, spreadsheets, database, presentation, e-mail, patient appointment scheduling, computer-based health records, billing, and financial management software. Laboratory specimens are sent out to a reference lab located at the county hospital. The lab has expressed interest in linking its lab results software to the new integrated system via its intranet. The lab manager indicates that the results can be transmitted in a format compatible with any relational database.

The administrative and clinical support employees are fairly stable, with an average personnel turnover rate of 8 percent and an average longevity of five years. The physicians on staff have only been with the clinic from six months to three years. The chief executive officer (CEO) has given the director of health information management the task of managing a project to convert existing systems to the new information management system.

Money available for the transition must be spent by the end of the fiscal year; there are 10 months left. The CEO also has indicated that all existing health records need to be scanned and loaded into the new system and expects to see this completed within the next two years.

Case Study Questions

1. Up to seven representatives from different departments can serve on the multidisciplinary project team. Prepare a list of types of individuals you would want to serve on this project team.

2. What departmental areas of the healthcare organization should be represented?

3. What specific skills, knowledge, and expertise should team members possess?

4. Draft a timeline showing the major phases of the project and the key tasks for each phase.

Project Application

The Microsoft Project (2010) provides information and demonstrates how to set up a project schedule and track its progress.

Other Web resources are available through searches using key words such as "timeline" or "project management" that provide access to tools such as Gantt and PERT charts.

Type the search words "project management software" or "timeline" into an Internet search engine. Explore and develop a list of sources that provide software for managing a project.

Review how you may apply project management methods to group projects in class or in the workplace.

Summary

Effective project management requires an understanding of the four phases a project team goes through in the life cycle of a project: initiation, planning, execution (or implementation), and closure. During each of the phases, the team completes a logical series of processes that are similar to the steps of the PI team process presented in chapter 1. Organizational behavior and group dynamics play an important role in the success or failure of a project. Commitment and support from organizational leadership also is critical to project completion and success.

References

Center for Project Management. n.d. http://www.center4pm.com.

Cheng, M., A. Dainty, and D.R. Moore. 2005. What makes a good project manager? *Human Resource Management Journal* 15(1):25.

Glacel, B.P. 1997. Teamwork's top ten lead to quality. *Journal for Quality and Participation* 20(1):12–16.

Globerson, S., and O. Zweifael. 2002. The impact of the project manager on the project management planning process. *Project Management Journal* 33(3):58–64.

Gunasekaran, S. 2008. Transformation diary. *Healthcare Informatics* 25(2):88.

Hersey, P., K.H. Blanchard, and D. Johnson. 2000. *Management of Organizational Behavior: Leading Human Resources*, 8th ed. Englewood Cliffs, NJ: Prentice-Hall.

Kaufman, D.S. 2005. Using project management methodology to plan and track inpatient care. *Joint Commission Journal on Quality and Patient Safety* 31(8):463–468.

Keeling, R. 2002. *Project Management: An International Perspective*. New York: St. Martin's Press.

Microsoft Project. 2010. http://www.microsoft.com/project/en/us/project-professional-2010.aspx.

Montebello, A.R., and V.R. Buzzotta. 1993. Work teams that work. *Training and Development* 47(3):59.

Project Management Institute. 2008. *A Guide to the Project Management Body of Knowledge*, 4th ed. Newtown Square, PA: Project Management Institute.

Zimmer, B.T. 1999. Project management: A methodology for success. *Hospital Material Management Quarterly* 21(2):83–89.

Resources

Ash, T. 1998. Seven reasons why Internet projects fail. *UNIX Review's Performance Computing* 16(11):15.

Federal Emergency Management Agency. 2011. Emergency Management Institute. http://training.fema.gov/EMI/.

Kerzner, H. 2009. *Project Management: A Systems Approach to Planning, Scheduling and Controlling*, 10th ed. New York: John Wiley & Sons.

Seidl, P. 2010. Project management. Chapter 26 in *Health Information Management: Concepts, Principles, and Practice*. Edited by LaTour, K.M., and S. Eichenwald, 3rd ed. Chicago: AHIMA.

Chapter 18
Managing the Human Side of Change

Learning Objectives

- To apply change management techniques to implement performance improvements
- To describe the three phases of change
- To identify key steps in change management

Key Term

Change management

Background and Significance

In today's world, there is no such thing as permanent stability. The processes and structures that worked last year may be ineffective this year. The products and services that are considered cutting edge quickly become obsolete. Similarly, healthcare delivery in the United States has been in a state of rapid and unpredictable evolution ever since the Medicare and Medicaid programs were implemented in the 1970s and the prospective payment system (PPS) was instituted in the 1980s.

The overarching reason for change in healthcare organizations today is the need to improve the quality of care while at the same time controlling the cost of services. Hospitals and other healthcare organizations have institutionalized performance improvement (PI) programs to meet this need. Systems, processes, and staff competencies undergo a circular cycle of change as improvements are made in the clinical, administrative, and governance areas of the organization.

PI is based on the quantitative analysis of data, processes, and structures, but PI efforts also have a very human side. After all, healthcare is provided by individuals working in extremely complex organizations, not by robots that can be reprogrammed or replaced when change is needed. Failure to consider the human side of PI and the impact of change can derail even the best-conceived improvement efforts.

Healthcare professionals have always understood the importance of what they do. Today, during an era of dramatic and ongoing change, most clinical and allied health professionals strive to improve patient care services and outcomes. In this era of rapid change in healthcare, we see a proliferation of "disruptive technologies and business models that may threaten the status quo but will ultimately raise the quality of care for everyone" (Christensen et al. 2000, 104). Still, most employees find it difficult to alter their work habits, and healthcare professionals are no exception.

The Three Phases of Change

Every change that affects individuals is experienced in three phases. Whether changing their dietary habits or the way they write a patient care plan, all individuals go through a similar process. In his research on human reaction to change, Kurt Lewin (1951) calls the three phases *unfreezing*, *changing*, and *refreezing*. Lewin observed that during each of these basic phases, forces in favor of change and forces that resist change work against each other. The analysis of such competing forces in the face of a particular planned change is often called a *force-field analysis*. These phases also have been referred to as *ending*, *transition*, and *beginning*. The ending phase is characterized by grief and letting go. The transition phase is characterized by confusion and creativity. The beginning phase is characterized by acceptance and hope for the future.

The three phases of change are not clear-cut steps. Rather, they overlap one another. At any particular point, one of these phases is likely to predominate, while the emotions and concerns associated with the other two phases fall to the background. The movement is gradual as one phase gives way to the next.

Grief is a natural human reaction to loss of any kind. Simply defined, grief is the conflicting feelings that come along with the end of something familiar or a change in an accepted pattern of behavior. Before individuals can go on to a new beginning, they need to let go of their old identity or their old way of doing things. According to William Bridges (2003), "the failure to identify and be ready for the endings and losses that change produces is the largest single problem that organizations [and individuals] in transition encounter. The organization institutes a quality improvement program, and no one foresees how many people will experience the 'improvements' as a loss of something related to their job."

Like change, grief occurs in stages. Some propose that the process consists of three stages: shock, despair, and recovery. Still others posit that the process includes four stages—denial, resistance, adaptation, and recovery (Kreitzer 1998). Whatever the number and names of the different stages, it is clear that a transformation in thinking and perception must occur.

Between the ending of the old and the beginning of the new lies a transitional zone. This transitional period is experienced regardless of the desire to change or whether the perception of the change is good or bad. The transitional phase is unsettling and uncomfortable. Individuals often report feeling confusion, anxiety, and unsteadiness in the midst of change. The old way of doing things is gone, but the new way of doing things still feels untried and uncomfortable.

Left to their own thoughts and feelings and without sufficient information during this phase of organizational change, individuals may decide to escape their discomfort and confusion by leaving the organization. When the change process is understood, however, the transitional period can be a time of renewal and creativity. Often certain individuals within a larger group are optimistic about change. Their enthusiasm is contagious, and a wise organization will recognize and capitalize on such individuals to infuse their optimistic attitude into groups and departments to build positive momentum for change (Blancett and Flarey 1998).

During the final phase of change, the beginning of the new way of doing things, the people who make up the organization settle into a more comfortable state. The new processes or staff structures become familiar, and individuals come to understand and accept their new roles. Some may still worry that the new way of doing things may not work or that it may even make things worse. Some may feel last regrets about the ideas or coworkers they had to leave behind. Some may even miss the freedom of the transitional zone and find settling back into a routine rather boring. A beginning also can be a disappointing time when changes seem to have been made for no discernible reason. Still, eventually, the new way of doing things becomes the accepted way. The unfamiliar new task often becomes automatic within the cycle of change:

> Whenever people learn something sufficiently well, they cease to be aware of it. When you look at a street sign, for example, you absorb its information without consciously performing the act of reading. Computer scientist, economist, and Nobelist Herb Simon calls this phenomenon "compiling"; philosopher Michael Polanyi calls it the "tacit dimension"; psychologist T.K. Gibson calls it "visual invariants"; philosophers Hans-Georg Gadamer and Martin Heidegger call it "the horizon" and the "ready-to-hand"; John Seely Brown [. . .] calls it the "periphery." All say, in essence, that only when things disappear in this way are we freed to use them without thinking and so to focus beyond them on new goals. (Weiser 1991)

Any organization, and especially a large healthcare organization, thrives when operating with established structures and processes. And when change is necessary, effective management of the phases of change enables an organization to successfully weather the transition.

Change Management

Like PI, change can be thought of as a process to be understood and managed. For the purposes of this chapter, **change management** can be defined as a group of techniques that help individuals understand the process of change and accept PI in work processes. One or more members of the PI team may become change manager(s) for the project, or a manager in the areas affected by the change may play this role. Many organizations hire consultants to handle the change management process when the planned changes will have a significant impact on employees and medical staff.

The steps in the process of change management are as follows:

1. Identifying the losses
2. Acknowledging the losses

3. Providing information and asking for feedback

4. Marking the endings

5. Managing the transition

6. Clarifying and reinforcing the beginning

7. Celebrating the successes

Nothing is as crucial for ensuring the success of a change plan as effective education and communication about change management. Often the best strategy for change is preparation. Training often gets overlooked or is not well planned. It is a good idea to educate your team on the principles of change management. This will better prepare them for the reactions of others to change and equip them with the skills to appropriately handle these reactions (Amatayakul 1999).

At Norton Healthcare in Louisville, Kentucky, Chief Information Officer Marilynn Black (2003) reported that during a time of heavy transition, the organization realized that communication and training were the keys to success. As the organization prepared to unroll an electronic health record system project titled "Carelink" at two hospitals, it appropriately managed the change process in the following ways:

- Educating leadership regarding the dependency of information technology (IT) project success on appropriate change management

- Establishing ownership and accountability of organization-wide operational leadership for the project early in the process

- Creating a steering committee composed of operational leaders from functional areas impacted by Carelink to govern implementation and identify and discuss operational risks

- Creating a vision and project management structure to support the change

- Creating a go-live plan to support the late adopters

- Building a training program to support the change

Furthermore, leaders at Norton Healthcare wholeheartedly embraced the task of training staff by doing the following:

- Implementing a variety of communication techniques to prepare staff and managers in a countdown to the day of transition

- Creating a job-specific training curriculum

- Constructing a learning center

- Constructing a training morale package of materials for staff to review

By all accounts, the transition was successful and went smoothly, thanks to the forethought and planning of leaders and to their attention to change management best practices.

Identifying the Losses

When a PI project is still in the planning stage, identifying the losses that will result from changes that need to be made may be difficult, especially if the change affects more than one area of the organization. The PI team should describe the proposed improvement in as much detail as possible. Using flow charts to map out processes may help the team identify all of the areas that will be involved. Changes made in one area may create the need for secondary changes in other areas. The task of the PI team is to identify all of the people who will need to let go of a current way of doing things before an improvement can be implemented. The team also needs to determine exactly what will need to come to an end for the project to be successful.

Identifying the losses after the improvement has been implemented is much easier. The PI team or change manager for the project need only ask affected people questions such as, "What is different for you now?" or "What don't you do anymore now that you used to do?" It is important to remember that no new process or structure can be implemented until its predecessor has ended. Ideally, identifying and acknowledging the losses necessitated by a change should come before the change is implemented, but the ending phase will happen whether it is planned for or not.

Acknowledging the Losses

Depending on the extent of the changes to be made, representatives of the PI team, department managers, or senior executives should explain the planned changes to the people who will be affected. The change manager should be prepared to accept and acknowledge the reactions that result, even if they seem like overreactions.

According to Susan Helbig (2003, 67), "how you frame your message is key to garnering interest, support or a firm commitment from various stakeholders." Even among those communicating in this way with staff, there are different roles for different purposes. Messengers simply provide information about the change. Advocates garner enthusiasm for change. Change agents manage the process and are available to answer more detailed questions. Each of these roles should be used at the appropriate time in the change process (Helbig 2003).

When endings take place, people may feel angry, sad, anxious, confused, or depressed. All of these feelings are normal reactions to loss. Allowing people to express their emotions openly is difficult but critical to success. Sometimes, even minor changes may become symbols of much more comprehensive changes that took place in the past but were never fully acknowledged. Minor changes also may be treated as harbingers of more drastic changes in the future. For example, a process redesign that will result in the elimination of one staff position may be seen by employees as the first of many layoffs to come. The key to effectively handling this step in the change management process is active listening: Ask questions about how people feel, and acknowledge the legitimacy of those emotions.

Providing Information and Asking for Feedback

The timing and content of communications should be carefully planned in advance as an element of project design. It is crucial that the proposed changes be described in specific detail early in the PI process. If people do not understand the purpose of a change, they will have difficulty accepting it. If they are not sure what the change will entail, they will come to their own conclusions about which processes will end and which will continue. If they are not told how the change will affect them, they may assume the worst.

The PI team or its representative must provide as much information as possible to the people who will be affected directly by the proposed change. Withholding information may lead to intense speculation about the changes to come, and such speculations often create feelings of helplessness and anger. Although some information may need to remain confidential, the change manager should never fabricate answers to questions that he or she cannot answer fully. Rather, the manager should acknowledge the questions and provide as much information as possible. Glossing over the potentially negative aspects of the change only creates mistrust.

Information about the change project should be communicated consistently and often. Repeating the information in a variety of ways will help people accept the change. Newsletters, special announcements, staff meetings, and other forms of communication can all be used to convey the message. The people affected by the change also should be kept up to date as proposed changes are developed, and they should be given an opportunity to provide feedback to the PI team.

The PI team should be sure to seek feedback during every critical stage of the project. They should ask for information about the concerns of stakeholders early in the project design phase. During testing, stakeholders should be asked for feedback on what is working well and what is not, and they should be directly involved in creating a detailed plan for implementation. During implementation, the people who apply the change should be asked to suggest refinements and improvements. After the project is complete, they should be asked to provide feedback on whether the goals of the project were met.

Marking the Endings

Actions always speak louder than words. The change manager should find some method to mark the ending of the old way of doing things. Removing old paper chart storage equipment in an organization that has transitioned to an electronic health record marks a symbolic end to the old way.

Managers sometimes make the mistake of criticizing the way things were done in the past as a way of introducing improvements. Creating negative pictures of the past is not effective. Instead, the past should be honored for the positive things accomplished and for the foundations laid for the future.

Managing the Transition

The length of the transitional period between old and new depends on the extent of the changes to be implemented. Obviously, the restructuring of a whole organization would require a much longer transition than the installation of a document imaging system. However, both would require that people become accustomed to a new way of doing things. In the first case, everyone in the organization would be affected, from clinical staff to administrative staff and nurses to health information managers. The installation of a new piece of diagnostic equipment, however, might affect only a small number of people. The technicians using the equipment would be affected most directly, but the change also might affect the nursing staff, the patient transport staff, and the medical staff working in that specialty area.

The transitional period is a difficult time for everyone. Productivity is likely to diminish as energy levels fall and people feel unsure of themselves and of the systems on which they depend to accomplish their work. Old resentments may resurface, and staff turnover may increase. During any transition, people tend to oppose the change, endorse the change, or reserve judgment. Interpersonal or interdepartmental conflict may result. Things can feel out of control and chaotic, and people may dread going to work.

The change manager's task is to help people understand that chaos is a necessary and normal part of change. It is during this period that people learn new skills, redefine their roles, and work through their questions about the new processes or structures to be implemented. Creative solutions to unforeseen problems are devised, and new relationships are forged. Special training in creative problem solving and team building may be helpful during this period.

The change manager also needs to ensure that nothing falls between the cracks. Temporary systems may be needed to maintain operations. For example, interim team leaders may be assigned to handle staff scheduling, or temporary record-handling procedures may be instituted during the transition between a paper-based and a computer-based health record system.

Above all, the change manager must keep the channels of communication open. Information about the progress of the project and the problems encountered during implementation must be shared among the areas affected, the PI team, and senior management. New policies and procedures should be developed, and position descriptions should be revised. Change managers may find it helpful to use storyboards to document and explain the improvements being made.

The purpose of the change or the problem that required resolution should be explained and repeated in every communication during the transitional period. The people affected by the change also should be involved in the development of a step-by-step plan for phasing in the new process. The plan should spell out the role that each individual is to play during the transition and after the new system has been fully implemented. The plan also should establish and communicate realistic target dates. As progress is made toward target goals, public acknowledgment is helpful for building positive momentum. Newsletters, group announcements, and posters all work well to accomplish this.

Clarifying and Reinforcing the Beginning

The arrival of a new manager, the installation of new equipment, or the move to new offices marks the beginning of long transitional processes. Before a beginning can be successful, the people affected by the change must go through both an ending and a transition. A true beginning confirms the end of the old way of doing things.

The PI team, the change manager, and other decision makers in the organization need to reinforce new beginnings on every level. Nothing will doom a change effort more quickly than conflicting messages. For example, an improvement that involves changing from traditional directive management to a self-managed team will not succeed unless the employees are delegated the authority to make decisions. If the former department manager continues to make every important decision, other people on the team will revert to silence.

Similarly, customer service initiatives will not survive if senior managers emphasize cost cutting over quality in their communications to staff.

Celebrating the Successes

People use ceremonies to mark beginnings as well as endings. The change manager should find a way to help people celebrate their successes in making meaningful changes in the way they perform their work. A ribbon-cutting ceremony at a new facility, an open house for a reorganized department, and a demonstration of new equipment for colleagues outside the department are some examples of celebrations that mark new beginnings. Even the accomplishment of a minor procedural improvement should be acknowledged with a sincere thank-you to all people involved in conceiving, planning, and implementing the change.

Case Study

Faced with rising costs and declining revenues, the board of directors for a community hospital located in a large East Coast city decided to combine its obstetrics and pediatrics units. The obstetrics service was located in the oldest part of the facility, and the labor and delivery rooms were cramped and inefficient. A large medical center nearby offered comfortable, family-centered accommodations and state-of-the-art equipment.

As a result of the more state-of-the-art equipment at the large medical center, several obstetricians had recently moved their practices from the community hospital to the medical center. The board was reluctant to discontinue obstetrics services, because the hospital had a long history of providing maternity care to the surrounding community. However, overhead costs for the underutilized and obsolete unit were skyrocketing, and the cost of replacing the unit was prohibitive.

The pediatrics unit, in contrast, was housed in the newest wing of the hospital. The hospital's emergency department was one of only two in the city equipped to provide pediatric trauma services, and a number of patients were admitted to the service through the emergency department. In addition, a large physician group that specialized in pediatric oncology admitted hundreds of patients to the facility each year. The physician group was recognized nationwide and handled referrals from pediatricians throughout a four-state area.

The consolidation of services made sense to the board on several levels. From a cost-control perspective, closing the obsolete facility would save the hospital millions of dollars in renovation expenses. The consolidation also made sense from a patient care point of view. Expectant mothers who were known to have high-risk pregnancies could plan to deliver their babies at a facility that specialized in treating pediatric patients. In addition, the head of the obstetrics unit was scheduled to retire soon, and the board saw an opportunity to make significant changes in the clinical area. The board believed that the obstetrics service should change its focus from handling routine deliveries to handling high-risk pregnancies and thus overcome the competitive disadvantage the hospital now faced when compared with the medical center. The board voted to seek funding for a new center of excellence for the care of high-risk mothers and newborns.

Combining the two units will require fundamental changes, as the units are managed in very different ways. The department head of the obstetrics unit is a traditionalist, and the obstetrics staff is accustomed to deferring to his judgment when problems arise. By contrast, the department head of the pediatrics unit believes in self-managed work teams, and her unit is structured into cross-functional teams with independent decision-making authority. There are other obvious differences as well: one unit treats adults and the other treats children. One unit treats women who stay in the unit for a day or two at most, while the other treats infants, children, and adolescents for conditions that require complex treatment regimens and long hospital stays. Parents often sleep in their children's rooms for weeks at a time. Each of the units has a separate identity, and a certain animosity has developed between the units over time.

Case Study Questions

1. How do you think the nurses who work on the two units will feel about the change? How will the department heads feel? Who will lose what? How could those losses be acknowledged?

2. Create a communications plan for the project. How would you describe the purpose of the change? What tools would you use to communicate information about the project?

3. Who do you think should act as the change manager for the consolidation?

Summary

PI initiatives sometimes fail when human factors in change are ignored or mismanaged. By recognizing the steps people go through to accomplish change and managing the transition from old to new, change managers can ensure the success of PI efforts.

References

Amatayakul, M. 1999. *The Role of Health Information Managers in CPR Projects*. Chicago: AHIMA.

Black, M. 2003. Carelink project report: Carelink critical success factor—Integrating change management into the IT implementation process. Norton Healthcare Internal Finance Committee Memorandum. Louisville, KY, April 24.

Blancett, S.S., and D.L. Flarey. 1998. *Health Care Outcomes: Collaborative, Path-Based Approaches*. Gaithersburg, MD: Aspen Publishing.

Bridges, W. 2003. *Managing Transitions: Making the Most of Change*. New York: Perseus Books.

Christensen, C.M., R. Bohmer, and J. Kenagy. 2000. Will disruptive innovations cure health care? *Harvard Business Review* (September–October):102–110.

Helbig, S. 2003. Communicating change with style. *Journal of AHIMA* 74(5):66–67.

Kreitzer, D.J. 1998. What I learned about change, I learned in practice, not from the literature. Proceedings of the 17th Annual Midwest Research-to-Practice Conference in Adult, Continuing, and Community Education. Ball State University, Muncie, IN, October 8–10.

Lewin, K. 1951. *Field Theory in Social Science: Selected Theoretical Papers.* Edited by D. Cartwright. New York: Harper and Row.

Weiser, M. 1991 (September). UBICOMP paper: The computer for the 21st century. *Scientific American.* http://www.ubiq.com/hypertext/weiser/SciAmDraft3.html.

Resources

Buckley, D.S. 1999. A practitioner's view on managing change. *Frontiers of Health Services Management* (Fall):38–43.

Centers for Medicare and Medicaid Services. n.d. http://www.cms.hhs.gov/.

Galpin, T.J. 1996. *The Human Side of Change.* San Francisco: Jossey-Bass.

Kohles, M.K., W.G. Baker, and B.A. Donaho. 1995. *Transformational Leadership: Renewing Fundamental Values and Achieving New Relationships in Health Care.* Chicago: American Hospital Publishing.

Kotter, J.P. 1995. Leading change: Why transformation efforts fail. *Harvard Business Review* (March–April):59–67.

Senge, P., A. Kleiner, C. Roberts, R. Ross, and B. Smith. 1994. *The Fifth Discipline Fieldbook: Strategies and Tools for Building a Learning Organization.* New York: Doubleday.

Chapter 19
Developing the Performance Improvement Plan

Learning Objectives

- To describe the areas that should be addressed in the development of a healthcare organization's performance improvement plan

- To identify how performance improvement activities are implemented and findings are communicated throughout the organization

Key Term

SWOT analysis

Background and Significance

Performance improvement (PI) in healthcare is most effective when it is well planned, systematic, and organization-wide, and all appropriate individuals and professions work collaboratively to plan and implement activities. When individuals from different departments representing the scope of care, treatment, and services across the organization are included in PI activities, complex problems and processes can be improved. Collaboration on PI activities enables an organization to create a culture that focuses on PI and to plan and provide improvements that endure. When planning PI activities, the organization should identify those areas needing improvement based on data collection and analysis and the desired changes that will lead to sustained improvements. This chapter introduces students to the process of developing a PI plan.

Strategic Planning

Planning for PI activities in healthcare organizations is an outgrowth of the organization's overall strategic planning process. The strategic plan is developed by the organization's senior leaders and board of directors, whom, as discussed in chapter 14, the public holds accountable for the quality of the organization's products and services. Strategic planning may include a process called **SWOT analysis,** in which the leaders complete an assessment of the organization's **S**trengths, **W**eaknesses, **O**pportunities, and **T**hreats. Findings from SWOT analyses are used to validate the mission of the organization as a whole and determine the direction the organization is going as a business entity during the coming year. In addition, the leaders carefully consider input from the community the organization serves, its scope of services, the available technologies, staff expertise, the needs and expectations of its customers, and outcome information from PI activities during the past year.

PI Plan Design

Key to the implementation of an effective PI program is a written plan that systematically describes the structure and approach the organization will follow in the continuous assessment and improvement of its important systems, processes, and outcomes of care. Figure 19.1 shows an example of an organization-wide PI plan. The Joint Commission (2008) recommends that the following activities be included in an organization's PI plan (although by 2011, its publications place greater emphasis on the collection and analysis of data concerning the organization's primary focus areas):

- The organization's leaders decide the scope and focus of performance monitoring and data collection activities, including factors that contribute to unanticipated adverse events or outcomes.

- These activities are planned, systematic, and organization-wide.

- The organization sets priorities for PI, ensuring that the scope of care, treatment, and services is represented across all disciplines.

- Data are systematically collected, aggregated, and analyzed on an ongoing basis.

- Improvement opportunities are identified, and changes are made that will lead to and sustain improvement.

The leaders are expected to select an organization-wide PI approach and clearly define how all levels of the organization will monitor and address improvement issues. As of 2008, the Joint Commission has stipulated many of the measures for which hospitals should collect data. For example, it now requires data on the following areas that possibly

Figure 19.1.   PI and patient safety plan, Community Hospital of the West

Community Hospital of the West is a 350-bed tertiary medical center with an inpatient and outpatient continuum of care that provides medical and surgical services to a community of approximately 250,000. The facility's scope of services includes cardiology, orthopedics, obstetrics/gynecology, oncology, and psychiatry. The Community Hospital of the West board of directors is committed to continually improving the delivery and effectiveness of the care and services provided and proactively monitoring and assessing care delivery, patient safety, and the satisfaction of its customers. The board supports an environment that encourages the identification of improvement opportunities from all sources throughout the organization and community and the provision of care and service that is reflective of the organization's mission and vision.

Mission

Community Hospital of the West is the preeminent regionally integrated healthcare delivery system in the Intermountain West dedicated to providing compassionate, quality, high-value healthcare services to the residents of our communities.

Vision

To provide leadership in patient-centered care, built on a foundation of knowledge, innovation, and human values.

Performance Improvement Approach and Model

An interdisciplinary, continuous performance improvement approach is recognized across our continuum of care and service areas utilizing a Plan-Do-Check-Act (PDCA) model. Patient care and safety, and all other important organizational functions, are continually monitored, analyzed, and improved.

Organizational Performance Improvement Structure and Expectations

The leaders of Community Hospital of the West (the board of directors, the medical staff officers, and the senior hospital administrators) are committed to the integration of performance improvement activities. All staff are educated in the principles of performance improvement and participate in identifying opportunities for improvement, data collection and reporting activities, performance improvement team activities, and ongoing education. The board of directors has overall responsibility for ensuring the quality of care and services provided to the community. The board has delegated implementation responsibility for the organization-wide continuous performance improvement activities to the Performance Improvement and Patient Safety Council.

Performance Improvement and Patient Safety Council

The Performance Improvement and Patient Safety Council is an interdisciplinary senior-leadership committee that provides oversight and direction for the design and implementation of the organization-wide, continuous performance improvement and patient safety program. The council annually reviews outcome data and survey information as part of its strategic planning and prioritization processes. The council reports monthly to the medical executive committee and quarterly to the board of directors any adverse outcomes, significant process variations, and actions taken to improve care and address patient safety issues, both proactively and reactively. Standing committees of the medical staff, clinical and department discipline meetings, and this council are responsible for managing and improving patient care and safety issues within their particular high-risk areas. Prioritized measures that include high-risk and problem-prone areas identified throughout the organization are trended, analyzed, and reported to the council by assigned committees/staff on a preestablished schedule. The performance improvement department coordinates the implementation of the performance improvement and patient safety plan. The department provides organization-wide support in the design of data collection tools, data display, statistical analysis, benchmark data research, and the preparation of council reports. The council is responsible for receiving findings and acting on recommendations from the board and all committees, departments, and performance improvement teams, as well as customer survey data, sentinel events, near misses, and other identified trends in areas such as risk management and infection control. The council also is responsible for the design of the organization-wide staff development program related to continuous performance improvement and patient safety, and for the assessment and assignment of an annual proactive risk reduction activity. At least annually, the council reviews the activities of the performance improvement program and makes recommendations for the continuous improvement of the performance improvement and patient safety plan to the board of directors. The council membership is composed of a physician chairperson, the chief executive officer, medical director, clinical and administrative service directors, performance improvement team members, and other invited staff and guests as appropriate. The council meets at least every other month and as needs indicate.

(Continued on next page)

Figure 19.1. *(Continued)*

Standing Committees of the Medical Staff

All standing committees of the medical staff are chaired by a physician with representation, as appropriate, from hospital leadership, department directors, and frontline staff. Reports are submitted to the Performance Improvement and Patient Safety Council, which in turn forwards critical events and findings to the executive committee and to the board of directors. Communication throughout the organization among the board, committees, councils, hospital departments, medical staff, employed and contract staff, and its patients/families is open and flows in all directions, as appropriate and as allowed by regulations.

Medical Executive Committee

An elected official from the medical staff, medical staff committee chairs, medical director, chief executive officer, clinical service director, compliance officer, and the chief financial officer are standing members of this committee. This committee meets monthly and coordinates the business of the medical staff (recommending changes to their bylaws, rules, and regulations; reviewing appointment and reappointment recommendations; and election of officers) and the integration of patient care and hospital support services. Significant performance improvement and patient safety-related issues forwarded from the Performance Improvement and Patient Safety Council are reviewed, discussed, acted upon, and forwarded to the board and, as appropriate, to other departments, committees, and staff.

Medical Staff and Specialty Department Meetings

Each clinical staff specialty department meets at least quarterly to review and discuss performance improvement activities, staff development issues, and other related planning and directing activities. The medical staff at large meets at least annually for the election of officers, bylaws review, and general staff education.

Ethics Committee

This committee is responsible for serving as a resource regarding medical/ethical issues that surface for patients, their families, and the organization's clinical care providers.

Credentials Committee

This committee is responsible for the design and implementation of the organization's credentialing process and includes reviewing applications for appointment and reappointment, defining privilege delineation criteria, and evaluating physical health issues. Recommendations on all credentialing-related issues are reported to the executive committee and forwarded to the board of directors for final approval.

Utilization and Documentation Standards Committee

This committee is responsible for the review of findings from the monitoring activities on patient-specific data and information, timeliness of clinical record entries, and appropriateness of admissions and continued stays. Significant findings and recommendations are reported to the Performance Improvement and Patient Safety Council, the executive committee, provider quality profiles, other committees, and departments and individuals, as appropriate.

Pharmacy and Therapeutics Committee

This committee is responsible for formulary review and development, policy setting, procedure development, medication-related safety education, and monitoring the safety and efficacy of medication use throughout the organization. Medication monitoring includes a systematic, ongoing process of reviewing prescribing/ordering, procurement and storage, preparation and dispensing, administration, and adverse drug reactions. This committee performs data collection, analysis of aggregate data for patterns and trends, recommendations for process/system changes, and reporting of significant findings and actions to the Performance Improvement and Patient Safety Council.

Environmental Safety Committee

This committee is responsible for planning and directing environmental services within all environments of care. It also is responsible for educating staff on environmental safety issues and performance monitoring, data analysis, and continuous improvement efforts. This committee meets monthly and reports data collection, analysis, and improvement initiatives to the Performance Improvement and Patient Safety Council at least quarterly. The committee submits an environmental safety report identifying and reviewing improvement goals to the board of directors annually. Committee representation includes individuals from hospital and medical staff leadership, engineering and maintenance, housekeeping, central processing, security, and employee health.

Figure 19.1.   *(Continued)*

Strategic Planning Process

The strategic planning process occurs annually prior to the start of the fiscal year and coincides with organization-wide plan/program reviews and the budgeting process. Performance improvement and patient safety program review is initiated by the council using findings from the leaders' strategic goals, the council's self-assessment, and staff survey data on the program's effectiveness. Additional information, such as aggregate outcome data from performance measures, effectiveness of corrective actions implemented as a result of process variations and adverse outcomes, input from customer surveys, status on past year's goals, findings and actions from the annual proactive risk assessment/reduction activity, and regulatory and hospital process changes, are all reviewed and considered in the planning process and in the prioritization of performance initiatives and measures for the upcoming year.

Criteria for Prioritization of Improvement Goals, Performance Measures, and Data Collection

- Does the improvement opportunity/measure support the organization's mission, scope of care, and service provided and/or population(s) served?
- Is the performance measure a required regulatory measure, and does it provide performance information on an important function?
- Does the opportunity improve patient safety?
- Does the opportunity relate to an event that resulted in a sentinel event or near miss?
- Does the opportunity reflect patient feedback on needs or expectations?
- What degree of adverse impact on patient care can be expected if the improvement opportunity remains unresolved?
- Does the opportunity reflect a high-volume, problem-prone, or high-risk process?
- Are resources available to conduct the improvement process?
- Does the opportunity involve changing regulatory requirements?

Performance Measurement

This organization collects data on key systems, processes, and outcomes to monitor its performance. Data collection is prioritized based on this organization's mission, scope of care, services provided, and populations served. Data collection is systematic and may be used to establish a performance baseline, describe process performance stability, identify areas for more focused data collection, and/or determine if improvement has been sustained. Available benchmark information for established performance measures is drawn from internal and external databases. Data collection, responsibilities, and reporting schedules are defined in an appendix to this plan. Data that are collected to monitor performance include the following:

- Performance measures related to accreditation requirements (core measures or ORYX)
- Patient safety issues, including the following error-prone areas: medication events, falls, blood events, procedure/treatment/surgical events, behavioral events, equipment events, and laboratory events
- High-risk processes that may have the potential to result in a sentinel event, including operative or other invasive procedures that place patients at risk, medication management, restraint use, seclusion use, blood and blood product use, and outcomes related to resuscitation
- Relevant clinical practice guidelines
- Adverse drug events (ADEs)
- Needs, safety concerns, expectations, and satisfaction of patients and their families
- Failed processes related to the Joint Commission's National Patient Safety Goals
- Utilization management activities
- Performance of new and modified processes
- Quality control activities in the clinical laboratory, diagnostic radiology, nutritional services, nuclear medicine, radiation oncology, and pharmacy
- Infection control surveillance and reporting
- Medical record documentation for quality of care and timeliness

(Continued on next page)

Figure 19.1. *(Continued)*

- Risk management information, including sentinel events, near misses, complaints, findings from inspections by regulatory agencies, and compensable events
- Environmental safety
- Efficacy of services provided through contract or written agreement
- Appropriateness and effectiveness of pain management
- Appropriateness of behavior management procedures
- Autopsy results, when performed
- Customer demographics and diagnoses
- Financial data
- Staff opinions and needs
- Measures established when performance improvement and patient safety teams are chartered to design/redesign a process
- Other measures that may warrant targeted study

Measurement Process and Tools

When clinical conditions or systems are evaluated, measurement includes the following components:

- Design and assessment of new processes
- Assessment of data from customer satisfaction surveys, financial analysis, clinical outcomes of care, and functional outcomes of care
- Development of indicators of care or service that are measurable and focus on processes or outcomes
- Utilization of benchmarks or thresholds for performance
- Identification of data sources
- Development of a method of data collection and organization of data measures
- Measurement of the level of performance and stability of important existing processes
- Aggregation and trending of data
- Use of established clinical practice guidelines as a framework for standards of care and practice, when applicable
- Evaluation of individual cases that have potential or actual risk to the patient (adverse event/sentinel event review)

Benchmarks/thresholds are based on current professional literature, national standards, clinical practice guidelines, or internal benchmarks for improvement. Thresholds are derived from retrospective data relative to previous measurements within the organization or from comparable organization data. A benchmark is a quantitative goal embraced by the organization and is reflective of best practices within the internal and/or external environment. These goals serve as a mechanism for acceleration of performance curves through the process of continuous improvement.

Data Sources and Sampling

Data sources include medical records, encounter data, satisfaction surveys, complaint information, and internal clinical databases (for example, information from the order-entry system, diagnosis and procedural coding system, departmental logs, observation, surveys, and interviews). Sampling methodology shall be relevant to the performance measures or study being conducted. For general review studies, a sample size of 5 percent or 30 cases, whichever is greater, may be utilized. When the statistical significance of a study is critical, a scientific methodology is recommended. Control charts are used to measure key indicators on an ongoing basis to assist in determining sustained improvement(s). Statistical process control methods are utilized to identify whether an indicator is in control.

Aggregation and Analysis of Performance Data

The results of systematic, ongoing measures are aggregated and analyzed to identify trends, variances, and opportunities to improve patient care and safety. Data analysis should answer the following questions:

- What is our current level of performance?
- How stable are current processes?
- Do any steps in the process have undesirable variation(s)?

Figure 19.1. *(Continued)*

- Have strategies to stabilize or improve performance been effective?
- Are there areas that could be improved?
- What should the improvement priorities be?
- Was there sustained improvement in the processes that were changed?

Data Review

Trended data are reviewed when:

- Trended performance measures significantly and undesirably vary from those of other organizations, requiring a more detailed review.
- Trended performance measures significantly and undesirably vary from recognized standards, benchmarks, or statistical process controls.
- The occurrence of an event is questionable or too infrequent to make judgments about patterns in care or to analyze statistical significance.

Event Definitions

Near miss is defined as an opportunity to improve patient safety–related practices based on a condition or incident with potential for more serious consequences. A root-cause analysis may be performed when a near miss occurs.

Reportable event is defined as an unintended act, either of omission or commission, or an act that does not achieve its intended outcome. An incident report is completed by staff and forwarded to the Performance Improvement and Patient Safety Council. Reportable events are trended quarterly. These events are reviewed by their respective committees and/or service area directors, and recommendations for corrective actions are reported to the Performance Improvement and Patient Safety Council.

Sentinel event is defined as an unexpected occurrence involving death or serious physical or psychological injury or the risk thereof. Serious injury specifically includes loss of limb or function. A root-cause analysis is performed when a sentinel event occurs. All Sentinel Event Alert publications from the Joint Commission will be reviewed for relevance to our organization.

Intensive review of an incident requires the review of medical records or other data elements to determine if process problems exist and if an ongoing performance measure should be established to monitor process stability. An intensive review is undertaken when:

- A significant adverse drug reaction or medication error occurs
- An external regulatory agency requests the review
- The Performance Improvement and Patient Safety Council requests the review
- An organization is performing proactive risk-reduction activities

Root-cause analysis is conducted when a significant negative deviation from expected outcomes occurs or when a near miss occurs and further study is recommended by the council.

Peer Review Process

Cases are referred to peer review when they meet criteria as defined in the medical staff peer review plan. Findings are referred to appropriate committees for review and action, as warranted, and to individual physician practice profiles and are reviewed as part of the reappointment process.

Performance Improvement Model

The model for performance improvement is Plan-Do-Check-Act (PDCA) and is defined as:

- **Plan** is based on the results of data collection or the assessment of a process. The plan should include how the process will be improved and what will be measured to evaluate the effectiveness of the proposed process change(s).
- **Do** includes the implementation of process changes. These changes may be tested before changing policies and procedure or conducting extensive education.

(Continued on next page)

Figure 19.1. *(Continued)*

- **Check** evaluates the effect of the action taken at a given point in time.
- **Act** is to hold the gain and to continue to improve the process.

Evaluation

The measurement, assessment, and evaluation processes will continue to provide the necessary information about the effectiveness of the improvement. If the identified problem continues to persist despite the planned improvements, the PDCA model will continue until sustained improvement is achieved. Any findings, conclusions, recommendations, actions taken, and results of the actions taken based on the performance improvement process are documented and reported to the appropriate individuals, departments, or committees. This information is used in the reappointment of providers, recontracting with agencies providing outsourced patient care services, and the employee evaluation process.

Patient Safety Risk Reduction Model

The model used to conduct the annual proactive risk assessment and reduction activity is the failure mode effects analysis (FMEA).

Communication

Performance improvement and patient safety activities are communicated through the established committee structure as well as through regular clinical, discipline, and staff meetings; e-mails; the annual storyboard fair; and the intranet. Members of the council are responsible for maintaining communication related to performance improvement and patient safety initiatives. The treating physician is responsible for informing patients and their families (when appropriate) about the outcomes of the patients' care, including unanticipated outcomes such as sentinel events, and for documenting such communication in the patients' clinical records.

Education

The organization's leaders and council members are responsible for ongoing educational activities related to the performance improvement and patient safety program. This includes orientation of new employees at hire, orientation of new board members, and annual education of all employees at the annual employee fair and through participation in performance improvement teams.

Staff Support

The Employee Assistant Program (EAP) is a resource to support staff involved in a sentinel event and other work-related performance issues. The EAP is a confidential employee service. The clinical leadership also is responsible for meeting with staff involved in sentinel events to provide a means for communication and support.

Confidentiality

All performance improvement and patient safety activities set forth in this plan, including minutes, reports, and associated work products, are confidential and may not be released or discussed with any person or agency except those mandated by hospital policy or state or federal law.

Annual Review

The performance improvement and patient safety plan is reviewed annually as part of the organization-wide strategic planning process. The plan review is based on the organization's mission, evaluation of goals from the previous year, data collection results, and external regulatory changes.

APPENDIX A: PERFORMANCE IMPROVEMENT INITIATIVES

Goal 1: To improve patient, physician, and employee satisfaction

    A. Patient Satisfaction: Improve patient satisfaction as measured by the Gallup Patient Satisfaction Survey

       Action Plan:

- Implement the caring model of nursing.
- Refine and improve the centralized scheduling process.
- Improve patient education and communication in the area of advanced directives.

Figure 19.1. *(Continued)*

Measurement:

- Patient responses on the Gallup Patient Satisfaction Survey will shift from satisfied or dissatisfied to increase the very satisfied category by 5 percent.
- The number of positive comments will increase by at least 5 percent.
- The number of billing complaints will decrease by at least 5 percent.

B. Physician Satisfaction: Improve physician satisfaction as measured by the biannual medical staff survey

Action Plan:

- Implement the caring model of nursing.
- Refine/improve the centralized scheduling process.
- Evaluate and downsize committee structure as appropriate.

Measurement: The results of the biannual medical staff survey will shift from satisfied or dissatisfied to increase the very satisfied category by 5 percent.

C. Employee Satisfaction: Improve employee satisfaction

Action Plan:

- Implement the caring model of nursing.
- Award/recognize employees for years of service.
- Review/improve the employee evaluation process.
- Implement a system of merit raises.
- Develop department-specific action plans based on employee survey results and exit interview feedback.

Measurement:

- The annual employee turnover rate will decrease by 5 percent.
- All employees will be surveyed in June/July at department meetings using Gallup Patient Satisfaction Survey questions.
- A system of performing exit interviews will be implemented.

Goal 2: To improve the infrastructure and systems used to collect, measure, and assess information so that information will be secure, accurate, appropriately accessible, useful, timely, and effective

Action Plan:

- Provide education in basic information management principles and provide tools, including software/hardware training, for leaders and other staff as needed.
- Improve/develop point-of-service data documentation with associated monitoring and evaluation of outcomes.
- Develop standing agendas for meetings to support appropriate flow of information throughout the organization.
- Develop standardized documentation measurement, including expansion of the organizational data dictionary.
- Improve communication pathways to provide information to, and encourage feedback from, patients, trustees, physicians, employees, and other customers.

Measurement:

- Performance improvement/risk and safety reports will be complete, accurate, and timely.
- Compliance with documentation requirements as measured by data quality monitoring program will increase.
- Communication as measured by employee, physician, and patient survey results and through unsolicited comments will improve.

(Continued on next page)

Figure 19.1. *(Continued)*

Goal 3: To improve leadership orientation, education, and performance

Action Plan:

- Revise/develop executive team and manager orientation and reference manual.
- Provide/attend at least two leadership education programs focusing on assessed needs for trustees, medical executive staff, executive team, and managers.
- Establish protocols for development, implementation, and review of standing physician orders.

Measurement:

- Educational program feedback surveys from participants will demonstrate program effectiveness.
- Trustee self-evaluation results will improve.
- Trustee evaluations of the CEO will improve.
- Survey results and self-evaluations will improve.
- Use and annual review of standing physician order protocols will be monitored.

Goal 4: To develop and improve employee competence and performance

Action Plan:

- Develop and administer an organization-wide educational needs assessment program, including feedback from physicians and employees as well as patient satisfaction surveys.
- Develop and implement educational programming to address prioritized needs, for example, mandatory staff education requirements, restraint protocols, confidentiality issues, universal precautions, and patient and family education process.

Measurement:

- Results of mandatory staff education posttests will demonstrate that competencies have been achieved.
- Employee perception that needs have been met will be measured by participant evaluations of the educational offerings and employee satisfaction surveys.

---

require improvement (the full list can be found in the appropriate accreditation standards manual):

- Medication management
- Blood and blood product use
- Restraint and seclusion use
- Behavior management and treatment
- Operative and other invasive procedures
- Resuscitation and its outcomes

Because most organizations identify more improvement opportunities than they can act on, priorities must be set. Criteria are helpful in setting priorities and may include:

- High-risk, high-volume, or problem-prone processes

- The degree of adverse impact on patient care that can be expected if an improvement opportunity remains unresolved

- The degree to which patient safety is improved

For example, at Community Hospital of the West, the managers and employees participate in organization-wide strategic planning. As part of strategic planning one year, they identified a list of their organization's important functions and processes in which they thought improvement opportunities existed. (See figure 19.2.) The participants used brainstorming techniques and nominal group techniques to identify and prioritize improvement opportunities. The prioritized ranking shows the number of points assigned to the various opportunities for improvement upon review by the entire organization. The prioritized opportunities were then reevaluated and regrouped by the hospital's board of directors and senior leaders in light of other available survey and outcome data. Using preestablished prioritization criteria, the leaders finalized the hospital's improvement goals, the results of which can be found in figure 19.1.

Many of the items in the strategic planning process document are related to patient care (see "Provision of care, treatment, and services" in figure 19.2). Before using strategic brainstorming, the organization had been collecting data using the Gallup® Patient Quality System. An in-depth analysis of the data revealed a negative trend in multiple indicators related to nursing care. The measures included the following:

- Overall quality of nursing care

- Staff showed concern toward patient

- Nurses anticipated patient needs

- Nurses explained procedures to patient

- Nurses demonstrated skill in providing care

- Nurses helped calm patients' fears

- Staff communicated effectively with patients

- Nurses/staff responded to patient requests

After considerable discussion of the brainstormed opportunities and of the Gallup Patient Satisfaction Survey data, the leadership decided to implement a new approach to nursing care in response to issues affecting that area.

Following considerable literature research, the leadership decided to implement Jean Watson's theory of human caring. The theory of human caring "recognizes the dignity and

Figure 19.2.   Example of a strategic planning document showing potential PI opportunities

Community Hospital of the West—Important Functions and Opportunities, Annual Strategic Planning	
Functions and Opportunities	**Priority Points**
Provision of care, treatment, and services	
• Define restraint protocol	22
• Provide physical therapy services on weekends	1
• Change menu service	4
• Improve patient transport process	10
• Develop community awareness program	12
• Expand patient and family education	48
• Improve discharge instruction and documentation procedures	25
• Improve education for surgical patients	16
• Expand blood donor program	9
• Define assessment process	34
• Code status on admission	55
• Do more complete assessment on pre-op patients	11
• Address regional psychiatric services support	12
• Target high-risk patients for preventive care	17
• Respond to changing regulations on authorized procedures	15
• Define proper follow-up call from hospital to patient	10
• Define proper protocol for standing orders	27
Ethics, rights, and responsibilities	
• Include discussion of patient rights as part of admissions process	23
• Educate staff, families, and patients about the function of the ethics committee	21
• Respect patient's right to privacy and treatment with dignity	22
Surveillance, prevention, and control of infection	
• Enforce universal precautions	58
• Develop infection-control program for home care	14
• Ensure that patient rooms are clean before assigning new patients to rooms	19
• Improve traffic control in patient care areas	18
Management of the environment of care	
• Develop master plan for remodeling patient care areas	22
• Refine role of housekeeping	26
• Look at complaints about waiting areas	22
• Develop a system for providing hazardous-spill carts	2
• Address after-hours and weekend security issues	25
• Remodel the operating room transitional area	3
• Upgrade operating room furniture and equipment	8

Figure 19.2. *(Continued)*

Improving organization performance	
• Develop plan to reduce medication errors	21
• Explore concurrent data collection and reporting processes	13
• Implement supply chain management	4
• Improve radiology and operating room scheduling process	18
• Support process improvement activities through development of teamwork	16
Leadership	
• Develop a physician-hospital organization to work with managed care	13
• Conduct a community needs assessment	7
• Build feedback from employee and physician satisfaction surveys into the strategic planning process	7
• Develop mission, vision, and organizational goals for each department/service	5
• Downsize the number of committees	9
• Clarify leadership's role in all important organization-wide functions	8
• Introduce staff to board of trustees and define board's expectations of staff	2
• Define protocol for charity care	1
• Define hospital's system for acknowledging patient deaths	2
• Clarify role of administrator on call	1
• Update and maintain all departmental policies and procedures	8
Management of human resources	
• Provide identity badges for all physicians	4
• Improve communications with key customers (patients, employees, physicians)	14
• Improve mandatory staff education process	20
• Develop and implement competencies/skills checklists for every department	18
• Improve system for designating PRN staff—who to call, how many, etc.	1
• Update physician directory	1
• Utilize intranet training	3
• Develop policy on lab testing for employees and physicians	2
• Develop staff cross-training program	10
• Decrease staff turnover	1
Management of information	
• Standardize organization of policies and procedures among departments	18
• Raise awareness of confidentiality issues	41
• Inventory the information the organization collects and determine what is necessary for quality control and leadership/governance needs	9
• Provide Internet access in the library	6
• Provide training and policy development on CMS coding rules	6

worth of individuals and that their responses to illness are unique; acknowledges the individual's right to continuous autonomy; helps individuals reach maximum capacity; recognizes that nursing takes place within a human-to-human caring relationship; and supports caring as the core of nursing practice, recognizing that caring is effectively demonstrated and practiced interpersonally" (Watson 1985). In Watson's theory, caring nursing is exhibited by five behaviors:

- Nurse introduces himself or herself to the patient and explains role in care that day

- Nurse calls the patient by preferred name

- Nurse sits at the patient's bedside for at least five minutes per shift to plan and review care

- Nurse shakes the patient's hand or touches the patient on the arm

- Nurse uses the mission and vision statements of the organization in planning care (Dingman et al. 1999).

Implementation of this care model became a PI initiative for improving patients' perceptions of nursing care. All other opportunities were aligned to this major initiative. The organization's intent was that changing the strategy for nursing care in this dramatic way would be evidenced in subsequent measures of nursing effectiveness by the Gallup Patient Satisfaction Survey.

The first part of the PI initiative document was organized to reflect the needs of the organization's mission, vision, and most important customers—patients, physicians, and employees. Opportunities were then listed beneath the customers to whom they pertained. A component of the organization's PI approach was to focus on, and maintain visibility of, the customer.

The rest of the PI initiative document focused on the important processes and functions of the organization that are most likely to affect high-risk, high-volume, and problem-prone outcomes. Each section identified an action plan and the means by which the efforts at improvement will be measured. These measurements should provide good data for the organization to assess itself and plan the following year's PI initiatives, thus maintaining a continuous PI philosophy and cycle in the organization.

Other important areas that should be addressed in an organization's PI plan include the following:

- Initial and ongoing education of the board, medical staff, and employed staff members on its PI process and annual improvement initiatives

- The expectations of all members of the organization in PI activities

- Annual review of the effectiveness of the organization's PI program

Implementing the PI Plan

The organization's leaders have a central role in initiating and maintaining the organization's PI priorities.

Implementation of the organization-wide plan for PI is a challenge at best. The plan should clearly delineate how members of the organization are educated on the PI process and what their roles and responsibilities are in carrying out the organization's plan. For example, Community Hospital of the West's PI and patient safety plan (figure 19.1) describes how the board of directors delegates plan implementation responsibility to the Performance Improvement and Patient Safety Council. The council, in turn, defines which committees, departments, and staff are responsible for collecting data, assessing and reporting findings, and performing other PI activities.

The scope and focus of what will be measured, which data will be collected and by whom, and the frequency and intensity with which the data will be collected and reported should be clearly defined by the healthcare organization. In chapter 16, figure 16.1 shows an example of one organization's data collection and reporting schedule. While healthcare organizations do have some control over what types of data they collect, healthcare regulations mandate some of what must be collected. For example, the organization collects data on patients' perceptions of care, treatment, and services, including their specific needs and expectations, how well the organization meets these needs and expectations, and how the organization can improve patient safety.

PI priorities should be data driven. That is, the data the organization collects about its own performance should be analyzed and considered when setting improvement priorities. Data should be aggregated and displayed in a way that provides for easy assessment of the findings. Establishing benchmarks on each measure the organization collects data on and displaying the benchmark information alongside the aggregate data measures are ways to quickly identify less-than-desirable outcomes in performance. Figure 16.1 provides one example of how an organization displays its outcome data. Historically, healthcare organizations have been referred to as "data rich" and "information poor," meaning they spent too much time collecting data and failed to turn the data into meaningful information or use it in setting performance priorities. Setting measurement and data collection priorities are newer standards that have evolved over the past few years to help organizations better identify, manage, and act on collected data.

In demonstrating the effectiveness of its PI model, a healthcare organization must show evidence that the entire cycle has been completed on each of its prioritized improvements. Often, organizations fail to complete the cycle. Data can be collected, aggregated, and analyzed, and an improvement priority can be established, but without providing evidence of an effective and sustained improvement, the cycle remains incomplete. It is not unusual for process changes to initially result in variations in performance or for an organization to find that a process change may not be the correct "fix" to an identified problem. The ongoing, systematic review of measurements identified to confirm process stability is the "check" step in the improvement cycle. Monitoring a process change for up to six months, with ongoing data checks (sampling at regular intervals) once stability is achieved, validates the improvement or the need for continued improvements (the "act" step) and completes the performance improvement cycle.

Case Study

Students should look at the list of functions and opportunities (figure 19.2) and the PI and patient safety plan for Community Hospital of the West (figure 19.1) and answer the questions listed below.

For school or work experience, students should draft a PI plan that identifies specific PI priorities, measures selected to monitor improvement priorities, possible corrective actions, and any other important information that describes the PI process.

Case Study Questions

1. How is the PI plan linked to the list of functions and opportunities identified during strategic planning?

2. Can you identify items in the prioritized strategic planning process document that are related to initiatives in the PI plan?

3. Note that the items in the strategic planning process document are very specific. Were related items from the list grouped into a more general category for the final PI initiatives?

4. Are the measurements identified for the initiatives truly quantifiable? That is, will the measurements actually lead to objective data that can be evaluated for evidence of improvement?

Summary

Planning the direction of a healthcare organization's PI program is a complex activity. The program must be created in concert with the organization's overall strategic plan. From the many potential improvement opportunities, the organization must prioritize the issues it will focus its improvement efforts on during the coming year.

PI program planning includes a review of the results from the strategic planning process, the organization's mission, community needs, customer expectations, and other related outcome data on the organization's performance. The planning document also may include a discussion of the educational initiatives to be developed to support the PI program, descriptions of the components of the program, the methodology, and other pertinent information.

References

Dingman, S.K., M. Williams, D. Fosbinder, and M. Warnick. 1999. Implementing a caring model to improve patient satisfaction. *Journal of Nursing Administration* 29(12):30–37.

Joint Commission. 2008. *2009 Hospital Accreditation Standards*. Oakbrook Terrace, IL: Joint Commission Resources.

Watson, J. 1985. *Nursing: Human Science and Human Care: A Theory of Nursing*. Norwalk, CT: Appleton-Century-Crofts.

Resources

Baker, S.K. 1998. *Managing Patient Expectations: The Art of Finding and Keeping Loyal Patients*. San Francisco: Jossey-Bass.

Joint Commission on Accreditation of Healthcare Organizations. 2000. *Improving the Care Experience*. Oakbrook Terrace, IL: JCAHO.

Plisek, P.E. 1995. Techniques for managing quality. *Hospital and Health Services Administration* 40(1):50–79.

Ransom, E., M.S. Joshi, D.B. Nash, and S.B. Ransom, eds. 2008. *The Healthcare Quality Book: Vision, Strategy, and Tools*, 2nd ed. Chicago: Health Administration Press.

Chapter 20

Evaluating the Performance Improvement Program

Learning Objectives

- To explain why performance improvement programs are evaluated

- To identify the aspects of the performance improvement program that should be evaluated

- To describe what organizations should do with the information gathered from the performance improvement program evaluation

Background and Significance

The processes of planning and evaluating a performance improvement (PI) program should mirror each other. Taken together, they are a cyclical activity: Planning leads to evaluation, and evaluation provides the impetus for new planning. The task of appraising the PI program is generally completed on an annual basis, and the results should be reported to the healthcare organization's board, management, employees, and medical staff.

PI programs are evaluated for four reasons:

1. *To determine whether the organization's approach to designing, measuring, assessing, and improving its performance is planned, systematic, and organization-wide.* Forethought and deliberation help the organization focus on important issues and lead to better results of program activities. Systematizing the PI program makes it possible for participants to understand what is expected and enables them to anticipate program requirements. Committing to the organization-wide nature of the program ensures that everyone in the organization is in concert with the program's objectives and understands

what they are expected to contribute. The PI evaluation process includes the participation of all employees, medical staff, and organizational leaders, from frontline staff to the board of directors. Involvement of the organization's staff in the evaluation process can be demonstrated through team or committee input, questionnaires and surveys, self-evaluation, suggestion boxes, and so forth. For example, each department in the organization can assess the educational competency of individual staff as it relates to PI knowledge. Department competency then can be compared with an established organization-wide PI competency goal.

2. *To determine whether the organization's approach and activities are carried out collaboratively.* PI activities should be multidisciplinary and should improve performance across department lines; in other words, they should be cross-functional or interdepartmental. Another expectation is that all factors that contribute to a problem will be remedied. For example, PI teams should be assessed in an annual evaluation of frontline staff or multidisciplinary team participation through documentation of regular attendance at meetings, data collection, and overall success of the team's improvement efforts.

3. *To determine whether the organization's approach needs redesign in light of changes in the strategic plan or organizational objectives.* If the organization's mission, vision, organizational structure, or strategic initiatives have changed since the PI program was planned, then new measures and assessment activities may have to be undertaken. For example, if an organization has a strategic initiative to add a new service, all departments, organization leaders, and the board of directors would be included in defining measures and assessment activities for the new service. Modifications should be implemented as soon as possible after major changes in organization objectives have been made. In addition, the organization needs to assess the adequacy of the human, information, physical, and financial resources allocated to support PI and safety activities.

4. *To determine whether the program was effective in improving overall organizational performance.* It is important to identify whether the PI program was responsible for important improvements in organizational performance or whether those improvements were due to other factors. It is also important to identify whether improvements were achieved and maintained. Review of program performance should identify whether program processes are efficient, effective, timely, and appropriately supported with personnel, budget, and other resources. Figure 20.1 shows survey questions used in one organization to assess the effectiveness of the different departments' PI programs. The results from the survey can be used to assess and then recommend changes to the organization's PI program.

Figure 20.1. PI staff survey questions

- How is PI used in your department/service?
- Are you asked for suggestions/ideas for processes that need to be improved in your area?
- Are you asked for suggestions/ideas for processes that need to be improved organization-wide?
- Have you been involved in any PI activities in the past year?
- Have the results of PI activities been communicated to you on a regular basis? If yes, how have they been communicated?
- Have you used the results of any PI activities in the delivery of patient care/service in the past year?
- Have PI activities improved patient care or service in your area in the past year?
- What PIs need to be made to improve the safety of patient care delivery?
- Do the staff in your work area understand PI activities?
- Which patient care process is strongest in your work area?
- Which process related to patient care is weakest in your work area?
- If you could improve only one patient process or outcome, which would you choose?
- Do you feel that your area has adequate resources to support PI and patient safety activities?

Components of Program Review

PI review is performed on an annual basis. The results from this evaluation are reported to the board of directors, medical staff, and leaders of the organization. During program review, each of the areas in which clinical and nonclinical services are provided should be examined for continued focus and relevance. Each area should document opportunities for improvement that were identified and PI goals that were met. Each area should document which problems remain unresolved from prior evaluation periods and which have not shown significant improvement. Each area should identify issues in the PI program that, if changed, would better support the organization's overall mission and PI efforts. Although the evaluation of the organization's PI program can be structured in any number of ways, the questions provided in figure 20.1 are typical.

Executive Summary

The executive summary section of the PI review summarizes the main points of the annual report. The summary should provide the reader with a snapshot of the year's best and most significant issues and should answer the question, "If readers looked at only one or two pages of the report, what would you want them to be aware of and remember?"

Overview

Information on collaboration, strategic planning, and operating goals related to PI should be reviewed in the overview section. This might include the organization's mission statement.

In general, the mission statement should continue to reflect the organization's key customers and long-term direction. Establishing direction and planning from organization leaders is essential in illustrating how PI is focused and prioritized from year to year. How and why teams or processes were identified for improvement should be discussed to provide a rationale for how organization leaders determine and prioritize areas for improvement and development. This section links the organizational goals identified by the board with the way the PI initiatives were operationalized.

PI Structure

The organizational structure that supports, directs, and coordinates all PI activities should be described, and any changes should be illustrated in the PI structure section. A key element is how findings from PI activities are shared with the board, hospital and medical staff leaders, and other staff. The report should review how well the organization routes, communicates, and shares performance-related information. Responses from the annual staff PI survey might include answers to the following questions:

- Does the organization's current PI methodology continue to support its PI activities and management style?

- Could some activities in the model be made more efficient or be simplified?

- Do all members of the organization understand the model and how it can help structure PI activities?

Improvement Opportunities

Trends from aggregate data analysis, interventions, corrective actions or improvements, or changes in policies and procedures may be highlighted in the improvement opportunities section using graphic representation and storyboard findings rather than detailed reports. Data should show evidence of continued and sustained improvement. System improvements may be broken into four areas: patient-focused improvements, organizational improvements, ongoing measurements, and comparative summary measurements.

Patient-Focused Improvements

The patient-focused improvements section focuses on clinical PIs that have affected patient care, treatment, and services. Patient care activities, such as medication management, patient rights, infectious disease management, and so forth, may provide an outline for addressing these improvements and prioritized opportunities. The efforts of patient care improvement activities are reviewed, as are team processes and areas of measurement. Examples may include the results of monitoring pain management on postsurgical patients, waiting times for emergency patients, and antibiotic administration times.

Organizational Improvements

The focus of the organizational improvements area is nonclinical and may deal with systems such as environment-of-care issues, staff development needs, and leadership development goals. Organizational improvements may include activities such as reengineering the admitting process, reducing the suspense days on unbilled accounts, or reducing staff injuries. The efforts of all organizational improvement activities are reviewed, as are process changes and areas of measurement.

Ongoing Measurements

Ongoing measurements and results are related to important systems, processes, and outcomes that are monitored on an ongoing basis. They include measurements that are required by regulatory agencies, such as staffing effectiveness, disease-specific monitoring, medication use, blood and blood component use, and customer satisfaction. Major results and impacts should be included for each function. Sentinel events and resulting root-cause analyses also should be presented, along with information related to near misses. The results of risk reduction assessments and strategies should be discussed here as well. Any ongoing variations noted in aggregate data findings would become a target priority area for ongoing improvement in the coming year's plan.

Comparative Summary Measurements

If internal or external comparative databases have been used in the organization's improvement activities to assess outcomes or determine areas for improvement, a synopsis of these critical measures and improvement results should be included and reviewed here. Information on key patient care issues related to the Joint Commission's Core Measure initiatives is an example of one external comparative database used by healthcare organizations.

PI Team Activities

The PI team activities part of the report should highlight the work of PI teams sanctioned by the organization's PI council and should provide answers to the following questions:

- Has the team's work resulted in measurable and sustained improvements?
- What process changes and training occurred to support and sustain the improvement(s)?
- Has the organization's staff assigned to PI team projects been effectively trained to work on PI teams?
- Is staff willing and able to take on the important roles in team activities?
- Does staff participate and interact well at team meetings to work through PI processes?
- Can they document important team milestones with appropriate tools?
- Have they implemented the organization's PI model appropriately?
- Have they learned to listen and question effectively in interpersonal communication?
- Can they effectively communicate the team's process and outcomes to the rest of the organization?

Other PI Review Topics

Other topics that may be addressed in the organization's PI plan review may include areas of focused change or improvement.

Customer Satisfaction

Have internal and external customers been identified for all PI projects? Have customers' requirements been identified in detail? Has customer satisfaction been measured objectively and with appropriate tools?

Risk Exposure and Patient Safety Assessment

Is adherence to procedures monitored and appropriate education undertaken when necessary? Are the right services always rendered to the right patient, at the right time, with the right procedure? Are adverse events always reported per policy and procedure? Are care processes modified when necessary to prevent injury to patients, visitors, and employees?

Human Resources

Are appropriate hiring, staffing, training, and competency assessment activities occurring in all departments? Are employees being screened for disease as required by state health regulations? Are required documents being maintained on all employees? Are required credentials and licenses being verified on all employed staff and licensed independent practitioners? Are appropriate competency reviews being performed on all staff? Are performance appraisal activities incorporated into the PI process?

Accreditation and Licensure

Is the annual periodic performance review being documented and are corrective actions implemented? Is the organization always ready for review by accrediting and licensing agencies? Have adverse outcomes from past regulatory surveys been corrected? Have new standards and changes to standards been implemented?

PI Program Effectiveness and Recommendations

The PI program effectiveness and recommendations section outlines the areas identified and prioritized for improvement, measurement, and data collection during the next year. In large part, these recommendations are based on the findings outlined in the annual report, as well as goals identified in the organization's strategic planning process.

Case Study

Look at the case study in chapter 3. The team at Western States University Hospital continued to work on the issue. During the ensuing months, the team elected a leader, found a facilitator, and constructed its vision statement: "Patient location is correctly identified in XYZ and ABC systems at all times." It tentatively identified process customers as nursing staff, patient accounting staff, admitting staff, and patients.

The team decided early in the process that it did not have sufficient data to make decisions about system capabilities or to recommend solutions to the problem. The team developed data collection activities to get a handle on the realities of patient location within the institution and then spent the first four months collecting data. It collected data on the number of patients admitted, discharged, and transferred within the system; examined the user procedure for entering the admissions, discharges, and transfers in the system; and finally, summarized the amount of admitting, discharging, and transferring that each user performed. It did observational studies of the patient transfer procedure, identifying how long the typical patient transfer took from one unit to another, the exact times of initiation and completion, and the time of transfer input into the information system. It identified the number and type of errors that occurred concerning patient admission, discharge, and transfer, and the effects those errors had on the census and in other departments.

At the end of the first four months of activity, the quality council of Western States University Hospital began its annual review of the important aspects of the PI program. The leader of the patient transfer team was asked to submit a one-page synopsis of the team's activities that included a brief description of team activities and a complete set of the data collected by the team.

Case Study Questions

1. If you were the leader of the patient transfer team, how would you summarize the team's accomplishments thus far?

2. If you were a member of the quality council, how would you assess the patient transfer team's accomplishments thus far?

3. What recommendations would you make with reference to the team's future activities?

Summary

The annual evaluation of a PI program ensures that the program focuses on opportunities for improvement that are truly important to the organization. The foundation of a PI program assessment includes how well the organization's leaders set expectations; developed plans; and managed processes to measure, assess, and improve the quality of the organization's operations (such as governance, management, clinical, and support activities).

Evaluation should encompass all areas of the program, including the organization's strategic goals, PI structure, and team training and functioning, as well as ongoing and comparative measurement monitoring of the results of established improvement priorities. The findings from the PI program evaluation are reported to the board of directors, medical staff, and organization leaders.

Resource

Bassett-Lathrop, C., et al. 1995. A structure for organizing a facility's annual performance review. *Journal for Healthcare Quality* 17(4):18–23.

Chapter 21
Understanding the Legal Implications of Performance Improvement

Learning Objectives

- To describe the legal aspects of performance improvement activities conducted in healthcare organizations

- To explain the significance and relationship of tort law to quality improvement activities

- To define the concepts of protection and privilege with respect to quality improvement activities

- To distinguish quality improvement activities from research activities

Key Terms

Breach of duty

Causation

Damages

Discoverable

Duty to use due care

Elements of negligence

Generalizable knowledge

Privilege

Protection

Research

Background and Significance

In healthcare organizations, performance improvement (PI) activities are affected by a number of laws, rules, and regulations. Because PI processes can be complex and, at times, controversial, understanding the legal context in which these activities are carried out is critical. This chapter addresses the legal implications of PI in relation to the following areas:

- Avoidance of risk from a malpractice perspective
- Tort law
- Four basic elements of negligence or malpractice
- The organized medical staff
- Peer review protection
- Immunity from liability
- Occurrence reports and sentinel events
- Responsibility for disclosing adverse events to the patient or patient's family
- Distinguishing quality improvement from research
- Public health activities

Avoidance of Risk from a Malpractice Perspective

The introduction to this book points out that healthcare professionals need to be concerned with PI because it is the key to ensuring high-quality yet cost-effective care that is desired by payers and consumers. The noble and positive pursuit of best serving patients and clients is the bedrock on which PI initiatives are based. Satisfied customers and the demand for services are the positive rewards for a successful PI program.

In addition to the pursuit of quality, healthcare organizations also want to avoid negative consequences. Failure to meet expected performance standards creates risk. In the healthcare setting, this risk is unsatisfied patients, loss of market share, and exposure to legal action in the form of malpractice litigation.

Particularly since the 1970s, technology has improved, costs have skyrocketed, the number of lawyers has grown, and lawsuits have proliferated. This increase in litigation has been particularly dramatic in the healthcare sector. Thus, part of the dedication to PI is driven not only by the benefits of high-quality care but also by the desire to avoid the increased malpractice risk associated with poor quality.

Tort Law

A tort is a wrongful act committed against a person or a piece of property. A tort is a civil action as opposed to a criminal act or a breach of contract.

Tort law in the United States is based on English law and provides a means for private parties to resolve disputes. Individuals, groups, businesses, corporations, and other nongovernmental organizations can bring many kinds of legal actions, or lawsuits, under the general heading of tort law in civil courts. In such actions, one party generally seeks monetary payment for harm or damages caused by another party.

In contrast, criminal actions are prosecuted by the government against an individual accused of committing a crime. In criminal actions, the result sought by the government is generally a jail sentence.

In healthcare, the most notable tort is the tort of negligence, also commonly referred to as malpractice. In malpractice actions, generally, providers or hospitals or both are sued for being careless and thereby causing an injury to a patient.

Four Basic Elements of Negligence or Malpractice

Four basic elements must be proved in a malpractice case:

1. **Duty to use due care:** A relationship must have been established between the parties in which one party has an obligation, or *duty*, to act as a reasonably prudent person would act toward the other. This duty exists in a physician's relationship with his or her patients. *Using due care* is acting as a reasonably prudent person would act under a given set of circumstances.

2. **Breach of duty:** In a malpractice action, the issue is whether a physician exercised a standard of care that a reasonably prudent physician would have exercised under those circumstances. Failure to exercise due care is a *breach of duty*.

3. **Damages:** The patient must show that actual harm, or *damage*, occurred.

4. **Causation:** There must be a connection between the breach of duty and the damage— evidence that the failure to exercise due care, or breach, *caused* the damage.

All four **elements of negligence** must be present to accomplish a successful malpractice action.

Hypothetical Situation 1. A physician carelessly administered the wrong drug to a patient, which caused the patient to lapse into a coma. All elements of a malpractice action are met. The physician has a duty to exercise due care in treating a patient, and the physician breached that duty by carelessly administering the wrong drug. As a result of that breach, the patient was harmed, ending up in a coma directly caused by administration of the wrong medication.

Hypothetical Situation 2. A physician carelessly administered the wrong drug to a patient, but the patient was not harmed by this medication error in any way. In such a case, a malpractice action should not succeed, because the element of damage is absent, as is causation since no ill effect was suffered.

One of the purposes of PI initiatives is to develop the best possible clinical practices. At a minimum, the organization must meet what is legally referred to as the "community standard of care," or the use of practices of care by the provider that are acceptable and expected by other reasonably prudent providers in similar circumstances in the same community. Most PI initiatives strive to exceed this minimum standard and to achieve "best practices," or the highest quality of care that the organization is capable of providing. However, it is important that the organization avoid the trap of setting standards it cannot meet.

Hypothetical Situation 3. State law requires the ratio of nurses to patients in a certain type of nursing unit to be 4 nurses to every 10 patients, and every hospital in the community complies with this standard. In an effort to promote itself as providing the highest quality of care in the community, Hospital X develops a written policy stating that it will provide 5 nurses for every 10 patients. However, shortly after the policy is approved, a significant number of nurses leave Hospital X for other jobs, and the hospital is unable to recruit enough nurses to meet the staffing ratio that it established. During this period, a patient falls and breaks her hip, and the accident is undiscovered for 30 minutes. In this case, Hospital X could be found negligent because it failed to comply with the standard set in its own policy, even though no other hospital provides such a high nurse-to-patient ratio.

There is a natural inclination for healthcare providers to draft policies and statements referring to the "highest" quality of care, or they set standards that they would like to reach rather than what they can reach. From a legal perspective, it is important to provide an acceptable standard of care, to strive to meet the best possible practice, but not to overreach when setting standards or drafting policies.

The Organized Medical Staff

The basis for the PI process is the organized medical staff. As described in chapter 13, the medical staff consists of individual practitioners who are permitted by law to provide patient care services without direction or supervision and within the scope of their license. Such independent practitioners commonly include physicians, dentists, clinical psychologists, and podiatrists. Additionally, other types of practitioners may be members of the medical staff or affiliated with the medical staff. They may include certified nurse-midwives, certified registered nurse-anesthetists, nurse-practitioners, physician's assistants, and pharmacists.

As discussed in chapter 13, it is important for organizations to have a well-defined recruitment process. At a minimum, the recruitment process generally includes a job announcement, job description, and minimum qualifications to be eligible to be considered for the position. These qualifications may include educational and licensure requirements as well as previous experience.

In the case of independent practitioners, they most likely will not respond to a job announcement or become employees of a hospital. Instead, they want to remain independent and may want to join a hospital's medical staff because it is close to their private office, because their practice group is associated with the hospital, or because they want to expand their practice by being able to treat patients at a hospital most convenient for their patients. Since there is not a traditional recruiting process for such independent practitioners, hospitals need to have a process for identifying these people and ensuring that they meet the hospital's qualifications for providing services to its patients. Accordingly, legal requirements were developed for organized medical staffs, that is, medical staff bylaws stipulating the rights and responsibilities of medical staff members, and credentialing and privileging processes of medical staff members. Chapter 13 set forth in detail the process for credentialing (verifying a practitioner's qualifications) and privileging (determining what services and procedures the practitioner is qualified to provide). As described in chapter 13, failure to ensure that a staff member's qualifications are consistent with his or her job responsibilities can be a significant problem. This is true for physicians, other healthcare providers, administrators, and staff.

The process for ensuring qualifications for medical staff members is unique because it is a peer review process, as opposed to a supervisor evaluating an employee. Providers review the credentials of other providers and determine whether they qualify for membership on the medical staff and what services and procedures they are qualified to perform. It has often been said that physicians are poor at policing each other. Difficulties with the peer review process are not surprising since peers are required to make decisions about one another that affect their reputations, futures, and livelihoods. It is awkward and difficult for one provider to tell another (who has spent years going to medical school and has completed an internship and residency program) that he or she is not qualified to perform a certain procedure. Additionally, providers may worry about destroying the reputation of a peer and incurring personal liability for voicing their opinions about another staff member.

Both state and federal legislators have tried to ease the difficulties in peer review by (1) providing protection for peer review materials and meetings, and (2) providing immunity from liability for medical staff members in carrying out their peer review responsibilities. The concepts of protection and immunity are discussed next.

Peer Review Protection

Peer review protection means that the discussions, deliberations, records, and proceedings of medical staff committees having responsibility for the evaluation and improvement of quality are kept confidential and are not subject to disclosure outside the medical staff process. This confidentiality protection generally applies to peer review and PI information regarding any member of or applicant to the medical staff, meetings of the medical staff, and meetings of standing and ad hoc committees created by the medical staff. The significance of this protection is that information from peer review proceedings, whether oral or written, generally is not **discoverable,** meaning that the information is shielded and cannot be introduced at trial to support a patient's malpractice action against a physician or hospital.

Most state legislatures have created a peer review protection for public policy purposes. It is accepted that effective PI activities, peer review, and consideration of medical staff applicants must be based on free and candid discussions within the quality improvement process. These state legislatures place a greater importance on effective PI than on an individual plaintiff's ability to obtain information on medical staff discussions that may pertain to a malpractice action.

A **protection** is often confused with a **privilege.** A privilege applies to discussions and correspondence between persons with a certain type of relationship that has been recognized as needing confidentiality. Examples of such relationships include those between a lawyer and a client, priest and penitent, husband and wife, and doctor and patient. In each of these cases, the person seeking some type of counsel holds the privilege (whether a client, penitent, spouse, or patient). *Privileged* information is not admissible at trial unless the holder waives the privilege. In contrast, documents and discussions generated by peer review and medical staff privileging activities are *protected* due to their nature. The individual subjects of the documents do not hold the protection and do not have the right or ability to waive the protection. By the very nature of what they are, these documents are not admissible as evidence in legal proceedings.

Immunity from Liability

The Health Care Quality Improvement Act (HCQIA) of 1986 (42 USC 11111, et seq.) is a federal statute designed to make the peer review process more effective by reducing the fear of legal liability on the part of participants.

This statute confers immunity from civil liability for damages under federal and state laws to the following individuals and entities for actions taken by peer review bodies:

- The professional body itself

- Any person acting as a member of or staff to the professional review body

- Any person under a contract or other formal agreement with the professional review body

- Any person who participates in or assists the professional review body with respect to the action (42 USC 11111[a][1])

This statute also provides protection from liability for individuals who provide information to professional review bodies during the medical staff appointment and reappointment process, including physicians and members of hospitals, medical schools, and insurance companies.

A professional review action is defined as:

An action or recommendation of a professional review body which is taken or made in the conduct of professional review activity, which is based on the competence or professional conduct of an individual physician (which conduct affects or could affect adversely the health or welfare of the patient or patients) and which adversely affects (or may affect) adversely the clinical privileges, or membership in a professional society, of the physician. (42 USC 11151 [9])

As with peer review protection, by providing immunity from civil liability for participants in the peer review process, the legislature has recognized the need for candor and the free flow of information for the peer review process to be effective.

The HCQIA also created the National Practitioner Data Bank, discussed in chapter 13.

Occurrence Reports and Sentinel Events

In addition to credentialing, privileging, and PI initiatives, peer review committees also review specific incidents through the occurrence reporting or sentinel event review process (occurrence reports and sentinel events were discussed in chapter 10). To foster an environment in which healthcare professionals can honestly and openly review and discuss issues involving the provision of care, including errors and systems that are not working well, the court protects these PI (or peer review) activities from being used as evidence in malpractice cases. However, the peer review protection applies only to the discussions and materials from peer review meetings.

In the event of a malpractice action, the facts of what happened must be disclosed. The patient will have access to his or her health record, which should include a full description of what happened from the perspective of the clinicians involved. Additionally, providers and staff involved in the incident at issue may be compelled to testify in a deposition and at trial as to their knowledge of what happened. Only the discussions and follow-up judgments in the context of the peer review meetings are protected from discovery.

The law makes a distinction between (1) the facts of what happened, which must be disclosed in court proceedings, and (2) an organization's analysis and response to the incident as an organizational peer review process, which are protected. This distinction is made to foster environments in which problems can be assessed and corrected without fear of having those corrections result in the organization's legal detriment.

Responsibility for Disclosing Adverse Events to the Patient or Patient's Family

Even though it is uncomfortable and may not be in a physician's or hospital's best legal interest, ethical standards require that adverse events be disclosed to the patient or the patient's family. Adverse events are negative clinical outcomes stemming from a diagnostic test, medical treatment, or surgical intervention. Adverse events may or may not be the result of clinical error. The treating physician is responsible for disclosure of an adverse event to the patient or the patient's family.

Disclosure should include the following elements:

- A factual explanation of the circumstances surrounding the adverse event

- An explanation of the impact of the adverse event on the patient's treatment, including treatment that may otherwise not have been necessary

- Steps that will be taken to correct or mitigate any injury

- An assurance that the physician and other members of the patient care team will remain available to discuss any concerns that the patient or family may have

Additionally, documentation should be added to the patient's health record that includes (1) a factual description of the adverse event (without conjecture as to the cause or attribution of fault); (2) a note outlining the substance of the discussion with the patient and family members about the adverse event, including the date, time, and who was present; and (3) a note describing any follow-up discussions with the patient and family members.

An occurrence report also should be filed for the adverse event, thereby triggering a review through the organization's PI process. The patient and family have a right to a factual explanation of the circumstances and treatment and the steps that will be taken in regard to the patient. The PI review process, including the occurrence report, discussion of individual fault, and corrective plans implemented to prevent similar errors in the future, are protected and do not need to be disclosed to the patient or the patient's family.

Distinguishing Quality Improvement from Research

Quality improvement initiatives and research studies are similar in that they typically are aimed at improving some element of care or testing the utility of some mode of care or process. However, it is important to distinguish quality improvement from research because they fall under different legal frameworks.

Quality improvement generally involves using data collection and analysis activities as management tools to improve the provision of services to a specific healthcare population. These activities are not intended to have any application beyond the specific organization in which they are conducted. In fact, organizations take measures to keep the results of quality improvement activities confidential so that they do not lose their peer review protection status.

In contrast, **research** is defined by Department of Health and Human Services regulations as "the systematic investigation, including development, testing and/or evaluation, designed to develop or contribute to generalizable knowledge" (45 CFR 160.510). In the context of research, **generalizable knowledge** means that the results of the activity may be applied to populations outside the population being studied. Participants in a research project may or may not benefit directly from the study, but a larger group may benefit from the knowledge obtained in the study. The investigator conducting the research usually intends to publish the results in a scientific or professional journal.

If an activity is research, federal regulations require the researchers to follow a variety of procedures to protect the human subjects involved. Most notably, research involving human subjects must be reviewed and approved by an Institutional Review Board (IRB) before the work may be undertaken. It is the responsibility of the IRB to ensure that subjects are protected from undue risk and from deprivation of personal rights and dignity. Two issues that are the touchstone of ethical research are (1) voluntary participation by the subjects as indicated by informed consent, and (2) an appropriate balance that exists between the potential benefits of the research to the subject or to society and the risks assumed by the subject. Additionally, pursuant to the Health Insurance Portability and Accountability Act (HIPAA) of 1996, patients must authorize the use or disclosure of their patient health information for research purposes. Alternatively, if obtaining authorization for access to patient health information is not possible or practical, healthcare organizations may waive the authorization requirement upon the approval of an IRB or Privacy Board (45 CFR, Parts 160 and 164).

Per the December 19, 2000 draft document by the National Bioethics Advisory Commission, "When the purpose of an activity is to assess the success of an established program in achieving its objectives and the information gained from the evaluation will be used to provide feedback to improve that program, the activity is not human participants research. The evaluation is a management tool for monitoring and improving the quality of the program. Information learned has immediate benefit for the program and/or clients receiving the program or services. When the activity involving human participants is undertaken to test a new, modified, or previously untested intervention, service, or program to determine whether it is effective and can be used elsewhere, the activity is research" (Johns Hopkins Medical Institutional Review Boards 2004).

Incorrect classification of investigations as quality improvement or research may have significant implications. On the one hand, research initiatives that are misclassified solely as quality improvement may be conducted without appropriate review, thereby violating federal regulations and potentially resulting in harm to patients and others or endangering federal grants-in-aid to a whole host of healthcare activities. On the other hand, if IRBs had to review all quality improvement initiatives, they would be so overburdened with additional work that they would become inefficient. Additionally, important quality improvement initiatives might be unnecessarily delayed or discarded due to the rigorous and time-consuming requirements for IRB review of proposed research (Casarett et al. 2000).

Public Health Activities

Public health departments are charged with conducting certain activities to protect the health of a population. Examples of such activities include disease surveillance, emergency responses, and program evaluations. They also may include activities to prevent and control disease, injury, or disability; provide information to the Food and Drug Administration regarding adverse drug events; track health-related products; enable product recalls; and conduct postmarketing product surveillance. These public health activities are neither quality improvement nor research.

Summary

PI activities in healthcare organizations are affected by a number of laws, rules, and regulations. Understanding the legal context in which performance activities are carried out is critical. It is important to know the legal protections offered to hospitals and providers for the peer review process to be effective. It also is important to be able to distinguish between quality improvement activities and other types of activities such as research and public health functions.

References

42 USC 11111, et seq.: The Health Care Quality Improvement Act (HCQIA). 1986.

45 CFR 160.510: Public welfare and human services. Ex parte contacts. 2007.

Casarett, D., J.H.T. Karlawish, and J. Sugarman. 2000. Determining when quality improvement initiatives should be considered research: Proposed criteria and potential implications. *JAMA* 284(17):2275–2280.

Health Insurance Portability and Accountability Act of 1996. Public Law 104-191.

Johns Hopkins Medical Institutional Review Boards. 2004. QI/QA guidance: Definition of research as it applies to clinical practice, quality improvement/quality assurance, and public health activities. http://irb.jhmi.edu/Guidelines/QI_QA.html.

National Bioethics Advisory Commission draft, December 19, 2000.

Chapter 22
Predicting the Future of Performance Improvement in Healthcare

Learning Objectives

- To describe new theories and models of performance improvement
- To consider the feasibility of the new theories and models and their potential for long-term impact on the healthcare system

Key Terms

Accountable Care Organization (ACO)

Affordable Care Act

American Recovery and Reinvestment Act (ARRA)

Continuous quality improvement (CQI)

Health Information Technology for Economic and Clinical Health (HITECH) Act

Meaningful use

Background and Significance

The introduction of this book provides a brief historical account of events and quality improvement models that brought the healthcare system to its current level of performance at the beginning of the 21st century. Although the healthcare system continues to improve, it still faces criticism regarding lapses in quality and patient safety. Healthcare professionals must deal with environmental changes, challenge paradigms that may no longer be effective, and look for trends and new developments that can continue to improve healthcare quality and performance in the future.

Differing Views on Performance Improvement in Healthcare

Some experts have very positive views of and expectations for the healthcare industry, as reflected in the following statement:

> Healthcare organizations are continuously looking for ways to improve quality, increase patient satisfaction, and reduce costs. By adopting practices used by centers of excellence—including a specialty-focused, coordinated, and multidisciplinary approach to care as well as a commitment to innovation—organizations can enhance their clinical and financial performance. (Wolf 2002, 23)

A counteropinion in a 1999 report from the Office of Inspector General (OIG) regarding accreditation of healthcare organizations stated that "while they matter enormously to hospitals, Joint Commission survey results fail to make meaningful distinctions among hospitals" (OIG 1999, 2). Another article expressed similar sentiments addressing the arguments and concerns raised in an Institute of Medicine Medical Practice Study that declared, "Between 44,000 and 98,000 people die in U.S. hospitals annually as a result of medical errors" (Leape 2000, 95).

Emerging Trends in Healthcare Performance Improvement

On March 1, 2001, the Institute of Medicine (IOM) published a two-part report, *Crossing the Quality Chasm*, that presented medical error as a chronic health threat that compares with breast cancer, motor vehicle accidents, and AIDS in its lethality. The IOM committee's report makes the following charge: "In its current form, habits, and environment, American health care is incapable of providing the public with the quality health care it expects and deserves" (Berwick 2002, 85). Information published in a previous IOM report, *To Err Is Human: Building a Safer Health System*, served as a foundation for more comprehensive research that made a compelling case for concern about the health and safety of patients entering the US healthcare system. The report asserts that existing systems are often unreliable and that attempts to fix what is broken in them would not do enough to correct the problem. In other words, the situation requires a major change in the entire healthcare system (Berwick 2002).

According to Thomas C. Dolan, president of the American College of Healthcare Executives, when the report was published, it "attracted a great deal of attention" from healthcare administrators and the public. The second part of the report provides "a blueprint for redesigning the healthcare system to improve care" (Dolan 2002, 4).

Time will tell whether changes in the healthcare system will result from modification of existing models or will emerge from creative innovations. The IOM committee recommends the following six core requirements on which healthcare organizations and professionals should focus and align in the 21st century. Care should be:

- Safe
- Effective
- Patient centered
- Timely

- Efficient

- Equitable

Ideally, the healthcare system will continue to seek out new areas of focus for performance improvement (PI). At the beginning of the 21st century, five primary areas are getting attention: information systems and information technology, payment systems, Six Sigma, systems thinking and learning organizations, and evidence-based medicine and management. These areas of focus have emerged or are emerging in the healthcare system, and questions remain regarding how effectively they will diffuse into the industry.

It may be helpful to consider new PI trends from the same perspective that Henry Mintzberg (1994) approaches strategic planning. The model in figure 22.1 depicts how managers plan to pursue an intended strategy, and as their intended strategy fails to be realized, how they adopt a more deliberate strategy. Meanwhile, conditions in the environment emerge that evolve into a realized strategy. The emergent strategy is neither planned nor intended but evolves out of trial and error.

For example, Mintzberg's emergent strategy model can be adapted to formulate a model for managed care. Originally, managed care was implemented with the intent of reducing costs and increasing profits. The sequence of events following the emergence of managed care can be diagrammed using Mintzberg's emergent strategy model.

Cost reduction and profit increase were partially met using supply-side control, but efforts to decrease demand for healthcare services were unrealized. The financial incentives to employ error prevention programs or seek less costly alternatives for healthcare services were not effectively built into the design of managed care plans. The shift in managed care focus began to narrow with greater attention to supply-side cost containment as an interim strategy. As other strategic forces have emerged in the economy, a new model for demand management strategy has evolved. Some of these forces include pressure for greater preventive measures, nurse advice, access to use of decision support technology, promotion of healthier lifestyles, and pursuit of **continuous quality improvement (CQI)**.

Figure 22.1.   Mintzberg's emergent strategy model

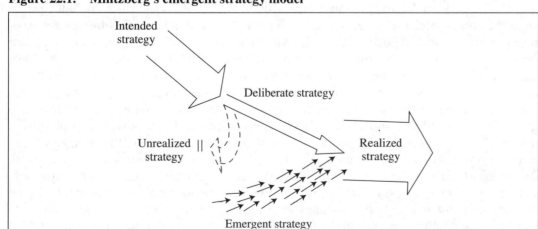

Information Systems and Information Technology

In the last two decades of the 20th century, information technology capability expanded exponentially. Computers have the capability to store and retrieve incredibly large amounts of data. However, in many cases they are merely used to perform functions that were done manually in the past. For example, Donald Berwick (1999), in his presentation, "Escape Fire," at the 11th Annual National Forum of Quality Improvement in Healthcare, noted the following reality, still present today in spite of recent technological advances in the handling of healthcare information:

> In the current model, information is treated generally as a tool for retrospection, a record of what has happened, a stable asset that sometimes we might or might not use to see the past, or to defend or prosecute a lawsuit.

Chapter 16 explains that PI is an information-intensive activity. Information management continues to migrate from paper systems to paperless systems that rely on computer technology for storage and retrieval of data. In the past, data were recorded into hard-copy records by hand or through the use of typewriter keyboards. For years, the only document regarding a patient's diagnosis and treatment that was legally admissible in a court of law was the paper health record.

There was a major shift in legal precedent when a physician's electronic signature became admissible in court. Some state governments were quick to embrace the idea. Accreditation agencies were more reluctant but have come to accept this as status quo.

The current trend in documentation is to move to a paperless environment. This trend has both pros and cons. Computer technology can speed up the transmission and retrieval of large amounts of information. It also makes information easily accessible to multiple individuals over wide areas. In many healthcare environments, providers have instant access to patient information and can consult with specialists around the world using the common tools that information technology makes available. Research and evaluation of healthcare practices has been expanded because researchers can retrieve information that was previously inaccessible from data repositories.

The **American Recovery and Reinvestment Act (ARRA)**—which includes provisions for health information technology in the **Health Information Technology for Economic and Clinical Health (HITECH) Act**—passed in 2009, requiring that healthcare organizations and providers make significant investments in information systems that have "**meaningful use.**" The objective of this concept is to focus the attention of healthcare organizations and providers on the attributes of healthcare information systems that will make the greatest positive impact on the care the organizations and clinicians provide to their patients, residents, and clients. Recognizing that these impacts will be primarily of a technological nature, it is important to also recognize that most will have a significant impact on quality as well (assuming their use by professionals and staff as projected). Examples of attributes that demonstrate meaningful use are the requirement to implement at least one clinical decision-support rule, to maintain demographic information in digital formats, to maintain allergy or no-allergy information in digital formats, and to submit data from clinical quality measures to the Centers for Medicare and Medicaid Services (CMS) and the states electronically (Kallem 2010).

Handheld Technologies

Are we looking at the end of handwritten data? Technology is already in place that converts handwriting into a digitized document. Many students currently attending universities have become accustomed to taking notes on personal digital devices and electronically transmitting data to other students and to their instructors. As they complete their college degrees, they will enter the workforce expecting their coworkers to be conversant in the same technology.

The use of handheld devices is becoming more and more prevalent in healthcare organizations. Many executives and professionals own personal digital assistant (PDA) tools and use them for both personal and professional purposes. Handheld devices that incorporate cellular telephone technology, Internet access, and personal computing are widely available and affordable to the average individual.

Cyborg Technology

Cyborg technology also is becoming a reality in daily life. No one thinks twice about cardiac pacemakers and defibrillators, which, when implanted, collect data about the heart that can be read by passing a wireless device over the patient's chest. Two million people have already received implants of this kind (Schonberg 2002). Cochlear implants have restored hearing to the deaf. Implanted chips for storing patient information and for physically locating individuals also are being developed and tested. Health information management (HIM) professionals continue to wrestle with the challenge of managing high volumes of patient information and data generated by cyborg technology as well as the legal and ethical implications associated with use of that technology.

Artificial Intelligence

Another area of information technology that continues to grow is artificial intelligence. Software using artificial intelligence that employs algorithm-directed decision making for healthcare professionals is emerging, especially in the area of triage. The implications of using artificial intelligence to make critical diagnostic and treatment decisions with or without human intervention have far-reaching legal and ethical consequences. Health information professionals will be heavily involved in this development because of the need to document the decision-making process.

Internet Use in Healthcare

The development of electronic health records (EHRs) is expanding the use of the Internet. Many organizations make clinical information available to providers over Internet connections from their homes or mobile technologies such as PDAs and smartphones. Another developing Internet-based technology is the provision of access to patients' personal health information through information portals via the Internet. The portals allow patients to go to an organizational Web site where they can query their online records, retrieve lab and radiology results, make appointments, and even e-mail their providers. This is just one aspect of the now-maturing personal health record, which is an aggregation of health data that the patients themselves develop and maintain for their personal use. This collection of personal data or personal health record is especially important to those who travel far from home and do not want to carry a lot of paper documents, as they can still have access to their health information if they become ill on a long road trip within the country or when traveling overseas.

Currently, there are four groups of barriers to adoption of Internet-based systems. First is the patients, who do not have universal access. Second, some physicians are reluctant to accept Internet-based systems, primarily because of time constraints and malpractice exposure. Third, for administration, the tempo of change in information technology increases cost, and there are concerns about allowing proprietary information to be available on the Internet. Finally, there are concerns about privacy and confidentiality. Until the Health Insurance Portability and Accountability Act (HIPAA) (1996) regulations are more clearly understood with respect to Internet-based personal health information, the consequences of failed security or inappropriate disclosure will continue to be a barrier to the adoption of Internet-based systems (Kerwin 2002). Berwick (1999) observes, "Total access 24-7-365 begins to be achievable only when we agree—scientists, professionals, patients, payers, and healthcare workforce—that the product we choose to make is not a visit. Our product is healing relationships, and these can be fashioned in many new and wonderful forms if we suspend the old ways of making sense of care. . . . The healthcare encounter as a face-to-face act is a dinosaur."

Payment Systems

Payment systems are an integral part of the healthcare delivery system. Healthcare expenditures make up a significant portion of the US economy. The payment system has evolved from a time when a country doctor may have been reimbursed through bartering to the development of fee-for-service reimbursement and managed care plans. Eggleston (2000, 173) notes:

> It has been recognized for a long time that how we pay healthcare providers and how we insure consumers against the risks of medical expenditures—that is, how we design health insurance payment systems—can have significant consequences for the equity and efficiency of a healthcare system.

Finally at the end of the first decade of the 21st century, the country's politicians have tackled the issues of payment and insurance discrimination with the passage of the **Affordable Care Act** of 2010. The major focus of the act has been on providing or improving access to healthcare services for millions of US citizens, including new restrictions on the abilities of payers to limit coverage on the basis of pre-existing conditions or developing costly health treatment needs of patients. Recognizing that access is a financial issue as well as a quality issue, the act also has requirements directly related to the issue of quality. For example, it requires establishment of a quality measures program for Medicaid in the states; requires long-term care, rehabilitation, and hospice facilities to submit quality data to CMS; and expands the quality reporting in the prospective payment system that can have a negative impact on reimbursement rates when the patient encounters adverse events or complications resulting from inadequate treatment by providers. As of publication of this text, however, significant opposition to the act has developed in Congress, so the ultimate configuration of the protections and requirements at the time of its eventual full effect in 2014 is unknown.

Managed Care and Prospective Payment Systems

Payment systems also may have a positive or negative impact on the quality of healthcare delivery. The implementation of managed care and prospective payment systems (PPSs) was hailed as a new way to cut costs and encourage healthcare consumers to make better demand-side decisions. Studies have confirmed that lack of choice of healthcare providers is a key source of consumer discontent with PPSs compared to fee-for-service plans (Simonet 2005). However, patient satisfaction may be influenced by other factors as well.

In their more than 25 years' experience as healthcare administrators, the authors of this chapter have observed the following phenomenon in healthcare: The farther an individual is removed from actual payment for a service, the less he or she values the service provided. Some research that compares satisfaction between patients paying for services and patients visiting a free clinic supports this premise. Niakis and Mylonakis (2005) conducted telephone interviews with 570 patients who had either visited a free clinic or paid cash for service, and found a higher degree of satisfaction among the paying patients.

In community health programs in particular, individuals who pay the least in out-of-pocket expenses for healthcare services tend to be the most vocal in their criticism of the system. One may assume that this trend carries through when comparing patients using fee-for-service plans with those covered by PPSs. Even when Medicare patients have received more services and increased expenditures, patient satisfaction has not improved. A study of Medicare spending in California revealed that quality, patient satisfaction, and outcomes did not significantly improve when "hospitals spent up to four times more than others to treat patients with similar conditions" (Benko 2005). However, with the shift from fee-for-service as the predominant payment system to a greater prevalence of managed care systems, such as HMOs, which require small copayments, the perception of the value and quality of healthcare also may shift.

Managed care systems also created new limits on access to care. Under the fee-for-service system, a larger number of patients could easily find access to a specialist rather than a primary care provider. Under managed care, an individual with a sore knee or twisted ankle cannot go directly to an orthopedist but must first see a primary care physician. Regardless of the quality of care delivered and the number of positive outcomes patients experience, patients have a tendency to perceive the care of an orthopedist as more specialized, and thus of higher quality, than that of a primary care provider.

Accountable Care Organizations

Proposed in the Affordable Care Act of 2010, an **Accountable Care Organization (ACO)** is a network of doctors and hospitals that shares responsibility for providing care to patients. An ACO would agree to manage all of the healthcare needs of a minimum of 5,000 Medicare beneficiaries for at least three years. "By focusing on the needs of patients and linking payment rewards to outcomes, this delivery system reform will help improve the health of individuals and communities while saving as much as $960 million over three years for the Medicare program. Under the proposal, ACOs—teams of doctors, hospitals, and other health care providers and suppliers working together—would coordinate and improve care for patients with Original Medicare (that is, those who are not in Medicare Advantage private health plans). To share in savings, ACOs would meet quality standards in five key areas:

1. Patient/caregiver care experiences
2. Care coordination
3. Patient safety
4. Preventive health
5. At-risk population/frail elderly health

The proposed rules also include strong protections to ensure patients do not have their care choices limited by an ACO" (HHS 2011).

Six Sigma

Benchmarking has long been practiced within the domain of the healthcare system. However, some healthcare organizations have begun to benchmark against other industries and are selecting models that may be adapted to the healthcare industry. For example, some healthcare organizations have begun applying the Six Sigma philosophy to their PI programs. Six Sigma is practiced widely in business sectors outside healthcare, and this philosophy is gaining acceptance in the healthcare industry (Shortell and Selberg 2002).

Six Sigma uses statistics for measuring variation in a process with the intent of producing error-free results. Sigma refers to the standard deviation used in descriptive statistics to determine how much an event or observation varies from the estimated average of the population sample. For example, a student who scores 130 on an IQ test would be considered to have a higher IQ than 97.5 percent of the population. The average IQ is considered to be 100, and the standard deviation for IQ is 15 points. Thus, a score of 130 is a variation of two standard deviations above the average. Only 2.5 percent of the population is estimated to have scores above two standard deviations.

Using this kind of statistic to measure quality variation in healthcare requires some refinement of Six Sigma. The ultimate goal of any PI program is to minimize error and, by extension, to decrease the number of errors occurring in any observation of a number of encounters or activities.

Six Sigma was chosen as a target statistic because even two or three standard deviations would not be acceptable in certain scenarios. A 2.5 percent error rate for making correct change at a movie theater may be acceptable, but that error rate for airlines avoiding fatal crashes is completely unacceptable, because airlines have hundreds of flights in the air on any given day. Even if there were only 100 flights per day, two or three fatal crashes per day would be devastating to the airline industry, not to mention the population as a whole. Therefore, it is important to keep this PI approach in proper perspective when it is applied to healthcare.

The Six Sigma measure indicates no more than 3.4 errors per 1 million encounters. Consider the challenge of achieving no more than 3.4 errors per 1 million prescriptions, surgeries, or diagnoses. In certain areas, this standard may seem unattainable; in others, it may not be rigorous enough. However, incorporating Six Sigma into PI requires considerable organizational change.

Six Sigma has become more formalized in recent years. Using the martial arts designation of belts, Six Sigma certifies managers as green belts and black belts. The American Society for Quality has established a forum for Six Sigma, and there is a growing body of literature regarding it. Although Six Sigma started in the electronics industry at Motorola® and has gained a substantial foothold in manufacturing, healthcare has been less enthusiastic to embrace its techniques. Black belts from outside the healthcare industry have discovered that their experience in manufacturing settings does not prepare them to understand the confusing role of physicians in healthcare organizations. "A decision to use Six Sigma as an improvement methodology will only work when the individual [black belt] understands the complexity of service delivery in healthcare and, more importantly, physicians' roles in the process" (Caldwell et al. 2005). Success will come only when consultants engage physicians.

Actually deploying Six Sigma in healthcare requires the identification of elements of a product line that are "critical to quality," or CTQs. Focus groups or interviews can be used to elicit CTQs from customers of the product. Typically in healthcare, customers are the patients and consumers and the providers and physicians. All others involved—the corporations, the payers, and the accreditors and licensers—are identified as stakeholders, entities with an important interest in the product that do not have consumer relationships to it. Underpinning the CTQs are elements "critical to process" (CTPs). These also can be identified by such techniques as focus groups or interviews and represent those aspects of the living process that make the accomplishment of CTQs possible.

For example, the American Diabetes Association (ADA) and the National Committee on Quality Assurance (NCQA) have joined together to promote a CTQ (http://www. ncqa.org/tabid/139/Default.aspx), "to provide physicians with tools to support the delivery and recognition of diabetes mellitus care" and to recognize those providers who are able to maintain the CTQ in their practices. The CTPs supporting this CTQ include the first 10 evidence-based measures of the diabetes care rendered (see table 22.1). In addition, the

Table 22.1. Diabetes care CTPs

Diabetes Recognition Measure	Threshold (% of patients in sample)	Weight
HbA1c Control >9.0%	≤15%	15.0
HbA1c Control <7.0%	40%	10.0
Blood Pressure Control ≥140/90 mmHg	≤35%	15.0
Blood Pressure Control <130/80 mmHg	25%	10.0
LDL Control ≥130 mg/dL	≤37%	10.0
LDL Control <100 mg/dL	36%	10.0
Eye Examination	60%	10.0
Foot Examination	80%	5.0
Nephropathy Assessment	80%	5.0
Smoking Status and Cessation Advice or Treatment	80%	10.0
Total Points		**100.0**
Points Needed to Achieve Recognition		**75.0**

program provides a computer application in which the provider can record the findings for each patient on a regular basis. The output of the application is forwarded to the ADA and the NCQA on a regular basis, and when validated by them, the provider is placed on a public recognition list as meeting these evidence-based criteria and thus offering superior care for diabetes mellitus. Patients win as customers. Providers win as customers. The ADA wins as a stakeholder in promoting better diabetes mellitus care. Payers win as stakeholders in identifying providers who use best practices in the management of diabetes mellitus.

Systems Thinking

Systems thinking continues to emerge in efforts to improve quality. Approaching quality from a systems orientation rather than a process orientation requires development of individual and collective skill sets. Peter Senge (1990) outlines the following five disciplines that individuals should master to become adept systems thinkers:

- A shared vision
- Team learning
- Personal mastery
- Mental models
- Systems thinking

A critical element of systems thinking is viewing an organization as an open system of interdependencies and connectedness rather than a collection of individual parts and professional enclaves. This approach sees interrelatedness as a whole and looks for patterns rather than snapshots of organizational activities and processes.

Process orientation traditionally has relied on measurements of cost, productivity, quality, and time to improve processes. There is a tendency to approach processes in a linear fashion, fixing one process at a time. In some cases, organizations have begun to incorporate organizational learning and human capital into measurement (Forsberg et al. 1999). The difference in systems thinking is that rather than relegating PI to teams, the five disciplines are implemented to help the entire organization learn and make changes in processes.

The traditional approach to education and learning in the United States has been heavily influenced by the thinking of Sir Isaac Newton, which views the world with a focus on single material objects rather than on relationships between objects or concepts (Wheatley 1994). By contrast, systems thinkers consider the world around them from a holistic point of view. They look at relationships rather than at the parts and pieces in isolation. "Systems thinkers do not find satisfaction in problem diagnosis alone . . . Rather, they are interested in the patterns of behavior and other variables that caused the problem and in creating long-term changes that permanently prevent the problem in the future" (Bierema 2003).

Anyone who has worked in a hospital or an integrated healthcare system should intuitively understand how systems thinking is more appropriate for managing complex organizations with very diverse professional staffs. PI efforts, such as quality control and quality assurance, have focused heavily on structure and compliance standards. But as PI efforts have begun to focus on process and outcomes, the need to understand and embrace systems thinking has become more apparent. Focusing on the outcome of a patient encounter forces all members of the healthcare team to consider a shared vision and to work as a cohesive unit rather than operating as individuals who only contribute their expertise and energies to patient care in an episodic and isolated manner.

The physician's role has always been crucial to healthcare delivery. Two important characteristics of the healthcare system have shaped the role of physicians. "The first is the legal system: Only physicians are permitted to provide certain services. Second, both patients and insurers lack the necessary information to make many medically related decisions" (Feldstein 2003, 37). In the past, health services organizations operated under the assumption that physicians possessed all the necessary medical knowledge and everyone should respond to their instructions. Then schools of nursing began to specialize, and nursing began to develop a body of unique knowledge and skills. Other areas of specialization, such as medical laboratories, pharmacy, radiology, physical therapy, and health information, also have developed their own unique bodies of knowledge. Few individuals, including physicians, are capable of retaining the extensive knowledge and understanding of all specialized areas in health services organizations. Out of necessity, a greater degree of interdependence has emerged among different health professions. There is a need for information to flow in many new directions rather than just from the physician to all others in the organization. Some healthcare leaders now consider Peter Senge's (1990) model for learning organizations a viable PI model.

Systems Engineering

In 2002, the IOM and the National Academy of Engineering (NAE) initiated a project to:

- Identify engineering applications that could contribute significantly to improvements in healthcare delivery in the short, medium, and long terms

- Assess factors that would facilitate or impede the deployment of these applications

- Identify areas of research in engineering and other fields that could contribute to rapid PI (Reid et al. 2005, vii)

The result was a report that addresses these issues and provides recommendations regarding communication and information technologies, systems engineering, and related organizational innovations that impact the "interrelated quality and productivity crises facing the health care system" (Reid et al. 2005, vii). HIM employees will find themselves at the nexus of converging technologies. The trend toward acquisition and implementation of EHRs will force HIM professionals to adapt to and embrace new technologies. According to Reid et al. (2005, 11), it is paradoxical that the "United States leads the world in medical science and technology," yet the US healthcare system has been lagging behind other manufacturing and service industries in the application of new technologies for measuring quality and productivity. "The gap between the rapidly advancing medical knowledge base and its application to patient care can best be described as a chasm" (Reid et al. 2005, 12).

The structure of the third-party payer system and lack of investment in information technology have worked against closing this gap. As healthcare leaders have begun to focus on closing the gap, they have become more willing to benchmark innovation in information technology to other sectors of the US economy. This is leading to the incorporation of systems engineering in the design and implementation of information infrastructure in healthcare. The collaborative effort between the IOM and the NAE identified three sets of systems engineering tools—systems design tools, systems analysis tools, and systems control tools—that can be used at one or more of four system levels of application: patient, team, organization, or the environment.

Systems Design Tools

Concurrent engineering and quality functional deployment (QFD) can be applied at the team and organizational levels. "Concurrent engineering can be thought of as a disciplined approach to overcoming silos of function and responsibility" (Reid et al. 2005). This requires individuals from different departments within a healthcare organization to consider the impact of their department's acts and decisions on the whole organization. A concurrent engineering team would include membership from the functional areas of an organization affected by change or new process implementation. QFD is a two-step process that helps "the concurrent engineering team identify (1) factors that determine the quality of performance and (2) actions that ensure the desired performance is achieved" (Reid et al. 2005, 13).

Human factors engineering is another design tool that can be used in all four system levels of application. This application seeks to simplify a system to "increase productivity and reliability by making it easier for humans in the system to operate effectively" (Reid et al. 2005).

The third area of systems design tools is failure mode and effects analysis (FMEA). "The purpose . . . is to identify the ways a given procedure can fail to provide desired performance" (Reid et al. 2005). FMEA can be useful when designing such systems as EHRs. The Veterans Health Administration (VHA) and the Joint Commission have promoted adaptation and application of failure analysis methodologies. The Joint Commission published a book about FMEA for healthcare (JCAHO 2002) and, as discussed in chapter 10, has required healthcare organizations to identify high-risk processes.

Systems Analysis Tools

Systems analysis can be applied at the team, organizational, and environmental levels. It involves four groups of analysis tools. The first group is modeling and simulation, which includes queuing methods and discrete-event simulation. Since queuing deals with waiting lines, this tool has enormous applicability to the healthcare system. Discrete-event simulation analyzes the independent variable of time against dependent variables such as patients, caregivers, administrators, inventory, capital equipment, and others (Reid et al. 2005, 37).

The second group of analysis tools is enterprise management tools. This group includes supply-chain management, game theory and contracts, systems dynamic models, and productivity measuring and monitoring. The complexity of business in the healthcare system lends itself to the application of mathematical tools used in other industries to manage networks of suppliers, distributors, and service providers. Vanderbilt University Medical Center used supply-chain management to redesign its perioperative services, and Deaconess Hospital of Evansville, IN, used the same tool to improve its drug distribution in the operating room. In both cases, the improvement reduced costs and improved processes (Reid et al. 2005, 40). Although these tools have not been widely used in healthcare, the potential for application is great. As the industry moves to widespread implementation of EHRs, data for measuring productivity will be easier to retrieve and analyze. Managers of health information systems should expect to be heavily involved in supporting systems analysis.

The third group of analysis tools is financial engineering and risk management tools. The inherent risks of using these tools in healthcare involve the patient, the organization, and the environment. Assessing financial risk at the organizational level has driven efforts to increase return on investment, reduce risk, and increase efficiency. Healthcare organizations can use stochastic analysis (statistical forecasting) and value-at-risk models to predict the risk of financial losses.

The fourth group of analysis tools is knowledge discovery in databases. This includes data mining, predictive modeling, and neural networks. Four different types of information can be retrieved through data mining: classifications, estimations, variability, and predictions (Reid et al. 2005, 44). This information also can be used to predict outcomes for a variety of actions through predictive modeling or neural networks.

Systems Control Tools

Systems control tools employ statistical process control and scheduling to monitor and ensure that processes are performing as expected. Statistical process control may be as simple as developing control charts, as discussed in chapter 4. Scheduling involves ensuring that the right amounts of resources are in the right place at the right time. Although this sounds simple enough, scheduling can be difficult to implement. Forecasting demand, assessing workforce size and skill mix, and setting service standards depend on good data analysis. Sufficient information technology support, however, is necessary to implement these kinds of tools for everyday use.

Evidence-Based Management

Evidence-based medicine was addressed in chapter 8, and an offshoot of this concept now addresses evidence-based management. "Evidence-based medicine is based on the principle that providers and patients should adopt those medical treatments that scientific clinical trials find to be safe and efficacious. It advocates that clinical practice should be grounded in scientific evidence and continually improved by the results of robust research" (Van de Ven and Schomaker 2002, 89). This movement aims to "introduce rationality into the adoption and diffusion of innovations" (Denis and Langley 2002, 32).

Professors of healthcare administration have been encouraged by Shortell (2002) to merge evidence-based medicine and evidence-based management into their curricula. This includes addressing the six aims that an IOM (2001) report suggests will make the services provided by healthcare organizations safe, effective, efficient, timely, personalized, and equitable. The following three overarching principles also must be applied: patient-centeredness, system-mindedness, and evidence-based. To apply these principles, Shortell (2002) raises 10 key issues:

- Care based on continuous healing relationships
- Customized care based on patient needs and values
- The patient as the source of control
- Shared knowledge and free flow of information
- Evidence-based decision making
- Safety as a system property
- The need for transparency
- Anticipation of needs
- Continuous decrease in waste
- Cooperation among clinicians

Where evidence-based medicine has focused on collecting data from large patient populations, looking for indicators, and assessing outcomes that indicate the need for clinical guidelines, evidence-based management will require a broader systems approach to identifying interdependencies between administrative and clinician activities. For example, precertification for certain procedures was implemented by insurance companies as an administrative procedure to reduce costs. A growing body of evidence has been identified that indicates the precertification process may adversely affect the quality of care provided to patients and, in some cases, actually may *increase* costs in the long run. Consider the cases in which a procedure that may have allowed early diagnosis and treatment of an aggressive cancer was delayed by the administrative precertification process and the patient was subjected to more expensive and invasive treatment with a prognosis of an early death.

Shortell (2002) also presents six challenges facing leaders in healthcare:

- Redesign of care processes
- Effective use of information technology
- Knowledge and skills management
- Development of effective teams
- Coordinated care longitudinally
- Performance and outcome measurement

In the same manner that clinicians have used scientific investigation, managers also must use scientific inquiry to produce evidence that supports shifts in policy and practice in health services management. Shortell (2002) also makes the point that the focus of evidence-based management must be organization-wide and must be applied to at least the following four levels of change to effectively improve quality: individual, group or team, organization, and larger system or environment.

Fiction, Fad, or Fundamental?

The challenge facing healthcare improvement professionals is to determine which new ideas regarding quality programs and models are trends that will last over time and which ones will fade into the background when new trends emerge. For example, Avedis Donabedian (1966) is often credited with the development of the three classes of quality assessment: structure, process, and outcome. The first two were more readily embraced by the health system; it was only in the latter years of the 20th century that outcomes have become a major focus of PI programs. The health system continues to shift toward a broader, systems-oriented PI approach.

Virtuoso Teams

Publications on PI have given much attention to teamwork. A book by Boynton and Fischer (2005) presents cases studying "virtuoso teams" that take a different approach to team membership and processes. The authors studied cases in businesses such as Ford® Motor Company, Cray® Computers, IBM®, and Microsoft (Boynton and Fischer 2005). Members of virtuoso teams were handpicked for their exceptional expertise in a particular field and given ambitious goals. Rather than selecting team members according to their availability and experience as is done with traditional teams, virtuoso teams "hire the best skills and recruit specialists for each position" (Anonymous 2005). Boynton and Fischer (2005) believe this group of handpicked elite experts "work best when members are forced together in cramped spaces under strict time constraints." "When virtuoso teams begin their work, individuals are in and group consensus is out" (Boynton and Fischer 2005). Leaders of these teams encourage collaboration and creative confrontation. Instead of relying on e-mail, phone calls, and occasional meetings, virtuoso teams engage in intense face-to-face conversations. Where politeness and repression of individual egos are the norm in traditional teams, members of virtuoso teams celebrate individual egos, compete, and create opportunities for solo performances (Boynton and Fischer 2005). Virtuoso teams operate on the assumption that members have a stake in their reputation and are therefore energized to create notable results. This book was recommended to healthcare executives shortly after its publication (Anonymous 2005), suggesting that healthcare executives should consider forming virtuoso teams for certain projects in the future. Leaders and participants in virtuoso teams will be expected to employ different skills and methods of interaction than they have experienced in previous team participation.

ISO 9000 Certification

If healthcare organizations expand into global entities, they will be required to deal with the same issues that other industries face when doing business outside the United States. ISO 9000 certification is part of a PI system that is required to conduct business in certain foreign countries. The International Organization for Standardization in Geneva, Switzerland, first published ISO 9000 standards in 1987. Into the 1990s, it was much more prevalent in European countries than in the United States. ISO 9000 sets specification standards for quality management with regard to process management and product control. In the healthcare setting, product control is quality control of patient care activities. Companies that document and demonstrate compliance with ISO 9000 standards can receive certification by independent ISO auditors.

In 1998, the Ministry of Public Health in Thailand announced that it planned to require state hospitals to meet ISO 9000 standards (*Bangkok Post* 1998). At the same time, a few hospitals in the United States moved to adopt ISO 9002 standards, an enhancement of the original ISO 9000 standards. The American Legion Hospital in Crowley, LA, dropped JCAHO accreditation and adopted ISO 9002. Pulaski Community Hospital in Virginia's New River Valley continued with JCAHO accreditation but also adopted ISO 9002 standards (Babwin 1998).

Whether other hospitals follow the lead of these two remains to be seen. Although the American Legion Hospital in Louisiana must undergo a state audit to continue receiving Medicare payments, adopting ISO 9002 certification and dropping Joint Commission accreditation reportedly has reduced its costs by $100,000 a year. Over the first decade of the 21st century, more facilities followed the lead of the American Legion Hospital. In particular, the National Integrated Accreditation for Health Care Organizations (NIAHCO), offered by DNV Healthcare, has attracted quite a few healthcare organizations to date for its accreditation processes incorporating the ISO 9001 standards. These organizations must comply or be certified as compliant with the ISO 9001 quality management standards (see below) as well as the NIAHCO standards for accreditation. These latter standards are very similar to those of the Joint Commission and incorporate the CMS requirements outlined in its *Conditions of Participation*. The actual survey process is also similar, and the NIAHCO uses the tracer methodology now familiar to all healthcare professionals who have participated in a Joint Commission survey (DNVHC n.d.). In the future, many other organizations may choose to continue Joint Commission accreditation and also adopt ISO standards. If this becomes a trend, healthcare professionals will need to become conversant in ISO standards and learn how to apply them to direct care clinical processes (Schyve 2000).

In 2000, ISO made a significant revision to its 9000-level standards, discontinuing its 9002 and 9003 standard sets and refocusing its attention on the 9001 2000 set. This is the current set that can be used for PI purposes in healthcare organizations. The actual requirements for certification begin in the fourth chapter of the standards (the first three chapters cover a variety of introductory and legalistic subjects):

- Chapter 4.1 Systemic Requirements sets forth standards for developing, implementing, and improving the quality management system; 4.2 sets forth standards for developing and maintaining quality system documents, manuals, and records.

- Chapter 5.1 sets forth standards for promoting and improving the quality management system; 5.2 sets standards for identifying, meeting, and enhancing customer expectations; 5.3 establishes the organization's quality policy and commitment to continual improvement; 5.4 requires a quality management system plan and objectives; 5.5 and 5.6 control and evaluate the quality management system.

- Chapters 6.1 through 6.4 provide for resources, personnel, infrastructure, and environment to support the quality management system.

- Chapter 7 is about making the quality management system a reality in terms of product or process development, purchasing, and operational activities.

- Chapter 8 is about monitoring and measuring product or process quality and identifying and making necessary quality improvements.

Theory of Constraints

Eliyahu Goldratt (1987) has become a widely recognized leader for his development of the theory of constraints (TOC) as a process of ongoing improvement. The TOC has been accepted in some sectors of the industry, although more so in manufacturing than in service. The service industries have been less accepting of TOC. The concept of throughput and identifying constraints in healthcare organizations is complicated by the complexity of the system and its accounting procedures:

> Throughput is the rate at which a system generates money through sales after reduction for material costs, commissions, and distribution cost. Under TOC, the objective is to maximize throughput while minimizing operating expenses for labor, sales, and administration and simultaneously minimizing investment outlays for inventory, plant, and equipment. The first step in applying TOC is to identify the constraining factor. For manufacturing concerns, the constraining factor is often but not always the time available on a certain machine or process. For companies that employ skilled workers, and for many service organizations, the constraint is often the time of one or a few key employees. (Bushong and Talbott 1999, 53)

In healthcare, little has been published on TOC, and what have been published are a "few single-institution case studies" (Breen et al. 2002, 46). This PI approach may have been an idea ahead of its time within the healthcare industry. Only in recent years, with a shift toward systems thinking and surveying chains of interdependencies, have healthcare managers become more accepting of the TOC model.

A constraint within the context of TOC is thought of as a bottleneck in a process. In the healthcare setting, an example of a constraint might be found in a clinic where a limited resource slows down the overall ability of the clinic to move patients in and out during the normal workday. A shortage of medical assistants, for example, could lead to delays in turning over exam rooms and prepping that back up patients in the waiting room until an exam room is ready. This delay would also impact physicians' time because they are waiting for patients to be placed in exam rooms before they can see them.

The human response to this kind of constraint is frustration, which leads to a tendency to rush things at the end of the clinic schedule. Patients wait longer than necessary to be seen, which increases the risk of errors because physicians are rushed. Thus, the constraint in a health clinic can be a function of the health professional's appointment schedule and efficient use of exam rooms or procedure rooms. However, the patient is an important factor in that he or she must arrive at appointments on time and at the same time must view each experience as a high-quality encounter.

To apply TOC, the following five focusing steps must be completed (Breen et al. 2002):

1. *Identify the system's constraint.* The challenge here is to conduct an effective root-cause analysis. When team members are skilled in systems thinking, they are better able to see relationships and interdependencies between organizational structures and processes. The flowcharting of processes is a useful tool for focusing on a system constraint.

2. *Decide how to exploit it.* Exploit a constraint by deciding how best to change structure, policies, or procedures to open the flow of goods or services through the constraint. In the example cited above, the shortage of medical assistants may be exploited in a number of ways. Although the solution many would select is to hire more medical assistants, other ways to exploit the constraint might include shifting some tasks and responsibilities currently assigned to medical assistants to other staff members. Another solution may be found by determining whether certain policies are creating inefficiencies by requiring tasks that might be eliminated or combined if the policy were changed.

3. *Prioritize and synchronize decisions above everything else.* It is important to remember that a decision to change the conditions of a constraint is likely to be met with resistance. If the decision is made to hire more medical assistants, the entire organization must be dedicated to recruiting, selecting, orienting, and training them. This means other hiring actions must not take priority over hiring medical assistants. At the same time, this decision must be synchronized with other activities in the organization. For example, work schedules would need to be coordinated to accommodate training schedules for new hires.

4. *Elevate the system's constraint.* This means investing in the constraint. If more funding is needed for new hires, facilities, or equipment, the organization must commit the needed funds. Although the focus in step 2 is to find ways to exploit the constraint without significant increases in spending, step 4 may require the commitment of more funding.

5. *If in the above steps the constraint has shifted, go back to step 1. Do not allow inertia to become the system's constraint.* If during the process of implementing steps 1 through 4 the constraint shifts, go back to step 1 and address the new constraint. This step-by-step process of TOC is, like another PI program, an ongoing process of continuous improvement.

TOC requires commitment from the entire organization but offers promise as a PI tool for healthcare organizations. "Of particular benefit is the method's focusing power by targeting the weakest link in a system or process. Improvement efforts can be costly, but TOC makes the most of any effort by aiming at the single improvement that will significantly affect the overall system" (Womack and Flowers 1999, 405). Whether it will ultimately be embraced as a new paradigm in healthcare is not yet clear. Any organization that chooses to implement TOC should assess whether the leadership team is ready to accept this new PI approach.

Case Study

In mid-2000, six members of the executive team of the Community Health Center were trained in TOC by a consultant. The purpose was to explore the potential for applying TOC to management of the health center. Much effort was focused on step 1, but the different levels of sophistication in systems thinking among the team members were problematic and made it difficult to get through step 2. Without a better understanding of the chain of interdependencies, deciding how to exploit a constraint was difficult. Until the team and the organization learned to embrace and understand systems thinking, it was clear that effectively using TOC was futile. Some members of the team were still operating under the mental model of classic healthcare that responds to occurrences as episodic and isolated. Furthermore, a lack of understanding of the chain of interdependencies made it virtually impossible for the organization to subordinate and synchronize everything to exploit an identified constraint.

Case Study Questions

1. What opportunity for PI can you identify in this case?

2. What was the fundamental problem preventing implementation of a new model for quality improvement at the health center?

3. If you were the chief executive officer of the health center, what steps would you have taken to better prepare the executive team for implementing TOC?

Summary

The healthcare system continues to evolve, and quality improvement professionals must embrace new approaches and ideas for improving performance. As EHRs become the norm, HIM professionals must learn to shift from knowledge and management of paper records to the world of computers and data management if they are to stay current. Information systems and information technology have become the next locus of power within many healthcare organizations. The capability of information systems to seamlessly interface between health records and payment systems is powerful. This makes information systems a key point of leverage with healthcare organizations. Systems administrators have become chief information officers and now are evolving into business strategists. In the past, they were perceived as midlevel technical managers of hardware and software, but as organizations have made huge capital investments in information systems and have become dependent on information systems to conduct day-to-day business, they have taken on a more powerful role. Access to health information is clearly linked to corporate information systems. Shifts in payment systems will continue and will require adaptation by the organization.

Six Sigma or ISO 9001 2000 may become a new paradigm in health organizations as they are challenged to significantly reduce errors. How the concepts are implemented will determine their acceptance. The models for systems thinking and learning organizations continue to be adopted throughout the healthcare system. Leaders will have to become literate and skilled in systems thinking. Acceptance of evidence-based medicine and management will depend on management's capability to access and conduct research.

TOC has been applied in a number of areas in healthcare in the United States and England (Breen et al. 2002). Whether the concept will be widely accepted has yet to be determined.

The innovative healthcare professional must be able to distinguish between new trends that are efficacious and those that are merely fads that will fade away when the excitement about them wanes. It is imperative that managers who lead the way continually seek to improve their knowledge and skills by learning about new ideas and approaches to PI.

References

Anonymous. 2005. Recommended reading: Virtuoso vs. traditional teams. *Healthcare Executive* 20(6):58.

Babwin, D. 1998. Move over, JCAHO. *Hospitals and Health Networks* 72(10):57–58.

Bangkok Post. 1998 (November 26). In brief: State hospitals aim for ISO 9000.

Benko, L.B. 2005. Big spending. *Modern Healthcare* 35(48):14.

Berwick, D. 1999. Escape Fire. 11th Annual National Forum of Quality Improvement in Healthcare, New Orleans.

Berwick, D.M. 2002. A user's manual for the IOM's "Quality Chasm" report. *Health Affairs* 21(3):80–90.

Bierema, L.L. 2003. Systems thinking: A new lens for old problems. *Journal of Continuing Education in the Health Professions* 23(2):S27 [Supplement 1].

Boynton, A., and B. Fischer. 2005. *Virtuoso Teams: Lessons from Teams That Changed Their Worlds.* Harlow, England: FT Pearson Education Ltd.

Breen, A.M., T. Burton-Houle, and D.C. Aron. 2002. Applying the theory of constraints in healthcare, part 1: The philosophy. *Quality Management in Healthcare* 10(3):40–46.

Bushong, J.G., and J.C. Talbott. 1999. An application of the theory of constraints. *CPA Journal* 69(4):53–55.

Caldwell, C., J. Brexler, and T. Gillem. 2005. Engaging physicians in lean Six Sigma. *Quality Progress* 38(11):42.

Denis, J.L., and A. Langley. 2002. Forum: Jean-Louis Denis and Ann Langley. *Healthcare Management Review* 27(3):32–34.

Department of Health and Human Services. 2011. News Release: Affordable Care Act to improve quality of care for people with Medicare. http://www.hhs.gov/news/press/2011pres/03/20110331a.html.

DNVHC. n.d. http://www.Dnvusa.com/focus/hospital_accreditation.

Dolan, T.C. 2002. Crossing the quality chasm with ACHE. *Healthcare Executive* 17(1):4.

Donabedian, A. 1966. Evaluating the quality of medical care. *Milbank Quarterly* 44(3):166–206.

Eggleston, K. 2000. Risk selection and optimal health insurance-provider payment systems. *Journal of Risk & Insurance* 67(2):173.

Feldstein, P.J. 2003. *Health Policy Issues: An Economic Perspective*, 3rd ed. Washington, DC: AUPHA Press.

Forsberg, T., L. Nilsson, and M. Antoni. 1999. Process orientation: The Swedish experience. *TQM Magazine* 10(4/5):S540–S547.

Goldratt, Eliyahu. 1987. *Essays on the Theory of Constraints.* Great Barrington, MA: North River Press.

Health Insurance Portability and Accountability Act of 1996. Public Law 104-191.

Institute of Medicine. 2001. *Crossing the Quality Chasm: A New Health System for the Twenty-first Century.* Washington, DC: National Academy Press.

International Organization for Standardization (ISO). 2011. http://www.iso.org/iso/home.htm.

Joint Commission on Accreditation of Healthcare Organizations. 2002. *Failure Mode and Effects Analysis in Health Care: Proactive Risk Reduction.* Oakbrook Terrace, IL: JCAHO.

Kallem, C. 2010. Analyzing clinical quality measures for meaningful use. *Journal of AHIMA* 81(11):56–59.

Kerwin, K.E. 2002. The role of the Internet in improving healthcare quality. *Journal of Healthcare Management* 47(4):225–236.

Leape, L.L. 2000. Institute of Medicine medical error figures are not exaggerated. *JAMA* 284(1):95–97.

Mintzberg, H. 1994. *The Rise and Fall of Strategic Planning.* New York: The Free Press.

National Committee for Quality Assurance. 2011. "Diabetes Recognition Program." http://www.ncqa.org/tabid/139/Default.aspx

Niakis, D., and J. Mylonakis. 2005. Choice of physician, private payment and patient satisfaction. Is there any relationship? *International Journal of Healthcare Technology & Management* 6(3):288.

Office of Inspector General, Department of Health and Human Services. 1999. The External Review of Hospital Quality: The Role of Accreditation. OEI-01-97-00051.

Reid, P.P., W.D. Compton, J.H. Grossman, and G. Fanjiang, eds. 2005. *Building a Better Delivery System: A New Engineering/Health Care Partnership.* Washington, DC: National Academies Press.

Schonberg, E. 2002. The cyborg known as you. *Business 2.0 Media Inc.* 3(8):33.

Schyve, P.M. 2000. A trio for quality: Accreditation, Baldrige and ISO 9000 can play a role in reducing medical errors. *Quality Progress* 33(6):53–55.

Senge, P. 1990. *The Fifth Discipline.* New York: Doubleday Currency.

Shortell, S.M. 2002. Crossing the quality chasm: What it will take to make the leap. Presentation at the Association of University Programs in Health Administration (AUPHA) 2002 Annual Meeting, Washington, DC.

Shortell, S.M., and J. Selberg. 2002. Working differently: The IOM's call to action. *Healthcare Executive* 17(1):6–10.

Simonet, D. 2005. Patient satisfaction under managed care. *International Journal of Health Care Quality Assurance* 18(6/7):424.

Van de Ven, A.H., and M.S. Schomaker. 2002. Commentary: The rhetoric of evidence-based medicine. *Healthcare Management Review* 27(3):89–91.

Wheatley, M. 1994. *Leadership and the New Science: Learning about Organization from an Orderly Universe.* San Francisco: Berrett-Koehler.

Wolf, E.J. 2002. Employing practices used by centers of excellence. *Healthcare Executive* 17(1):20–23.

Womack, D.E., and S. Flowers. 1999. Improving system performance: A case study in the application of the theory of constraints. *Journal of Healthcare Management* 44(5):397–407.

Resources

Burton, L.R. 1998. Implementing medical call centers for demand management in healthcare organizations: A model for internal installation or outsourcing. Unpublished.

Fischer, B., and A. Boynton. 2005. Virtuoso teams. *Harvard Business Review* 83(7,8):116–123.

Gold, J. 2011. Accountable care organizations, explained. *National Public Radio*. http://www.npr.org/2011/04/01/132937232/accountable-care-organizations-explained.

Lipshitz, R. 2000. Chic, mystique, and misconception: Argyris and Schon and the rhetoric of organizational learning. *Journal of Applied Behavioral Science* 36(4):456.

PR Newswire. 1999 (April 8). Investing in the new economy: The convergence of the healthcare, biotechnology, electronics, computer, and telecommunications industries.

Praxiom Research Group, Ltd. 2008. ISO 9001 2000 translated into plain English. http://www.praxiom.com.

Ransom, S., M. Joshi, and D. Nash, eds. 2004. *The Healthcare Quality Book*. Washington, DC: AUPHA Press.

Glossary and Index

Glossary

Absolute frequency: The number of times a score or value occurs in a data set.

Accountable Care Organization (ACO): Proposed in the Affordable Care Act of 2010, an Accountable Care Organization (ACO) is a network of doctors and hospitals that shares responsibility for providing care to patients. An ACO would agree to manage all of the healthcare needs of a minimum of 5,000 Medicare beneficiaries for at least three years.

Accreditation: The act of granting approval to a healthcare organization on the basis of whether the organization has met a set of voluntary standards developed by an accreditation agency.

Accreditation standards: An accrediting agency's published rules, which serve as the basis for comparative assessment during the review or survey process.

Action plan: A set of initiatives that are to be undertaken to achieve a performance improvement goal.

Adverse drug events (ADEs): Patient injuries resulting from a medical intervention related to a medication, including harm from an adverse reaction or medication error (Joint Commission 2011).

Adverse drug reaction (ADR): A noxious and unintended response to a medicinal product that occurs at doses normally used in humans for the prophylaxis, diagnosis, or treatment of disease or for the restoration, correction, or modification of physiological or psychological function (Joint Commission 2011).

Affinity diagram: A graphic tool used to organize and prioritize ideas after a brainstorming session.

Affordable Care Act: Mandated increased quality measure reporting by payers and providers at all levels of care by implementing penalties for poor care in terms of reimbursement and by improving access for the millions of Americans who, prior to the act's implementation, had nowhere to turn but the nation's emergency departments. New quality measure reporting would establish a quality measurement program for Medicaid and require long-term care and hospice facilities to submit data on their quality of care for the first time.

Agenda: A list of the tasks to be accomplished during a meeting.

All hazards approach: When hospitals have a sound understanding of their response to the six critical areas of emergency management (communications; resources and assets; safety and security; staff responsibilities; utilities management; and patient, clinical, and support activities), they have developed an "all hazards" approach that supports a level of preparedness sufficient to address a range of emergencies regardless of the cause (Joint Commission 2008).

American Recovery and Reinvestment Act (ARRA): Focused funding on the expansion of the healthcare workforce by stimulating investment in the information systems infrastructure of professional practices, clinics, and hospitals; included the HITECH Act.

Bar graph: A graphic data display tool used to show discrete categories of information.

Benchmarking: The systematic comparison of the products, services, and outcomes of one organization with those of a similar organization; or the systematic comparison of one organization's outcomes with regional or national standards.

Blitz team: A type of performance improvement (PI) team that constructs relatively simple and quick fixes to improve a work process without going through the complete PI cycle.

Bloodborne pathogen: An infectious disease such as HIV or hepatitis B or C that is transported through contact with infected body fluids such as blood, semen, and vomitus.

Brainstorming: An idea-generation technique in which a team leader solicits creative input from team members.

Brand name: A patent for a new drug that gives its manufacturer an exclusive right to market the drug for a specific period of time under a brand name.

Breach of duty: In a malpractice action, the issue is whether a physician exercised a standard of care that a reasonably prudent physician would have exercised under those circumstances. Failure to exercise *due care* is a *breach of duty.*

Case management: The principal process by which healthcare organizations optimize the continuum of care for their patients.

Causation: In a malpractice action, there must be a connection between the breach of duty and the damage—evidence that the failure to exercise due care, or breach, *caused* the damage.

Cause-and-effect diagram: An investigational technique that facilitates the identification of the various factors (that is, *Manpower*, *Material*, *Methods*, and *Machinery*) that contribute to a problem; also called a fishbone diagram.

Certification: The act of granting approval for a healthcare organization to provide services to a specific group of beneficiaries; also, the act of granting a healthcare professional approval to practice. *See also* Credential.

Change management: A group of interpersonal and communication techniques used to help people understand the process of change and accept improvements in the way they perform their work.

Check sheet: A data collection tool used to identify patterns in sample observations.

Clinical guidelines: The descriptions of medical interventions for specific diagnoses in which treatment regimens and the patient's progress are evaluated on the basis of nationally accepted standards of care for each diagnosis.

Clinical Laboratory Improvement Amendments (CLIA): The 1988 reenactment of the 1967 Clinical Laboratory Improvement Act, the federal regulations outlining the quality assurance activities required of laboratories that provide clinical services.

Clinical practice standards: The established criteria against which the decisions and actions of healthcare practitioners and other representatives of healthcare organizations are assessed in accordance with state and federal laws, regulations, and guidelines; the codes of ethics published by professional associations or societies; the criteria for accreditation published by accreditation agencies; or the usual and common practice of similar clinicians or organizations in a geographical region.

Clinical privileges: The accordance of permission by a healthcare organization to a licensed independent practitioner (physician, nurse-practitioner, or another professional) to practice in a specific area of specialty within that organization.

Community needs assessment: An assessment tool used by HMOs to become acquainted with a community; identify the community as a client; and assess that client by collecting and analyzing information about community healthcare needs, targets for interventions, and its interest in change.

Community-acquired infection: An infection that was present in a patient before he or she was admitted to a healthcare facility.

Compliance: The process of meeting a prescribed set of standards or regulations to maintain active accreditation, licensure, or certification status.

Compulsory reviews: The examinations of a healthcare facility and its processes and infrastructures as required by state laws and regulations.

Conditions of Participation: A set of regulations published by the Centers for Medicare and Medicaid Services (CMS) to outline requirements of approved programs providing healthcare services to beneficiaries of Medicare and Medicaid programs.

Continuous data: Data that may have an infinite number of possible values in measurements that can be expressed in decimal values.

Continuous monitoring: The regular and frequent assessment of healthcare processes and their outcomes and related costs.

Continuous quality improvement (CQI): A component of total quality management (TQM) that emphasizes ongoing performance assessment and improvement planning.

Continuum of care: The totality of healthcare services provided in all settings, from the least extensive to the most extensive; the emphasis is on treating individual patients at the level of care required by their course of treatment.

Control chart: A data display tool used to show variation in key processes over time.

Core measures: Sets of patient care characteristics that the Joint Commission and Centers for Medicare and Medicaid Services (CMS) have determined to reflect the quality of care an organization can provide for important diagnoses.

Core processes: The acts of assessing, planning, providing, and coordinating the care, treatment, and services provided to patients.

Cost: The amount of financial resources consumed in the provision of healthcare services.

Credentials: A formal agreement granting an individual permission to practice in a profession, usually conferred by a national professional organization dedicated to a specific area of healthcare practice; or the accordance of permission by a healthcare organization to a licensed independent practitioner (physician, nurse-practitioner, or other professional) to practice in a specific area of specialty within that organization. This agreement usually requires an applicant to pass an examination to obtain the credential initially and then to participate in continuing education activities to maintain the credential thereafter.

Credentialing process: The examination of an independent healthcare practitioner's licenses, specialty credentials, and professional performance upon which a healthcare organization bases its decision to confer or withhold permission to practice (privileges) in the organization.

Critical pathway: A multidisciplinary outline of anticipated care within an appropriate time frame to aid a patient in moving progressively through a clinical experience that ends in a positive outcome. The case manager identifies, in conjunction with the treatment team, the actions to be taken when the patient's care is not proceeding optimally.

Cross-functional: A term used to describe an entity or activity that involves more than one healthcare department, service area, or discipline.

Customers: Individuals who receive a product or a service from an organizational process. *Internal* customers are those individuals within the organization who receive products or services from an organizational unit or department; *external* customers are those individuals from outside the organization who receive products or services from an organizational unit or department.

Damages: In malpractice terms, the patient must show that actual harm, or *damage*, occurred.

Dashboard: The regular presentation of concise, appropriately displayed monitoring data for hospital boards of directors. Similar to a dashboard of a car, this type of presentation provides minute-to-minute data in an organized, comparative format that maximizes the use of the board's time and assists its members in accomplishing [its oversight] activities in an efficient and effective manner (Dye 1991).

Data collection: In healthcare organizations, this falls into one of three categories: patient-specific, aggregated, or comparative.

Deemed status: The term used for the assumption by the Centers for Medicare and Medicaid Services (CMS) that an organization meets the Medicare and Medicaid *Conditions of*

Participation as a result of prior accreditation by the Accreditation Association for Ambulatory Health Care (AAAHC), the American Osteopathic Association (AOA), the Commission on Accreditation of Rehabilitation Facilities (CARF), or the Joint Commission.

Direct observation: A means of gathering data about a process in which participants in the process are observed.

Discoverable: Information that is not shielded and can be introduced at trial to support a patient's malpractice action against a physician or hospital.

Discrete or **count data**: Numerical values that represent whole numbers, for example, the number of children in a family or the number of unbillable patient accounts; discrete data can be displayed in bar graphs.

Diversion: The removal of a medication from its usual stream of preparation, dispensing, and administration by personnel involved in those steps in order to use or sell the medication in a nonhealthcare setting.

Document review: An in-depth study performed by accreditation surveyors of an organization's policies and procedures, administrative records, human resources records, performance improvement documentation, and other similar documents, as well as a review of closed patient records.

Drug pedigree: An FDA requirement under the Prescription Drug Amendment (2007) requiring drug manufacturers, wholesalers, repackagers, and pharmacies to maintain a record of the chain of custody of a drug as it moves through the supply chain from the manufacturer to the pharmacy.

Due process: The right of individuals to fair treatment under the law.

Duty to use due care: A relationship must have been established between the parties in which one party has an obligation, or *duty*, to act as a reasonably prudent person would act toward the other. This duty exists in a physician's relationship with his or her patients. *Using due care* is acting as a reasonably prudent person would act under a given set of circumstances.

Effectiveness: In the language of the Joint Commission (2008), the degree to which care is provided in the correct manner, given the current state of knowledge, to achieve the desired or projected outcome(s) for the individual.

Efficiency: In the language of the Joint Commission (2008), the relationship between the outcomes (results of care) and the resources used to deliver care.

Elements of negligence: Four basic elements that must be proved in a malpractice case: *duty to use due care*, *breach of duty*, *damages*, and *causation*.

Emergency: A natural or human-made event that significantly disrupts the environment of care.

Emergency operations plan (EOP): The organization's written document describing the process it would implement for managing the consequences of natural disasters or other emergencies that could disrupt the organization's ability to provide care, treatment, and services.

Evidence-based medicine: The care processes or treatment interventions that researchers performing large, population-based studies have found to achieve the best outcomes in various types of medical practice.

Exit conference: A meeting that closes a site visit during which the surveyors representing an accrediting organization summarize their findings and explain any deficiencies that have been identified; the leadership of the organization is allowed an opportunity to discuss the surveyors' perspectives or provide additional information related to any deficiencies the surveyors intend to cite in their final reports.

Expectations: Characteristics that customers want to be evident in a healthcare product, service, or outcome.

External customers: Individuals from outside the organization who receive products or services from within the organization.

Facility quality-indicator profile: A report based on the data gathered using the Minimum Data Set for Long-Term Care that indicates what proportion of the facility's residents have deficits in each area of assessment during the reporting period and, specifically, which residents have which deficits. The profile also provides data comparing the facility's current status with a pre-established comparison group.

Failure mode and effects analysis (FMEA): A technique that promotes systems thinking, FMEA includes defining high-risk processes using flow charts; identifying potential failure points in current processes; and scoring each potential failure by considering factors such as the frequency of failure, potential harm, and the likelihood that the failure will be detected before it reaches the patient. Potential failures with the highest criticality scores become the focus of process redesign (Joint Commission 2008).

Fishbone diagram: *See* Cause-and-effect diagram.

Flow charts: Analytical tools used to illustrate the sequence of activities in a complex process.

Formulary: A list of drugs approved for use in a healthcare organization; the selection of items to be included in a formulary is based on objective evaluations of their relative therapeutic merits, safety, and cost.

Functional: A term used to describe an entity or activity that involves a single healthcare department, service area, or discipline.

Gantt chart: A data display tool used to schedule a process and track its progress over time.

Generalizable knowledge: In the context of research, this term means that the results of the activity may be applied to populations outside the population being studied. Participants in a research project may or may not benefit directly from the study, but a larger group may benefit from the knowledge obtained in the study. The investigator conducting the research usually intends to publish the results in a scientific journal.

Generic: Once a patent for a brand drug expires, other manufacturers may copy the drug and release it under its pharmaceutical or "generic" name.

Ground rules: An agreement concerning attendance, time management, participation, communication, decision making, documentation, room arrangements, cleanup, and so forth that has been developed by performance improvement team members at the initiation of the team's work.

Hazard vulnerability analysis (HVA): An assessment to help an organization identify potential hazards, threats, and adverse events and their impact on the care, treatment, and services that must be sustained during an emergency.

Health Information Technology for Economic and Clinical Health (HITECH) Act: This bill accomplishes four major goals that advance the use of health information technology (HIT), such as electronic health records, by: 1. Requiring the government to take a leadership role to develop standards by 2010 that allow for the nationwide electronic exchange and use of health information to improve quality and coordination of care; 2. Investing $20 billion in HIT infrastructure and Medicare and Medicaid incentives to encourage doctors and hospitals to use HIT to electronically exchange patients' health information; 3. Saving the government $10 billion, and generating additional savings throughout the health sector, through improvements in quality of care and care coordination, and reductions in medical errors and duplicative care; and 4. Strengthening federal privacy and security law to protect identifiable health information from misuse as the healthcare sector increases use of HIT (Committee on Ways and Means 2009).

Healthcare Integrity and Protection Data Bank (HIPDB): A national database that maintains reports on civil judgments and criminal convictions issued against licensed healthcare providers.

Healthcare-associated infection (HAI): An infection occurring in a patient in a hospital or healthcare setting in whom the infection was not present or incubating at the time of admission; or the remainder of an infection acquired during a previous admission.

Histogram: A bar graph used to display data proportionally.

Icons: Graphic symbols used to represent a critical event in a process flow chart.

Incident report: *See* Occurrence report.

Indicator: A performance measure that healthcare organizations use to monitor the outcomes of a process; also called a criterion.

Information management standards: One chapter of the Joint Commission's *Hospital Accreditation Standards* (2011) that promulgates the Joint Commission's requirements regarding the data and information used for various purposes in hospital organizations.

Internal customers: Individuals within the organization who receive products or services from an organizational unit or department.

Interview: A discussion of the qualifications and experiences of a job applicant with respect to the employment process; or a discussion about an organization with its leadership during the accreditation or licensure survey process.

Leadership: The senior governing, administrative, and management groups of a healthcare organization that are responsible for setting the mission and overall strategic direction of the organization.

Licenses: The legal authorization granted by a state to an entity that allows the entity to provide healthcare services within a specific scope of services and geographical location. States license both individual healthcare professionals and healthcare facilities; usually requires an applicant to pass an examination to obtain the license initially and then to participate in continuing education activities to maintain the license thereafter.

Licensed independent practitioner (LIP): Any individual permitted by law to provide healthcare services without direction or supervision, within the scope of the individual's license as conferred by state regulatory agencies and consistent with individually granted clinical privileges.

Licensure: The process of granting a healthcare organization or an individual healthcare practitioner a license to practice.

Likert scale: A measure that records level of agreement or disagreement along a progression of categories.

Line chart: A data display tool used to plot information on the progress of a process over time.

Material safety data sheets (MSDSs): Documentation maintained on the hazardous materials used in a healthcare organization. This information outlines the common and chemical names, family name, and product codes; risks associated with the material, including overall health risk, flammability, reactivity with other chemicals, and effects at the site of contact; descriptions of the protective clothing that should be worn and the protective equipment that should be used to handle the material; and other similar information.

Mean (M): The average value in a range of values, calculated by summing the values and dividing the total by the number of values in the range.

Meaningful use: The Medicare and Medicaid EHR Incentive Programs provide a financial incentive for the "meaningful use" of certified EHR technology to achieve health and efficiency goals. By putting into action and meaningfully using an EHR system, providers will reap benefits beyond financial incentives, such as a reduction in errors, availability of records and data, reminders and alerts, clinical decision support, and e-prescribing and refill automation (CMS 2011).

Median: A measure of central tendency that shows the midpoint of a frequency distribution when the observations have been arranged in order from lowest to highest.

Medication administration record (MAR): The record used to document each dose of medication administered to a patient.

Medication error: A mistake that involves an accidental drug overdose, administration of an incorrect substance, accidental consumption of a drug, or misuse of a drug or biological during a medical or surgical procedure.

Medication reconciliation: The process of identifying the most accurate list of all medications a patient is currently taking and then comparing the list against the physician's orders at each transition point (admission, transfer, and discharge) along the continuum of care.

Minimum Data Set (MDS) for Long-Term Care: The data set that the Centers for Medicare and Medicaid Services (CMS) requires long-term care facilities to collect on all residents who are federal program beneficiaries.

Mission statement: A written statement that sets forth the core purpose of an organization or performance improvement team. It is simply an expression of what already exists. The generation of a mission statement usually precedes the formation of the organization's overall goals.

Multiple drug-resistant organisms (MDROs): Bacteria of any kind that has become resistant to many different antibiotics.

National Incident Management System (NIMS): A nationally standardized incident management system that provides guidelines for common functions and terminology to support clear communication and effective collaboration in an emergency situation.

National Practitioner Data Bank (NPDB): A federally sponsored national database that maintains reports on medical malpractice settlements, clinical privilege actions, and professional society membership actions against licensed healthcare providers.

Near miss: An opportunity to improve patient safety–related practices based on a condition or incident with potential for more serious consequences.

Nominal data: Values assigned to name-specific categories; also called categorical data.

Nominal group technique: A quality improvement technique that allows groups to narrow the focus of discussion or to make decisions without becoming involved in extended, circular discussions.

Occurrence report: A structured data collection tool that risk managers use to gather information about potentially compensable events; also called an incident report.

Opening conference: A meeting conducted at the beginning of the accreditation site visit during which the surveyors outline the schedule of activities and list any individuals whom they would like to interview.

Opportunity for improvement: A healthcare structure, product, service, process, or outcome that does not meet its customers' expectations and, therefore, could be improved.

Ordinal data: Values assigned to rank the comparative characteristics of something according to a given set of criteria; also called ranked data.

Outcome: The results of care, treatment, and services in terms of the patient's expectations, needs, and quality of life, which may be positive and appropriate or negative and diminishing.

Outcome measure: A measure that indicates the result of the performance (or nonperformance) of a function or process.

Pareto chart: A bar graph used to determine priorities in problem solving.

Patient-centered care: Care that involves the patient and the patient's family in care decisions; a respect for the patient's values, preferences, and expressed needs; and an emphasis on the provider's cultural competence.

Peer review: Review by like professionals, or peers, established according to an organization's medical staff bylaws, organizational policy and procedure, or the requirements of state law; the peer review system allows medical professionals to candidly critique and criticize the work of their colleagues without fear of reprisal.

Performance improvement council: The leadership group that oversees performance improvement activities in some healthcare organizations.

Performance improvement (PI) team: Members of the healthcare organization who have formed a functional or cross-functional group to examine a performance issue and make recommendations with respect to its improvement.

Performance measurement: The indicator of a healthcare organization's performance in relation to a specified process or outcome.

Performance measure: A quantitative tool (for example, a rate, ratio, index, or percentage) that provides an indication of an organization's performance in relation to a specified process or outcome.

Pharmacy and therapeutics (P and T) committee: The multidisciplinary committee that oversees and monitors the drugs and therapeutics available for use, the administration of medications and therapeutics, and the positive and negative outcomes of medications and therapeutics used in a healthcare organization.

Pie chart: A data display tool used to show the relationship of individual parts to the whole.

Pivot table: A Microsoft Excel tool used "to summarize data according to categories. Pivot tables also provide flexibility for the end user or analyst to organize and filter data in various ways before finalizing the analysis" (AHIMA 2011, 10).

Potentially compensable events (PCEs): Occurrences that result in injury to persons in the healthcare organization or property loss.

Privilege: A legal principle that applies to discussions and correspondence between persons with a certain type of relationship that has been recognized as needing confidentiality. Examples of such relationships include those between a lawyer and a client, priest and penitent, husband and wife, and doctor and patient. In each of these cases, the person seeking some type of counsel holds the privilege (whether a client, penitent, spouse, or patient). The privileged information is not admissible at trial unless the holder waives the privilege.

Process: The interrelated activities of healthcare organizations—including governance, managerial support, and clinical services—that affect patient outcomes across departments and disciplines within an integrated environment.

Process measure: A measure that focuses on a process that leads to a certain outcome, meaning that a scientific basis exists for believing that the process, when executed well, will increase the probability of achieving a desired outcome.

Process redesign: The steps in which focused data are collected and analyzed, the process is changed to incorporate the knowledge gained from the data collected, the new process is implemented, and the staff is educated about the new process.

Protection: Peer review protection means that the discussions, deliberations, records, and proceedings of medical staff committees having responsibility for the evaluation and improvement of quality are kept confidential and are not subject to disclosure outside the medical staff process. This confidentiality protection generally applies to peer review and performance improvement information regarding any member of or applicant to the medical staff, meetings of the medical staff, and meetings of standing and ad hoc committees created by the medical staff. The significance of this protection is that information from peer review proceedings, whether oral or written, generally is not *discoverable*.

QI toolbox techniques: Tools that facilitate the collection, display, and analysis of data and information and that help team members stay focused, including cause-and-effect diagrams, graphic presentations, and others.

Quality assurance (QA): A term commonly used in healthcare to refer to quality monitoring activities during the 1970s and 1980s, at which time it connoted a retrospective review of care provided with admonishment of providers for substandard care.

Quality improvement organizations (QIOs): Private or public agencies contracted by the Centers for Medicare and Medicaid Services (CMS) to undertake examination and evaluation of the quality of healthcare rendered to beneficiaries of federal healthcare programs.

Relative frequency: The percentage of times a characteristic appears in a data set.

Research: As defined by the Department of Health and Human Services regulations, this term refers to "the systematic investigation, including development, testing and/or evaluation, designed to develop or contribute to *generalizable knowledge*" (45 CFR 160.510). In research, the results of the activity may be applied to populations outside the population being studied. Participants in a research project may or may not benefit directly from the study, but a larger group may benefit from the knowledge obtained in the study. The investigator conducting the research usually intends to publish the results in a scientific journal.

Retrospective payment system: Healthcare providers are paid for services provided to patients in the past; also called fee-for-service payment.

Risk: A formal insurance term denoting liability to compensate individuals for injuries sustained in a healthcare facility.

Root-cause analysis: Analysis of a sentinel event from all aspects (human, procedural, machinery, and material) to identify how each contributed to the occurrence of the event and to develop new systems that will prevent recurrence.

Sampling: The recording of a smaller subset of observations of the characteristic or parameter, making certain, however, that a sufficient number of observations have been made to predict the overall configuration of the data.

Sentinel event: An unexpected occurrence involving death or serious physical or psychological injury, or the risk thereof. The phrase "or risk thereof" includes any process variation for which a recurrence would carry a significant chance of serious adverse outcome (Joint Commission 2011).

Site visit: An in-person review conducted by an accreditation survey team; the visit involves document reviews, staff interviews, an examination of the organization's physical plant, and other activities.

Standard deviation (*SD*): A statistic used to show how the values in a range are distributed around the mean.

Standard precautions: The application of a set of procedures specifically designed to minimize or eliminate the passage of infectious disease agents from one individual to another during the provision of healthcare services.

Standards of care: An established set of clinical decisions and actions taken by clinicians and other representatives of healthcare organizations in accordance with state and federal laws, regulations, and guidelines; the codes of ethics published by professional associations or societies; the criteria for accreditation published by accreditation agencies; or the usual and common practice of similar clinicians or organizations in a geographical region.

Storyboard: A graphic display tool used to communicate the details of performance improvement activities.

Storytelling: The act of relaying the performance improvement (PI) process in a structured manner to support learning and organization-wide PI.

Strategic plan: The document in which the leadership of a healthcare organization identifies the organization's overall mission, vision, and goals to help set the long-term direction of the organization as a business entity.

Structure: The foundation of caregiving, which includes buildings, equipment, technologies, professional staff, and appropriate policies.

Survey team: A group of individuals sent by an accrediting agency to review a healthcare organization for accreditation purposes.

Survey tools: Research instruments used to gather data and information from respondents in a uniform manner through the administration of a predefined and structured set of questions and possible responses.

SWOT analysis: Strategic planning that includes a process in which the leaders complete an assessment of the organization's **S**trengths, **W**eaknesses, **O**pportunities, and **T**hreats. Findings from SWOT analyses are used to validate the mission of the organization as a whole and to determine the direction the organization is going as a business entity during the coming year. In addition, the leaders carefully consider input from the community the organization serves, its scope of services, the available technologies, staff expertise, the needs and expectations of its customers, and outcome information from performance improvement activities during the past year.

Systems: The foundations of caregiving, which include buildings (environmental services), equipment (technical services), professional staff (human resources), and appropriate policies (administrative systems).

Team charter: A document that explains the issues the team was initiated to address, describes the team's goal or vision, and lists the initial members of the team and their respective departments.

Team facilitator: A performance improvement (PI) team role primarily responsible for ensuring that an effective PI process occurs by serving as advisor and consultant to the PI team; remaining a neutral, nonvoting member; suggesting alternative PI methods and procedures to keep the team on target and moving forward; managing group dynamics, resolving conflict, and modeling compromise; acting as coach and motivator for the team; assisting in consensus building when necessary; and recognizing team and individual achievements.

Team leader: A performance improvement (PI) team role responsible for championing the effectiveness of PI activities in meeting customers' needs and for the *content* of a team's work.

Team member: A performance improvement team role responsible for participating in team decision making and plan development; identifying opportunities for improvement; gathering, prioritizing, and analyzing data; and sharing knowledge, information, and data that pertain to the process under study.

Team recorder or **scribe**: A performance improvement team role responsible for maintaining the records of a team's work during meetings, including any documentation required by the organization.

Timekeeper: A performance improvement (PI) team role responsible for notifying the team during meetings of time remaining on each agenda item in an effort to keep the team moving forward on its PI project.

Total program approach: *See* All hazards approach.

Total quality management (TQM): A management philosophy developed in the mid-20th century by W. Edwards Deming (1986) and others who encouraged industrial organizations to focus on the quality of their products as their paramount mission.

Tracer methodology: A process [Joint Commission] surveyors use during the on-site survey to analyze an organization's systems, with particular attention to identified priority focus areas, by following individual patients through the organization's healthcare process in the sequence experienced by the patients. Depending on the setting, this process may require surveyors to visit multiple care programs and services within an organization or within a single program or service to "trace" the care rendered (Joint Commission 2011).

Transfusion reaction: Signs, symptoms, or conditions suffered by a patient as the result of the administration of an incompatible transfusion.

Value-based purchasing: Seen primarily in the public sector, a "system in which purchasers hold providers of healthcare accountable for both the costs of healthcare and its quality" (Casto and Layman 2011, 264). In the private sector, pay-for-performance programs are more common and base provider payments on performance and incentives.

Values statement: Describes the values and standards governing the operation of the organization and its relationship with customers, suppliers, employees, the local community, and other stakeholders.

Vision statement: Describes what the organization or performance improvement (PI) team initiative will look like in the future; also describes some milestone the organization or PI team will reach in the future.

Voluntary reviews: Examinations of an organization's structures and processes conducted at the request of a healthcare facility seeking accreditation from a reviewing agency.

References

45 CFR 160.510: Public welfare and human services. Ex parte contacts. 2007.

AHIMA. 2011. Health data analysis toolkit. Chicago: AHIMA. Web only.

Casto, A., and E. Layman. 2011. *Principles of Healthcare Reimbursement*, 3rd ed. Chicago: AHIMA Press.

Center for Medicare and Medicaid Services. 2011. EHR meaningful use overview. https://www.cms.gov/EHRIncentivePrograms/30_Meaningful_Use.asp.

Clinical Laboratory Improvement Act of 1967. Public Law 90-174.

Clinical Laboratory Improvement Act of 1988. Public Law 100-578.

Committee on Ways and Means. 2009. Title IV—Health Information Technology for Economic and Clinical Health Act. http://waysandmeans.house.gov/media/pdf/110/hit2.pdf.

Deming, W.E. 1986. *Out of the Crisis*. Cambridge, MA: MIT Press. First published in 1982 as *Quality, Productivity, and Competitive Position*.

Dye, C. 1991. Quality assurance data management: The trustees' role. Chapter 7 in *Quantitative Methods in Quality Management*. Edited by Longo, D.R., and D. Bohr. Chicago: American Hospital Publishing.

Joint Commission. 2008. *2009 Hospital Accreditation Standards*. Oakbrook Terrace, IL: Joint Commission Resources.

Joint Commission. 2011. *Hospital Accreditation Standards*. Oakbrook Terrace, IL: Joint Commission Resources.

Prescription Drug Amendment of 2007. Public Law 110-85.

Index